The Pharmacy
Informatics Primer

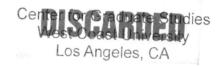
DOINA DUMITRU, PharmD, MBA
Pharmacy Operations Manager
Harris County Hospital District
Houston, Texas

With a Foreword by Karl Gumpper

American Society of Health-System Pharmacists®
BETHESDA, MARYLAND

Any correspondence regarding this publication should be sent to the publisher, American Society of Health-System Pharmacists, 7272 Wisconsin Avenue, Bethesda, MD 20814, attention: Special Publishing.

The information presented herein reflects the opinions of the contributors and advisors. It should not be interpreted as an official policy of ASHP or as an endorsement of any product. The information contained in this program, and the companion workbook, are to be used as guidance.

Because of ongoing research and improvements in technology, the information and its applications contained in this text are constantly evolving and are subject to the professional judgment and interpretation of the practitioner due to the uniqueness of each pharmacy's role in compounding sterile preparations and the handling of hazardous drugs. The editors, contributors, and ASHP have made reasonable efforts to ensure the accuracy and appropriateness of the information presented in this document. However, any user of this information is advised that the editors, contributors, advisors, and ASHP are not responsible for the continued currency of the information, for any errors or omissions, and/or for any consequences arising from the use of the information in the document in any and all practice settings. Any reader of this document is cautioned that ASHP makes no representation, guarantee, or warranty, express or implied, as to the accuracy and appropriateness of the information contained in this document and will bear no responsibility or liability for the results or consequences of its use.

Acquisitions Editor: Hal Pollard
Director, Special Publishing: Jack Bruggeman
Senior Editorial Project Manager: Dana Battaglia
Editorial Resources Manager: Bill Fogle
Cover and Page Design: DeVall Advertising
Compositor: Carol A. Barrer

Library of Congress Cataloging-in-Publication Data

The pharmacy informatics primer / [edited by] Doina Dumitru.
    p. ; cm.
 ISBN 978-1-58528-166-4
1. Medical informatics. 2. Pharmacy. 3. Information organization--Computer programs.
I. Dumitru, Doina.
 [DNLM: 1. Clinical Pharmacy Information Systems. 2. Information Storage and Retrieval.
3. Medical Records Systems, Computerized. 4. Safety Management. QV 26.5 P536 2008]
 RS122.2.P44 2008
 362.17'820285--dc22
                        2008036537

ISBN: 978-1-58528-166-4

Dedication

To Razvan, Matei, and Calin—their patience and support during this process has been my inspiration. And to my dad, Iosef Ciuca—he would have been so proud.

Acknowledgments

The writing and editing of *The Pharmacy Informatics Primer* could not have been accomplished without the tireless energy, enthusiasm, patience, and cooperation of my contributors. Each of them took time of away from their lives to write on topics that are key to the future of pharmacy practice. Their dedication to the profession is truly inspiring, and it has been an honor to work with each of them.

Hal Pollard at ASHP, who encouraged me to follow my dream and make a lasting contribution to our profession.

Dana Battaglia and the ASHP editorial team were instrumental in keeping the project on task. Their experience and patience dealing with unforeseen circumstances made the entire process smooth.

Lynn Boecler, who inspired me to enter the pharmacy informatics field in the first place. At the time I was a new pharmacy graduate, and she took a chance and gave me the opportunity of a lifetime. She also taught me to never forget that I was a pharmacist first, regardless of where my career path would take me.

Stan Kent, who suggested I go back to school for a management degree. I am very thankful for his timely advice and mentorship. He led me down the management path, and I have never regretted it.

My friends and former (unofficial) colleagues at Epic Systems: Jeff Krueger, Tony Brummel, Brian Eith, and Marc Mroz. They taught me more than I ever wanted to know about information systems, interfaces, and hardware. They also taught me how to approach project management from an engineering point of view. That skill has been invaluable to me over the years.

Table of Contents

Preface

In doing informatics presentations at various pharmacy and information system vendor conferences, I have been frequently struck by the commonality of questions that are asked by audiences after each presentation. Regardless of the topic on which I was presenting, the same questions would often be asked after each presentation. Further, in reviewing published pharmacy informatics literature, I had often been frustrated by the lack of practical application pearls. Too often, the literature presents abstract ideas that are difficult to visualize and operationalize in a health-system setting. By the fall of 2005, I had concluded that someone should write a book that captures the answers to those questions and provides real informatics application tips to pharmacy managers. When I was approached by ASHP in late 2005 to submit my ideas for a book to them, I was thrilled. I submitted a proposed table of contents that addressed the general categories of pharmacy informatics issues, corresponding to the questions I had received over the years. I just did not anticipate that the unknown author/editor of such a publication would be me. After much encouragement from ASHP, I agreed to work on the project, and I am very grateful to their team for the opportunity. I believe that *The Pharmacy Informatics Primer* will fill a much-needed void in pharmacy management literature.

The intended audience is primarily pharmacy managers and pharmacy information technology (IT) project managers. However, the book is also an excellent resource for pharmacy students exposed to pharmacy informatics for the first time, especially since pharmacy schools add informatics to their curricula. The intent of the publication is to provide readers with practical knowledge that can be applied immediately within their organizations.

The concepts presented in *The Pharmacy Informatics Primer* are meant to be used every day, in real-world situations. Although each chapter provides an introduction to the technology or management issue being presented, the core information focuses on practical implementation and technology usage issues. This information is what is often obtained in informal discussions with project and operations managers at conferences or dinners. To facilitate the use of the practical concepts presented, main points of each chapter are also summarized in a Pearls section in each chapter. This can serve as a quick reference for a busy pharmacy manager who needs a bottom-line answer to "how do I deal with bar coding?"

I recommend that pharmacy managers, IT project managers, and students utilize the following steps in applying the principles presented in the chapters:

1. Read the chapter that focuses on the technology you will be implementing or with which you are having issues.

2. Review the Pearls table and make a copy that can be placed on your bulletin board for daily review.

3. Compare the concepts/ideas presented in the chapter with your own organization. What are the similarities? What are the differences? What will work at your institution? What needs to be changed?

4. Plot your own course of action, based on the answers to the questions above. If you reach an impasse or have trouble answering those questions, team up with other managers in your organization to help facilitate discussion and brainstorming sessions. You may also contact the author of the chapter or myself for further guidance.

My goal is that pharmacy managers and pharmacy IT project managers will no longer feel that they must "reinvent the wheel" with each new IT project implementation. In most cases, other organizations have gone before you, and your organization can learn much from someone else's experience. I also hope that this publication will inspire a new generation of pharmacists to enter the informatics field. As more technology is developed to support clinical workflows (as opposed to reworking clinical workflows to support limited technology), there is a great need for experienced clinicians and managers to bring their knowledge to the informatics field. I hope that students will consider this as a future career path.

Doina Dumitru, PharmD, MBA
Pharmacy Operations Manager
Harris County Hospital District
LBJ Hospital–Pharmacy Administration
5656 Kelley Street
Houston, TX 77026
August, 2008

Foreword

As a clinical pharmacist, I have found many uses for technology in my practice. As a pediatric practitioner, I have used technology to compound parenteral nutrition solutions and to verify the safe prescribing of medications for our smallest patients. The use of technology in patient care is quickly evolving. Whether a clinical practitioner or a manager, today's pharmacist must rely on technology to perform his or her job duties effectively and efficiently.

Pharmacists have been routinely utilizing computers and automation since the 1980s to complete many tasks in providing care to patients. As the medication use process becomes more complicated, technology and automation may help make this system safer and more efficient. In 2006 the ASHP Board of Directors approved the formation of the Section of Pharmacy Informatics and Technology, which provides a membership community to ASHP members who work with information systems and technology in hospitals and health systems. The section has quickly grown to meet the needs of its members in all areas of pharmacy informatics. Members represent a broad spectrum of backgrounds and experience from pharmaceutical industry, academia, manufacturing, consulting, and hospitals and health systems. Members are pharmacy clinicians, managers, directors, technicians, analysts, students, and residents.

Many are interested in pharmacy informatics as a growing subspecialty in pharmacy, as evidenced by expanded requirements for our schools of pharmacy and growth of PGY-2 pharmacy informatics residencies. There is a need to better educate all healthcare workers about healthcare information technology and informatics. The medical and nursing professions are involved in defining the role of physicians and nurses in the development and implementation of health information systems. *The Pharmacy Informatics Primer* will help define some of the primary issues that all disciplines need to consider and work together.

The Pharmacy Informatics Primer is designed to be a starting point for pharmacists, residents, and students to explore the changing environment that many practitioners are experiencing. The authors have provided practical examples to illustrate the use of specific technologies in caring for patients in both an inpatient and outpatient environment.

As pharmacy moves forward, each pharmacist will need to evaluate where technology and automation will fit into his or her institution's practice model. The way pharmacists and technicians work at present may be entirely different in the future. Careful planning should be considered during the acquisition, implementation, and maintenance of these systems to ensure the system provides an optimal level of safety. This primer provides sound advice to the reader to evaluate not just the technology being considered for deployment but also the medication use process in its current and future states. When considering the deployment of a CPOE system, the institution must evaluate the impact of that system on the physician, nurse, pharmacist, and even practitioners that do not typically handle medications.

All healthcare institutions must begin evaluating the need for technology and automation in their environments. Those hospitals and health systems that have made the investment in technology should be expected to pave the way for other institutions by sharing their experiences with the profession and others. The reader of the primer will gain an appreciation for the complexities of these information systems. The use of CPOE, BCMA, CDSS, eRx, and robotics are available in many institutions. There is no right or wrong implementation strategy, but all institutions should be encouraged to start planning.

With the complexities of patient care that are evolving in gene therapy and genomics, the use of technology should aid the pharmacist to ensure appropriate therapies are ordered and provided to the patient to optimize his or her care. The integration of these technologies at the point of care will also allow for a greater access of information that will ensure safe and effective care. Since there are many companies providing these solutions, these systems must be interoperable and function without fail.

The Pharmacy Informatics Primer is an excellent resource for the novice and seasoned practitioner alike and is a reference in planning for the acquisition of technology or the enhancement of existing technologies. As expected, the use of technology will continue to grow and change at a rapid pace. When you think about the initial size of computers taking up whole rooms compared to today's tools being held in your hand, the rapid change in technology is mind boggling. One must keep in mind that research needs to be continuously conducted to demonstrate the value of technology on patient care. Remember, the introduction of technology is not without its positive and negative consequences and should always be implemented with patient safety foremost in the minds of pharmacists.

Karl F. Gumpper, RPh, BCNSP, BCPS, FASHP
Director, Section of Pharmacy
    Informatics and Technology
American Society of Health-System
    Pharmacists
August, 2008

Additional Resources

Koppel R, Wetterneck T, Telles JL, Karsh B-T. Workarounds to barcode medication administration systems: their occurrences, causes, and threats to patient safety. *J Am Med Inform Assoc.* 2008;15:408–423. PrePrint published April 24 2008; doi:10.1197/jamia.M2616.

Ash JS, Sittig DF, Poon EG, Guappone K, Campbell E, Dykstra RH. The extent and importance of unintended consequences related to computerized provider order entry. *J Am Med Inform Assoc.* 2007;14(4):415–423. PrePrint published July 1, 2007; doi:10.1197/jamia.M2373.

Contributors

Lynn Boecler, PharmD, MS
Senior Director, Pharmacy Services
Evanston Northwestern Healthcare
Evanston, Illinois

Kevin C. Borcher, PharmD
Pharmacy Informatics Coordinator
Nebraska Methodist Hospital
Omaha, Nebraska

Doina Dumitru, PharmD, MBA
Pharmacy Operations Manager
Harris County Hospital District
Houston, Texas

Helen T. Giannopoulos, PharmD
Pharmacy Clinical Manager
Children's Healthcare of Atlanta
Atlanta, Georgia

Karl F. Gumpper, RPh, BCNSP, BCPS, FASHP
Director, Section of Pharmacy Informatics and
    Technology
American Society of Health-System
    Pharmacists
Bethesda, Maryland

Chad Hardy, PharmD, MS
Pharmacy Informatics Manager
Harris County Hospital District
Houston, Texas

Patricia J. Hoey, RPh
Clinical Applications Coordinator
VA Puget Sound Health Care System
Seattle, Washington

Michael A. Jones, BS, PharmD
Pharmacy Informatics Specialist
University of Colorado Hospital
Aurora, Colorado

Stanley S. Kent, MS, FASHP
Assistant Vice President
Evanston Northwestern Healthcare
Evanston, Illinois

Kevin C. Marvin, RPh, MS, FASHP
Pharmacy Informatics Consultant
Burlington, Vermont

Scott R. McCreadie, PharmD, MBA
Strategic Project Coordinator
Clinical Assistant Professor
Department of Pharmacy Services
University of Michigan Health Center
Ann Arbor, Michigan

Michael E. McGregory, PharmD, BCPS
Strategic Projects Coordinator
University of Michigan Health System
Department of Pharmacy Services
Ann Arbor, Michigan

Joel Melroy, PharmD, MS
Manager
Ashley River Tower Pharmacy Services
Medical University of South Carolina Hospital
    Authority
Charleston, South Carolina

Alicia S. Miller, RPh, MS
Practice Manager
Eclipsys Corporation
Westerville, Ohio

W. Paul Nichol, MD
National Director Medical Informatics, Patient
    Care Services
Veterans Health Administration, Department
    of Veterans Affairs
Washington, DC

Associate Chief of Staff for Clinical
    Information Management
VA Puget Sound Health Care System
Seattle and Tacoma, Washington

Clinical Associate Professor of Medicine
Division of General Internal Medicine
School of Medicine
Clinical Associate Professor of Health Services
School of Public Health and Community
    Medicine
University of Washington
Seattle, Washington

Eric Rose, PharmD
Corporate Pharmacy Informatics Liaison
Orlando Health
Orlando, Florida

Steve Rough, MS, RPh
Director of Pharmacy
University of Wisconsin Hospital and Clinics
Madison, Wisconsin

Robert Silverman, PharmD
Pharmacy Informatics Specialist
Hines VA Hospital
and VA Pharmacy Benefits Management–
    Strategic Healthcare Group
Hines, Illinois

Michael Sura, PharmD
Director of Clinical Informatics
Froedtert Memorial Lutheran Hospital
Milwaukee, Wisconsin

Marc Young, PharmD, MS, BCPS
Lieutenant Commander, U.S. Navy
Pharmacy Informatics Advisor

CHAPTER 1

Computerized Provider Order Entry

Patricia Hoey, W. Paul Nichol, and Robert Silverman

KEY DEFINITIONS

Alert—a patient- and context-sensitive warning presented to the ordering provider at the time an order is being entered. Used to inform the provider of a clinical concern relevant to the patient and order being placed. Alerts are called "order checks" in some EHR systems.

Clinical Reminder—a context-sensitive electronic prompt to the provider to perform an intervention or procedure, based on the patient's specific clinical data as applied to a set of logical conditions.

Computerized Provider Order Entry—direct entry of medical orders into a healthcare system's EHR by licensed independent practitioners or other staff with specific ordering privileges, and not by clinical or administrative support staff.

Corollary Orders—orders entered as adjuncts to a primary order, e.g., orders for laboratory tests to monitor effects of a medication order, orders for special diets in preparation for a medical procedure.

Downtime—the period of time during which the healthcare facility's computer system is unavailable and electronic order entry is not possible.

e-Iatrogenesis—patient harm caused at least in part by the application of health information technology.[1]

Electronic Health Record (EHR) systems—software programs designed for use by healthcare systems to electronically place, store, and retrieve clinical orders, results, notes, reports, and other information related to the care of patients.

File Architecture—also referred to as the *medication masterfile,* a compilation of interconnected files and records that contain data elements that compose the medication and clinical information presented for use in an EHR system.

Notification—a patient- and context-sensitive prompt to the ordering provider, attending physician, primary provider, or care team to alert them of new information (i.e., abnormal lab result) or tasks in need of completion (i.e., unsigned order or note).

Order Menu—a listing of orders from which clinicians may select individual orders, organized to support a specific purpose, ordering environment, or type of order.

Order Set—a group of medication and procedure orders that can be accessed and ordered from a single source in the EHR, to facilitate entry of multiple orders and standardize ordering for a specific purpose. These are analogous to pre-printed paper order forms.

Quick Order—a pre-configured order in which the components (e.g., medication, dose, route, schedule, amount, number of refills, etc) are specified, allowing for faster order entry and limiting opportunities for entry errors. These are sometimes referred to as order sentences and may be maintained and standardized across an institution or created by individuals as personal quick orders, user preferences or preference lists.

Introduction

The Institute of Medicine's landmark 2000 report, *To Err is Human: Building a Safer Health System*, found that as many as 98,000 people die each year in the United States due to medical errors, and propelled Congress, the Joint Commission on Accreditation of Healthcare Organizations, healthcare professions, and the public towards a renewed commitment to patient safety. A central theme of the report is that bad systems cause most errors, not bad people, and this idea has fostered dramatic advances in clinical systems engineering with safety foremost in design, including "no-blame" error reporting and a call for widespread use of electronic health records.[2] Subsequent IOM reports, *Crossing the Quality Chasm: A New Health System for the 21st Century*, and *Patient Safety: Achieving a New Standard for Care*, emphasized the need for "a national health information infrastructure to provide real-time access to complete patient information and decision-support tools for clinicians and their patients, to capture patient safety information as a by-product of care, and to make it possible to use this

information to design safer delivery systems."[3,4] In the Medicare Modernization Act of 2003, Congress mandated the Institute of Medicine to "carry out a comprehensive study of drug safety and quality issues in order to provide a blueprint for system-wide change." This study resulted in the 2007 IOM publication *Preventing Medication Errors: Quality Chasm Series*, in which the Betsy Lehman cyclophosphamide overdose case is used to illustrate how an inferior medication-ordering and delivery system involving minimal double-checks, lack of attending physician oversight, ambiguous protocols, and different dosing expressions in the same order contributed to a tragic patient death; and then how the healthcare system responded, in part by designing a first-class computerized provider order entry interface featuring automatic dose-checking and associated warnings requiring interdisciplinary overrides, extensive point-of-care on-line references, and peer-reviewed templates and protocols.[5] The report further explores sources of medication errors such as gaps in medication knowledge and the lack of timely, easily accessible, and pertinent drug information at the point of ordering; incomplete medication and allergy histories which lack over-the-counter and herbal product information or prescription information from other heath care providers; illegible orders; and unavailability of relevant diagnosis and laboratory results at the point of ordering. CPOE has the potential to dramatically reduce these sources of order errors and significantly improve patient care overall.

What Is Computerized Provider Order Entry?

The term *computerized provider order entry* (CPOE) denotes the direct entry of clinical orders into a healthcare system's electronic health record (EHR) by licensed independent clinicians or others with ordering privileges. The acronym CPOE has different interpretations, including computerized prescription order entry, computerized physician order entry, and computerized provider order entry. We use the latter to emphasize that orders may be entered by physicians, physicians' assistants, nurse practitioners, and other licensed independent practitioners as well as other clinical staff whose scope of practice or protocols grant specific prescribing privileges. A healthcare system can have a comprehensive electronic health record maintained by pharmacists, laboratory and radiology technologists, nurses, dietitians, therapists, medical records specialists, and ward secretaries—all important clinical and administrative staff who are not ordering providers. The full benefits of CPOE accrue only when orders are directly entered by responsible providers and are not

placed or scribed by others on the healthcare team on behalf of ordering providers. Orders may include medications, laboratory tests, radiology requests, diets, nursing orders, consultation requests, procedures, equipment, or any other item or service that may have previously been ordered in a paper system.

This chapter will focus primarily on medication orders and corollary orders, such as lab tests, that may be indicated to monitor safe use of a given medication. Most EHR systems use some type of structured order entry format to ensure consistency, completeness, and accuracy of the order. For example, in the Department of Veterans Affairs' Computerized Patient Record System (CPRS), this is referred to as an order dialog box (Figure 1-1). The order

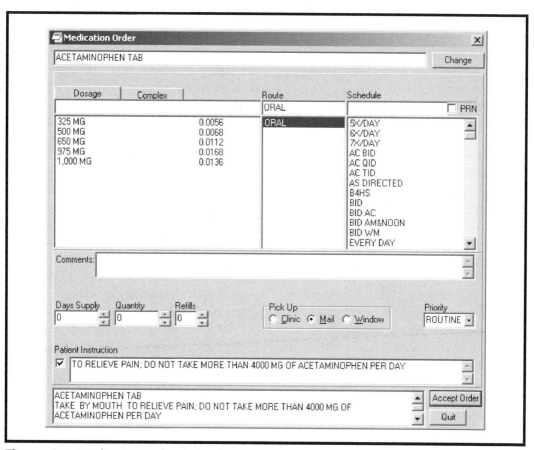

Figure 1-1. Medication order dialog box in VA's CPRS.

dialog includes a pick list for the item to be ordered, as well as the dosage, route of administration, schedule or administration frequency, prescription quantity, refills, and additional instructions for the patient, the nurse administering the medication, or for the pharmacist completing the prescription. A completed dialog for commonly used orders may be saved as a "quick order" or "order sentence" and subsequently retrieved to expedite future entry of the same order. Items frequently ordered together, such as medications and monitoring laboratory tests, may be grouped together into an order set to both facilitate the ordering process as well as enhance patient safety by prompting the provider to order these corollary items. Quick orders and order sets may be grouped together in order menus to facilitate navigation to the correct orders. Once entered, electronically signed, and released by the provider, the order is immediately available to the pharmacist or other receiving service, thereby eliminating transmittal time and misrouting errors as well as the opportunity for errors in transcription or miscommunication.

Many facilities claim to be proponents of CPOE, however, on closer inspection they employ a system whereby pharmacists, nurses, ward secretaries, laboratory personnel and other staff transcribe orders from handwritten paper orders, orders printed from a stand-alone order-writing program, or dictated verbal orders.[6] While insulating clinicians from the possibility of technical problems inherent in the clinician-computer interface, these systems bypass the fundamental benefits of CPOE: the promotion of patient safety and clinical decision support. Progressive EHR systems represent much more than an electronic replacement for the traditional paper medical record: they have come to serve as a comprehensive repository for clinical histories from multiple, diverse healthcare facilities; a compendium of evidence-based order menus and order sets organized to support the latest practice guidelines, responsible resource use, and rapid order entry; a vast library of primary and secondary references organized for rapid access through web links at the point of ordering; and the hub of time-sensitive results and other critical information constantly being updated by clinical ancillary systems such as pharmacy, laboratory, and imaging. The intersection in time at which the busy clinician interfaces with the continually dynamic EHR for the purpose of writing orders represents a unique opportunity to leverage all these capabilities, if well presented, to better inform the clinician of patient-specific factors, guidelines, and the latest research that can improve clinical decision-making for that patient.

Why Is Computerized Provider Order Entry Important?

Impressive patient safety benefits can be achieved with a CPOE system. Illegible hand-written prescriptions are a problem of the past, and CPOE can remind the ordering clinician of a patient's allergy to a specific medication and suggest alternatives or how to manage a reaction. It can alert the clinician of drug-drug interactions, educate on the severity and mechanism of action, and provide advice on managing them. It can check dosages against the patient's physical parameters, laboratory parameters, and previous dosing history and then warn the clinician of potential problems and how to alter a course of therapy. A CPOE system for medications that is integrated with diet orders and diagnoses can alert providers of dangerously incongruent ordering scenarios such as ordering insulin for an NPO patient or teratogenic drugs in a pregnant patient. It can facilitate appropriate monitoring with any potentially risky therapy, such as linking orders for liver function tests with thiazolidinediones and reminding ordering providers to monitor tardive dyskinesia in patients on neuroleptics. It can promote safety at the point of order selection, by detaching "sound-alike" drugs into separate order menus organized by pharmacological class or clinical indication, or by displaying drug names in "tall man" lettering (Figure 1-2). Medication histories, even from multiple healthcare facilities, can be more easily and in some systems automatically maintained, with all of the attendant benefits of medication reconciliation. These are examples of how CPOE can significantly enhance patient safety.

As a result of *To Err is Human*, the Leapfrog Group was convened. This organization is a consortium of purchasers of healthcare plans whose members base their purchases on quality improvement and consumer involvement as evidenced by four "leaps," or recommended practices: computerized provider order entry; evidence-based hospital referral; use of ICU specialists or "intensivists"; and adherence to the Leapfrog Safe Practices Score.[7] Included in the Safe Practices Score is a set of recommended alerts and clinical reminders which healthcare systems are encouraged to employ in their EHR:

1. drug-allergy alert
2. drug-drug interaction alert
3. drug-laboratory result alert (e.g., digoxin level, lithium level, theophylline level, INR, creatinine)
4. drug-monitoring laboratory test alert (e.g., LFTs with statins, TSH with amiodarone, electrolytes with angiotensin converting enzyme inhibitors)
5. drug-diagnosis alert (e.g., pregnancy, G6PD deficiency)

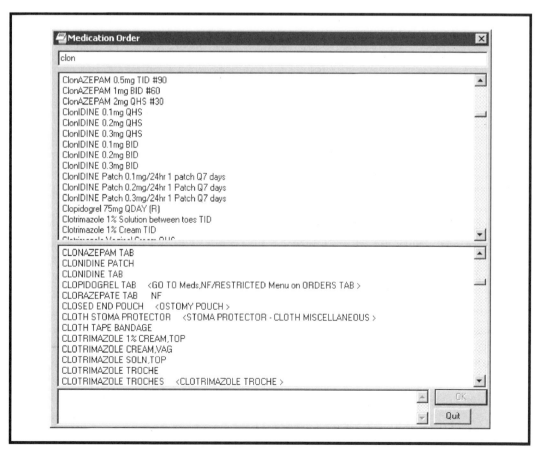

Figure 1-2. An example of "tall man lettering" in VA's CPRS.

6. drug-diet interaction (including NPO, TPN)

7. individual dose checking

8. cumulative dose checking

9. physical incompatibilities (e.g., calcium and ceftriaxone)

10. preventative health clinical reminders

As described previously, in addition to quick orders and order sets, most CPOE programs offer a structured order entry interface or "order dialog" that references an architectural system of interrelated files of order elements, and allows providers to build an order de novo by selecting from various order components. This file architecture is referred to as the *medication masterfile* in other chapters. Careful consideration of how the order dialog interacts with the underlying file architecture can be an important safety aspect of computerized provider order entry, especially for medications. Once a drug is selected, the order dialog should not allow the provider to make ambiguous or dangerously contradictory selections in dosage, routes of administration, or administration frequency, but rather offer appropriate, safe choices to ordering clinicians first, according to the drug selected. For example, it should not be possible to indicate an intravenous route for a medication intended to be administered intramuscularly only. Indications should be easily selected for inclusion in prescription directions for the patient or administering nurse, and should not be merely selectable text that appears in the directions but computable data that can be searched and aggregated for medication use evaluations, billing purposes, and research.

In addition to promoting safe ordering, CPOE can realize other benefits for the healthcare system. Through the use of electronic access and signature codes, electronically-enabled identification cards, and biometric devices utilizing optical or fingerprint scanners, CPOE can verify the identity of the ordering provider and prevent order forgery and other sources of diversion and fraud. It can cross-check the ordering provider's privileges and scope of practice against the orders he or she is attempting to place, and limit the provider to types of orders within his or her clinical specialty, licensure, and privileges. In large health systems or at an agency level, aggregated order data can be analyzed with clinical outcome data, the comparison of such data can lead to clinical practice guideline development, and the result can be fed back into the ordering interfaces to improve patient care for large populations. Studies have shown that CPOE, though initially expensive, can realize significant net savings to healthcare systems over time, due to better drug and staff time utilization, and fewer adverse drug events.[8] The organization and presentation of order menus can help promote hospital-preferred, evidence-based order selection. It can standardize ordering practices, when appropriate, and improve order entry efficiency by grouping orders for common ordering scenarios such as hospital admissions or medical procedures. This is only true, however, if both ordering providers and order receivers are closely involved in the menu design phase, and the health system commits to continuous improvement in its order menu content.[9,10]

Consideration must be given to how and where clinicians place orders, and menus must be designed to support and enhance that action in varying scenarios and by clinicians of different levels of clinical and technical expertise.[9,10] The master order menu architecture might include menus of quick orders sorted by ordering scenario as mentioned above; by ordering location such as the emergency room, women's clinic, or surgical ICU; by order-receiving service (pharmacy, laboratory, radiology, etc.); by chronic and acute diseases; and by listing orderable items alphabetically (Figure

1-3). Menus of order sets and quick orders organized around common and uncommon procedures can assist providers in entering orders quickly in familiar and unfamiliar scenarios according to the health system's accepted guidelines. The menu design could have hospital-approved links to relevant drug information or other resources for clinicians at the point of ordering, references, clinical calculators, patient education print-outs, and community resources. Such links are most efficiently maintained and retrieved via the internet but can reside within the EHR internally if staffing is available to update them. Finally, the component order menus in the master menu infrastructure should ideally be cross-linked, similar to the links in the web pages that form "Wikipedia," so that providers of differing specialization or expertise needing to address unfamiliar co-morbidities from varying ordering locations can quickly navigate to the other menus in the system with minimal clicks.

Key Considerations

Administrative Oversight

An order menu system as described above can promote the use of evidence-based,

---

Example of Integrated Master Order Menu Architecture

I. Outpatient Order Menus:

  A. Orders by Indication Menu:

    1. Diabetes Order Menu:

      a. Diabetes Medication Menu:

      b. Diabetes Laboratory Menu:

      c. Diabetes Consult Menu:

      d. Diabetes Guidelines and Web Links:

      e. Diabetes Clinic Menu:

      f. Hypertension Clinic Menu:

        i. Antihypertensive Medication Menu:

      g. Lipid Management Clinic Menu:

        i. Antilipidemic Medication Menu:

      h. Ophthalmology Clinic Menu:

        i. Podiatry Clinic Menu:

      j. Neurology Clinic Menu:

        i. Antidepressant Medication Menu:

        ii. Anticonvulsant Medication Menu:

        iii. Analgesic Medication Menu:

    2. Neuropathic Pain Order Menu:

      a. Antidepressant Medication Menu:

      b. Anticonvulsant Medication Menu:

      c. Analgesic Medication Menu:

      d. Diabetes Clinic Order Menu:

      e. Neurology Clinic Menu:

  B. Orders by Clinic Menu:

    1. Diabetes Clinic Order Menu:

    2. Neurology Clinic Order Menu:

    3. Hypertension Clinic Order Menu:

    4. Lipid Management Clinic Order Menu:

    5. Podiatry Clinic Order Menu:

    6. Ophthalmology Clinic Order Menu:

  Medication Orders by Drug Class Menu:

    Diabetes Medication Menu:

    Antihypertensive Medication Menu:

    Antilipidemic Medication Menu:

    Antidepressant Medication Menu:

    Anticonvulsant Medication Menu:

    Analgesic Medication Menu:

Figure 1-3. Example of integrated master order menu architecture.

clinically accepted guidelines that simultaneously educate providers and encourage responsible resource utilization, by making the preferred course of therapy foremost in the design (i.e., the easy default choice), and less preferred therapy available through decision-support algorithms. It is vital to have the support and concurrence of the healthcare system's clinical leadership in the selection of the guidelines and the design of the menus. Some healthcare systems charter a clinical guidelines committee comprised of clinical leaders, researchers, and medical informaticians to establish order menu content based on the latest evidence. For medications, many facilities charge the pharmacy and therapeutics committee with this responsibility, which documents the sponsor, discussion, and date of review of each guideline and menu in its meeting minutes. Ideally the date of the minutes and the menu's sponsors are also displayed on the order menus, making this information available to users. This allows questions or concerns to be directed appropriately. Other facilities convene a successor to the paper "forms" committee, charged with reviewing and sanctioning order sets and templates as the electronic descendants of pre printed paper ordering forms. Ad hoc committees can perform this task, however, the lack of continuity in membership can contribute to a lack of overall vision, a lack of adequate documentation which may be needed for audits, and lead to disruptive changes in menus that can confuse providers.

Build Considerations

An order menu design may involve thousands of quick orders and order sets and hundreds of order menus. For consistency, continuity, and ease of maintenance, the components should be the same, i.e., the same quick order for acetaminophen 650 mg PO Q6H PRN should be a component of the alphabetical drug menu, the non-narcotic analgesic drug class menu, the surgical ward admission order set, and the emergency room medication menu, so that when a change in the quick order is warranted the change can be made at the atomic level and be expressed in multiple menus. Such "object-oriented" design allows a component quick order to be created once but used many times, thereby increasing efficiency and consistency. However, it also significantly increases risk if a component quick order is not built correctly, without full knowledge of the myriad menus where it might occur, or there is a change in the file architecture on which the quick order is based (e.g., a change in the drug, schedule, or route files). This is an example of a *tightly coupled* system, one which responds to changes rapidly and efficiently, but catastrophically if the change is not well-planned and well-executed.[11] It is crucial to successful CPOE that order menus are maintained according to the latest formulary changes and newest clinical practice guidelines, by information systems analysts who possess both the clinical and technical knowledge necessary to safely manage tightly coupled systems.

Understanding Workflow

In addition to programmers, network managers, and technical support, most successful CPOE programs require information systems analysts who are able to act as liaisons between the clinical user community and the technical support staff. They typically are responsible for configuring the EHR and the order entry interface to meet the needs of the clinical users, training the users, and providing support if they have questions. In the Department of Veterans Affairs, these analysts are known as clinical application coordinators (CAC), but this sobriquet is not entirely accurate, since they do much more than coordinate applications. The more knowledgeable these staff members are regarding the clinical policies, procedures, workflow demands, regulatory pressures, organizational culture, and mission of their healthcare system, in addition to the technical aspects of their EHR, the more effective they will be. They understand and can speak in both clinical and technical terms and can serve as translators between clinical users and technical staff. They have first-hand knowledge of the workflow and processes in patient care areas and can both suggest and implement better ways to accomplish clinical tasks through their intimate knowledge of the EHR. Clinical users are often more receptive to an analyst whom they know has been "in the trenches" and can appreciate through personal experience the daily challenges they face. For that reason, staff with prior patient-care experience such as physicians, pharmacists, and nurses are well-suited for this role and must maintain their clinical competency in order to retain their relevance and credibility as they simultaneously acquire new skills, terminology, and contacts in the technological domain.

Professional user support with staff such as CAC's "at the elbow" brought in expressly for that purpose is very helpful during CPOE implementation, but as institutional CPOE experience grows, some support can be shifted to collegial, peer-to-peer support. The healthcare system can plan for that shift by formally recognizing and training front-line "superusers," clinical users whose affinity for technology can assist their peers in adopting the new tools. Likewise, CPOE can be sustained long-term if staff expectations with respect to training and user support are managed from the beginning, through the use of training milestones and accompanying "service level agreements" between the clinical users and the implementation staff. Service level agreements are contractual arrangements between the clinical users and information technology staff that establish the scope of training and user support that meets the needs of clinical users at a level that is sustainable long-term for the information technology staff. Administrative support at the departmental level to reliably

manage provider accounts in advance of the providers' arrival will make CPOE function smoothly. Many facilities have linked the need for user support and training, a continual requirement in academic medical centers with high trainee turnover, to succession planning for information technology (IT) professionals. Recognizing the value of first-hand clinical experience to CPOE, they have established a career track whereby "superusers" on the front line can train and support their colleagues while preparing to become information system analysts through formal coursework, then advance to more senior IT positions by undertaking more complex initiatives.

Implementation and Maintenance Strategies

Institutional Leadership

Much has been written regarding the components of a successful CPOE implementation.[6,12] In order for a healthcare system to realize the benefits of computerized provider order entry and not merely replace its paper-based charting system with an electronic version, successful CPOE implementations have found that organizational leadership and an unfaltering commitment throughout the healthcare system to improving patient safety and the quality of care are essential from the beginning. Of all the CPOE implementation and maintenance strategies in the literature and that we can offer herein, enthusiastic and ongoing clinical and administrative support at the highest levels, in terms of funding for equipment and staff, as well as establishing a vision of patient care for all staff, is fundamental to success.

Communication

Communicating changes in CPOE applications, policies, and new initiatives during the implementation phases of CPOE and beyond is critically important, but can be challenging in large organizations with frequent staff turnover, such as academic medical centers. Usually a healthcare system must employ a variety of communication methods to reach the widest possible audience. Electronic and paper newsletters, e-mail bulletins, a regular "CPOE minute" at departmental staff meetings, regular attendance at new staff orientations, participation in morning rounds as well as conducting separate "CPOE rounds" are techniques that have proven to be successful. Posting new information in a designated place on hospital and departmental websites and in team rooms, break rooms, charting rooms, elevators, stairwells, and even staff restrooms is another effective technique. CPOE information of a time-sensitive nature can be posted on websites, broadcast via overhead announcements, sent by high-priority e-mail, delivered by text pagers, and communicated via phone cascades.

Training

Training in basic computing competencies and the healthcare system's EHR of choice should be mandatory but need not be painful. Some facilities initiate their CPOE implementation by encouraging staff to play hospital-sanctioned computer games specifically designed to improve typing, mouse use, and web navigation skills. Short classes with subsequent refresher sessions are better tolerated and generally more effective than a single, marathon training session. New staff should receive their access codes only after they have successfully completed training, whether in the classroom, one-on-one with a trainer, or via the internet. Brief, interactive CPOE training modules available on the web allow incoming staff to prepare in advance of their arrival and existing staff to refresh their knowledge whenever it is convenient.

Infrastructure (Hardware, Software, Configuration)

Adequate hardware in terms of terminal devices, printers, servers, routers, system speed, memory, and reliability are absolutely vital to CPOE, during implementation and afterwards. The implementation and subsequent maintenance plan should accommodate network managers, programmers, technical support staff, help desk personnel, an education plan and staffing, and the aforementioned clinical/technical liaisons who link the clinical, technical, and administrative domains. Planning must include not only the ordering clinicians who will initially interact with the system but also each order-receiving department and the medical records staff, for orders properly placed but not carried out as intended and not adequately documented will quickly derail the implementation effort. Just-in-time training for new staff and the development of a "critical mass" of experienced front-line staff who can provide new staff with on-the-spot help is crucial for making the implementation self-sustaining.

Successful CPOE implementation is a multidisciplinary effort, and the selection of EHR software to fully support this concept should not be overlooked. Ideally, the components of the EHR software should be fully integrated, including the order entry interface, documentation interface, pharmacy interface, as well as adverse reaction tracking, laboratory, dietetics, imaging, nursing, vital signs, surgery, medical procedural, and consult components. This must be done in such a way that it is not necessary for the ordering clinician, pharmacist, laboratory technologist, or other clinical user to log in to a separate program to access different sections of the EHR, and data is fully transferable between components. For example, laboratory results should be as easily retrievable within the pharmacy component as within the order entry interface, and pharmacy data easily retrieved within the dietetics component. The inpatient and outpatient ordering and results review environments must likewise be integrated, to facilitate the continuum of care as it occurs in real life. As mentioned before, healthcare systems are realizing the importance of integrating not only the components of their EHRs, but also the ability to exchange data from their EHRs with other systems' EHRs, to better care for itinerant patients or those who have multiple providers.

Many facilities initially implement computerized provider order entry with electronic replacements for pre-printed paper orders and long, alphabetical lists of pre-configured quick orders organized around the order-filling service: pharmacy, laboratory, dietetics, radiology, and nursing. While these have a place in the overall order menu design, these facilities discovered they were not used by ordering providers to the extent anticipated.[9,10] Multi-layered order menus requiring multiple clicks to reach the desired order and lengthy menus requiring scrolling down the screen were deemed too time-intensive to navigate. Menus of quick orders organized around order-filling services were of limited help to providers needing to quickly place groups of orders intended for different departments, such as medications, laboratory tests, imaging orders, and consults for an emergency procedure. Involving providers in the design and configuration of CPOE tools is critical to success and helps avoid wasted effort.

Clinical/Technical Liaisons

As described previously under "Understanding Workflow," dedicated implementation staff, i.e., those not having direct patient-care responsibilities, who have first-hand knowledge of clinical workplace processes as well as technical aspects of the EHR are critical to implementation efforts. Such personnel ideally should be readily accessible around the clock, by telephone if not in person, during the introductory phases of a CPOE implementation. As the implementation matures, as baseline informatics skills in the healthcare system reaches a critical mass, and CPOE becomes engrained in the workflow, user support can migrate to the aforementioned "superusers." Other forms of user support can involve "help desk" staff available at a standard phone number or

through a computerized problem reporting system. The latter can be a simple e-mail message sent to a group of clinical application coordinators, or it can involve sophisticated software programs that triage a problem, alert the most appropriate IT professionals to resolve it, monitor its resolution, and electronically escalate the problem if needed. Similarly, procedures to escalate problems encountered during evening, weekend, and holiday shifts by telephoning on-call IT staff should be developed and widely distributed.

Mature CPOE programs have found it is just as crucial to plan for the return to system availability after a period of downtime as it is to plan for the initial downtime, especially with regard to medication reconciliation.[10] Medications may have been discontinued on paper during the downtime, yet the order may remain active in the computer and prompt for administration until it is discontinued electronically. New medications ordered on paper during the downtime will not appear in the computer for administration upon its return to availability until they are entered, potentially causing errors of omission. Laboratory and radiology results, changes in diet orders and nursing care orders must be entered into the computer as soon as possible, sometimes necessitating overtime or additional staff to enter the data, since the EHR is dynamic and clinical decisions depend on an up-to-date patient record. Policies and procedures for system unavailability and return to normal operations are ideally multi-disciplinary and should accommodate every aspect of the order placing, order receiving, order administration, and order documentation process.

Unexpected Consequences and Unique Challenges

Changes in Workflow Patterns

CPOE can change workflow patterns and communication between members of the patient care team. By placing desktop computers in provider offices, resident team rooms, charting rooms, satellite pharmacies, and even providers' homes, providers, nurses, and pharmacists are physically separated as they interact with the EHR, and attempts to communicate with each other clinically through the EHR cannot match the face-to-face communication that formerly existed when the hard chart in the nursing station was everyone's point of reference.[13,14] However, with the increasing use of wireless mobile computing via tablet PCs and PDAs; medical teleconferencing; and secure, asynchronous provider-to-provider messaging, professional communication is rapidly improving.

e-Iatrogenesis

This term was recently coined in the literature to describe adverse events caused at least in part by the use of health information technology in patient care that would not have happened with non-electronic health delivery systems.[1] For example, an e-iatrogenic event can involve CPOE errors of commission or omission due to an erroneous click due to too many unfiltered choices, erroneous assumptions of how providers interact with an ordering screen, or unexpected changes in order routing.

The concept that computerized provider order entry can solve all of a hospital's ordering problems is obviously wishful thinking. In reality, what often happens is that one problem is resolved as a new issue is created. Examples abound at the Department of Veterans Affairs medical facilities, which have employed CPOE and addressed these issues incrementally for nearly 15 years. With the introduction of CPOE for medication ordering, instantly gone were illegible orders, non-existent hand-written drug names, imaginary routes, and nonsensical schedules. The process by which CPOE notifies the pharmacy department of new orders created a new concern, however. Take for example the following series of orders which, as hand-written orders, would have been faxed together on one sheet to the pharmacy:

1. Mark chart for allergy to ampicillin/sulbactam

2. D/C Unasyn IVPB

3. Solumedrol 60 mg IVPB X1

4. Benadryl 25 mg IV Push X1

In a written system, the combination of the above orders is indicative of an allergic reaction. Pharmacy department policies would likely result in the documentation of an observed reaction, with resulting reports made to the pharmacy and therapeutics committee. To contrast, in an electronic system that distributes orders to various order-filling departments, the pharmacy may only receive orders #3 and #4 (#2 would occur without explicitly notifying the pharmacy). The ordering clinician may have overlooked the importance of entering order #1 (for documentation in the chart). The result is that it is much harder for the pharmacist to take note of this case as indicative of an allergic reaction, and it might be interpreted as a premedication order for a procedure.

CPOE cannot completely remove sources of medication errors. Consider for example the case of two patients with similar names and medical record identifying numbers. In a paper-based system, the patient's ID may be stamped onto an order sheet or progress note form using an addressograph card. The selection of cards available to the prescriber may also be limited to the patients currently admitted to the hospital unit. The transition to CPOE often brings with it the availability of the system's entire patient database, increasing the chances of selecting the incorrect record. Of course, it is possible for these two patients to actually be admitted to the same unit at the same time, and it is similarly possible for the pharmacy system to introduce the same potential for error in the transcription phase of a paper-based system. For this reason, using a second identifier, such as verifying the patient's date of birth, is a recommended step to ensure selection of the correct record.

As described previously, EHRs can incorporate "tightly coupled" systems to increase ordering efficiency; for example, employing the same medication quick order in multiple order menus allows updates to the quick order to be expressed in many locations. However, if the quick order is updated erroneously, the error is also expressed in many locations, multiplying the possibility for adverse patient events. Similarly, some EHRs allow entry of discrete, computable vital sign data concurrently with the entry of text-based electronic progress notes. This increases user efficiency by accomplishing two documentation requirements with one action: the textual progress note and vital sign data. However, if a progress note and embedded vital sign data are entered for the wrong patient, it is critical that both the note and embedded data be retracted, since computable vital sign data, especially patient weight, can be automatically incorporated into weight-based dosing order algorithms elsewhere in the EHR.

How human beings interact with technology to produce results either expected or not expected by the technology designers is the basis of the field of human factors engineering, and has great consequence to CPOE. For example, early versions of the VA's order entry dialog for medications employed for provider convenience use a completion-text matching technology, which allowed clinicians to enter a few characters of a lengthy drug name for which they may not have known the correct spelling and the CPOE dialog would complete the entry. However, the auto-completed entry may not have been the drug intended by the clinician. A clinician could desire to order "Procardia," a calcium-channel blocker, and enter "Procar," not realizing that the closest match to his/her entry is "Procarbazine," an antineoplastic agent, since the "b" in Procarbazine comes before the "d" in Procardia in the drug file. Another example occurred when the Joint Commission for Accreditation of Healthcare Organizations prohibited

the abbreviation of "QD." To comply, VA facilities changed their "QD" schedule entries to "Daily," however, ordering clinicians initially persisted in attempting to enter "QD" with their orders. Since "QD" was no longer on file, completion matching retrieved and offered the closest match: "Q12H." In both examples, if the clinician failed to notice the erroneous auto-completed components, the subsequent orders could result in serious harm to the patient. VA resolved these issues by disabling the completion matching feature and requiring the ordering clinician to actively and purposefully select each of the order components. It is of fundamental concern that the design of the CPOE interface not contribute to the commission of errors, but instead guide the clinician to safe choices.

Computer Unavailability (Downtime)

With successful implementation of an EHR and CPOE comes increasing dependence on computer based resources to support clinical care processes. This creates a unique challenge when these resources become unavailable, and strategies and procedures must be in place for both planned and unexpected computer down times which are inevitable even in the best of circumstances. Back-up procedures using paper, local non-networked or alternative computer resources, or a combination of the two must be clearly defined and communicated to all system users in advance. Most large healthcare systems keep files on independent storage media in a physically separate location in the event of a catastrophic outage, and automatically "push" copies of time-sensitive clinical information across the local area network to selected workstation hard drives every 30 minutes to 4 hours to provide a back-up clinical record in the event of lesser outages. Many facilities have found maintaining a "downtime folder" containing paper order forms and instructions for use in each clinical area to be very useful in minimizing disruption when regular computer resources are unavailable. Mature healthcare systems which have completely replaced paper order forms with electronic order menus involving decision-supported algorithms should consider including paper copies of order menus in the downtime kit as well. Having a web-based application that can access back-up read-only data when regular resources are not available has also been a significant asset. Close communication between clinical and technical staff is important in assessing the likely severity and duration of the unplanned downtime leading to the decision of whether and when to go to paper. Communication can occur via overhead loudspeaker, notice on non-EHR computer resources if still operational, telephone cascades, as well as through in-person visits to key clinical areas. Many facilities have adopted a monthly 4–6 hour pre-scheduled, pre-announced downtime to perform preventative maintenance on the hardware, which also affords the opportunity to conduct a computer disaster drill for front-line staff providing patient care. Disruption from planned downtimes can be minimized by sensitivity to clinical processes and close coordination with clinical service leaders. For instance, the time between 7 and 9 a.m. is typically a peak period for medication administration and clinical rounds in inpatient settings and a particularly bad time for planned computer outages. Scheduled planned downtime late in the day on a week end seems to strike the best balance of availability of technical staff and minimizing clinical process disruption. Once computer systems are again available, back entry of orders and documentation created during the down time is generally required to ensure that computerized records are accurate, up to date, and reflect the most current state of patient care. Communication between pharmacy and nursing is especially critical in inpatient settings to ensure that medication administration records are synchronized to avoid duplicate or missed medication doses. Computer downtimes will happen, but careful planning, preparation, and good communication can greatly minimize the impact on both patients and staff.

Information Overload and Desensitization of Ordering Providers

We have previously described how the point in time at which the clinician interfaces with the EHR for the purpose of placing orders represents a "golden" opportunity to leverage an enormous amount of information about the patient at hand and a vast web of clinical decision support tools, references, and research to assist the provider in making better-informed order choices. However, bombardment of uncoordinated and non-prioritized alerts, warning flags, notifications, and reminders at that golden moment quickly leads to alert fatigue and desensitization, effectively negating any benefit these tools might have offered to improving patient safety and decision support. It is important to establish institutional parameters that are above individual departmental agendas to control the application of attention-seeking electronic tools, if the healthcare system wishes to realize the benefits they were intended to provide. Often alternative systems of notification can be devised, such as surveillance reports run at the departmental level, to relieve providers of alerts of a less time-sensitive nature. Likewise, the specificity and usefulness of warnings and reminders must be deemed valuable to the provider if the healthcare system wishes the information to be integrated into the care of the patient, and not discounted and overridden as quickly as possible.[15,16] Cross-sensitivity warnings should have a logical and specific pharmacological basis; drug interaction warnings should include the mechanism of action; and warnings should provide information on severity and management advice with accompanying order menus.

Technology Outpaces Policy

In 2007, the Department of Veterans Affairs began displaying remote drug-allergy, drug-drug interaction, and duplicate drug alerts in all of its 172 healthcare facilities, i.e., the agency's EHR began warning ordering providers of potential order incompatibilities or duplicate therapy based on information on file at distant VA facilities where patients were treated previously. In the future drug-lab result and drug-diagnosis alerts may be added. This capability represents a significant enhancement in patient safety, especially for co-managed and itinerant patients, as well as an advance towards medication reconciliation, the Joint Commission's recent Patient Safety Goal, across the agency. However, this new information created an unanticipated logistical problem for providers. Because clinical privileges are facility-specific, a provider cannot legally, nor does VA's EHR provide the technical means to, discontinue a medication at a remote site even if the patient has been instructed to discontinue it, and therefore cannot support medication reconciliation across the agency. As is often the case where information technology intersects with healthcare policy, the technology and the policy were not initially aligned in their planning, development, or release, yet turned out to be serendipitously synergistic. The details of inter-facility transferring of prescriptions, reconciling remote prescription profile discrepancies, and cross-agency safety initiatives such as anticoagulation management, as well as with non-VA community partners, still need to be elucidated. The implementation of a standard medical nomenclature, including drug names, normalized lab results, etc., that can be shared, interpreted, and calculated equivalently in any EHR system and a basic national EHR architecture to facilitate that data sharing, will be instrumental in moving CPOE to the next phase of improving patient safety and quality patient care.

Future Trends

In the future medication reconciliation and real-time sharing of medical records across diverse healthcare systems employing very different EHRs will be available, with the development of a standardized medical nomenclature and a national health information infrastructure. Inter-facility EHR cross-referencing is especially important for patients who are co-managed by multiple healthcare systems, for itinerant patients such as "snowbirds," and for patients who are transferring their care in large numbers from one healthcare system to another such as military personnel transferring from the Department of Defense to the Department of Veterans Affairs.

Most CPOE systems, even those which are highly integrated, offer different order dialogs for the inpatient and outpatient ordering environments as well as the different order-filling departments (pharmacy, laboratory, imaging, dietetics, nursing, etc.). This is easier to program and makes sense from the standpoint of the order-filling departments, many of which have been using computer programs for their internal workload for years, and onto which CPOE was overlaid. Providers encountering CPOE for the first time, however, are not accustomed to having to search for and select different order dialogs for inpatient and outpatient medications, or for recording the OTC, herbal, and outside medications a patient is taking, then repeat the search for the laboratory order dialog, then for the imaging dialog. A well-designed order menu infrastructure comprised of pre-configured quick orders and order sets for a variety of ordering scenarios alleviates some of the searching and delays inherent in a menu-based system, but to the novice user, this system is personally more time-consuming (though safer and time-saving to the healthcare system overall) than scribbling a series of orders on a paper form. It can, however, contribute to new types of errors, e.g., attempting to order an outpatient medication with the inpatient order dialog or the OTC/herbal/outside med dialog. For safety, consistency, and intuitiveness, order dialogs should be similar in appearance, and to the extent it is reasonable, they should be combined, thereby reducing the need to search for and select the right order dialog. For instance, the inpatient and outpatient medication order dialogs could be combined with those used for ordering medications for use in clinic procedures as well as documenting OTC and herbal products the patient is taking. The combined medication order dialog could feature selectable components (e.g., dosage, schedule, route of administration, prescription quantity, number of refills, and purpose of the order) configured internally in the underlying file architecture to successively offer only safe, logical, and context-sensitive choices for each order component based on the selections of previous components.

An alternative approach to offering multiple order entry dialogs for different types of orders arranged in menus is to design a single "natural language" CPOE interface whereby providers type orders just as they would write them on a paper order, and the dialog references the file of pre-configured order menus, quick orders, and order sets.[17] The dialog retrieves entries by name, and offers the closest matches to the provider for selection and subsequent editing as appropriate. The file entries could be as simple as a quick order for "acetaminophen 650 mg PO Q6H PRN outpatient prescription" or as lengthy and complex as a multi-order "cardiac surgery post-op ICU" order set. File entries should be sanctioned by the healthcare system's clinical management, carefully named and managed with human factors engineering in mind, and continually updated according to approved guidelines. This design may make hunting

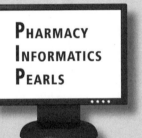

COMPUTERIZED PROVIDER ORDER ENTRY

PHARMACY
INFORMATICS
PEARLS

Provider Order Entry

- Direct entry of orders into an electronic health record system by a licensed independent practitioner with ordering privileges.
- Allow provision of time and patient-sensitive warnings and clinical decision support at the point of order placement.

Patient Safety Advantages

- No illegible orders.
- Allergy and adverse drug reaction warnings at the point of ordering.
- Drug-drug, drug-food, drug-lab, and drug-diagnosis interaction warnings.
- "Tallman" lettering.
- Remind or automatically order corollary monitoring e.g., LFTs.
- Individual order and cumulative dose checking
- File architecture can ensure that inappropriate dosage forms, routes, and schedules are not selectable.

Other Advantages

- Verify identity of prescriber and prescriber's ordering privileges.
- Standardize therapy when appropriate according to accepted guidelines.
- Provide opportunity for decision support.
- Enable aggregation of ordering and outcome data, analysis, and creation of new guidelines.
- Facilitate maintenance of medication history from multiple heath care systems.

Order Menus

- Commit time and staffing to providing up-to-date, clinically evidence-based order menus that providers will use.
- Provide administrative oversight via clinical guidelines committee, pharmacy and therapeutics committee, or electronic forms committee.
- Integrate menus supporting different ordering locations, order receiving services, levels of ordering providers, diseases, and orderable items to fully support continuum of care.

Implementation Issues

- Institutional leadership and support is critical.
- Need adequate infrastructure in terms of hardware, software, technical staff, administrative staff.
- Clinical/technical liaisons are crucial for user support, training, and system configuration that optimizes the business of healthcare. Develop an IT career track to ensure connection is maintained.
- Plan for "superusers," peer-to-peer support, service level agreements.
- Develop multi-disciplinary plans for ongoing communication, training, user support, downtime contingencies, security and confidentiality, and EHR content.

Unintended Consequences

- Changes in traditional paper-based communication patterns and workflow can lead to ordering errors.
- Beware of ramifications of "tightly coupled" systems (high efficiency increases scope of errors).
- Be alert to human factors engineering: assumptions and time-savers can lead to ordering errors.
- Plan for scheduled and unscheduled downtime.
- Beware of information overload from unmanaged warnings, reminders, alerts from providers' perspective.
- Foresee how technology can outpace policies, procedures, and practices, and plan for it.

Future Trends

- Medical information sharing across healthcare systems with diverse EHRs via national health information architecture and standardized nomenclature. Adopt and support standards as often as possible.
- Natural language order entry interface obviates need for navigating order menus.

---

for the correct order entry dialog or navigating order menus in search of the correct quick order or order set obsolete, thereby decreasing order entry time, reducing selection errors, and through careful management of the file entries it could significantly enhance clinical decision support and resource management with minimal impact on the ordering providers.

Conclusion

Throughout this chapter, we have asserted that computerized provider order entry is

an essential component of any electronic health record implementation, and the moment at which a provider interacts with the computer to personally place orders represents a golden opportunity to leverage considerable resources towards improving patient safety and applying evidence-based clinical care. Government, regulatory organizations, and patient advocacy groups are calling for "a national health information infrastructure to provide real-time access to complete patient information and decision-support tools for clinicians and their patients, to capture patient safety information as a by-product of care, and to make it possible to use this information to design even safer delivery systems," and CPOE is an integral part.[5] We have offered strategies for implementing and maintaining CPOE, and warned of unexpected consequences. Finally, we offered some suggestions for CPOE interfaces that would make it even more intuitive. When software makes the "right thing to do" also the "easiest way," CPOE will truly have realized its potential.

References

1. Weiner JP, Kfuri T, Chan K, Fowles JB.. "e-Iatrogenesis": The most critical unintended consequence of CPOE and other HIT. *J Am Med Inform Assoc.* 2007;14:387–388.

2. Committee on Quality of Health Care in America. *To Err is Human: Building a Safer Health System.* Washington, DC: National Academy Press; 2000.

3. Committee on Quality of Health Care in America. *Crossing the Quality Chasm: A New Health System for the 21st Century.* Washington, DC: National Academy Press; 2001.

4. Committee on Data Standards for Patient Safety. *Patient Safety: Achieving a New Standard for Care.* Washington, DC: National Academy Press; 2004.

5. Committee on Identifying and Preventing Medication Errors. *Preventing Medication Errors: Quality Chasm Series.* Washington, DC: National Academy Press; 2007.

6. Ash JS, Fournier L, Stavri PZ, Dykstra R. Principles for a successful computerized physician order entry implementation. *AMIA Annu Symp Proc.* 2003:36–40.

7. Leapfrog Group. http://www.leapfroggroup.org.

8. Kaushal R, Jha AK, Franz C, et al. Return on investment for a computerized physician order entry system. *J Am Med Inform Assoc.* 2006;13:261–266.

9. Payne TH, Hoey PJ, Nichol P, et al. Preparation and use of pre-constructed orders, order sets, and order menus in a computerized provider order entry system. *J Am Med Inform Assoc.* 2003;10(4):322–329.

10. Payne TH. *Practical Guide to Clinical Computing Systems: Design, Operations, Infrastructure.* Amsterdam, The Netherlands: Elsevier; 2008.

11. Perrow C. *Normal Accidents: Living with High-Risk Technologies.* New York: Basic Books; 1984.

12. Eslami S, Abu-Hanna A, de Keizer NF, et al. Evaluation of outpatient computerized physician medication order entry systems: a systematic review. *J Am Med Inform Assoc.* 2007;14:400–406.

13. Ash JS, Sittig DF, Poon EG, Guappone K, Campbell E, Dykstra RH, et al. The extent and importance of unintended consequences related to computerized provider order entry. *J Am Med Inform Assoc.* 2007;14:415–423.

14. Campbell EM, Sittig DF, Ash JS, Guappone KP, Dykstra RH, et al. Types of unintended consequences related to computerized provider order entry. *J Am Med Inform Assoc.* 2006;13:547–556.

15. Grizzle AJ, Mahmood MH, Ko Y, et al. Reasons provided by providers when overriding drug-drug interaction alerts. *Am J Managed Care.* 2007;10:573–580.

16. Payne TH, Nichol WP, Hoey P, Savarino J, et al. Characteristics and override rates of order checks in a practitioner order entry system. *Proc AMIA Symp.* 2002:602–606.

17. Lovis C, Chapko MK, Martin DP, et al. Evaluation of a command-line parser-based order entry pathway for the Department of Veterans Affairs electronic patient record. *J Am Med Inform Assoc.* 2001;8(5):486–498.

CHAPTER 2
ePrescribing

Kevin Marvin

KEY DEFINITIONS

ASC X12N—Accredited Standards Committee X12; creates standards for the cross industry electronic transmission of business information. ASC X12N standards are used for insurance eligibility and prior authorization communication.

ePrescribing—commonly defined as "ambulatory computerized provider order entry" or ambulatory CPOE. There are many variations on this definition based on the needs of the definer. According to Department of Health and Human Services Centers for Medicare & Medicaid Services (CMS), the definition of ePrescribing is "The transmission, using electronic media, of prescription or prescription-related information, between a prescriber, dispenser, PBM, or health plan, either directly or through an intermediary, including an e-prescribing network." This definition does not specify who does the data entry or how the data is handled when received by the organizations. It only specifies that the information is sent electronically. It is generally assumed that in order to fully realize the advantages of electronic prescribing, the data should be entered by the prescribing practitioner and the electronic data should not be manually transcribed into the receiving systems. Few current ePrescribing installations currently realize this goal.

ePrescription—according to CMS, a prescription is not an ePrescription unless it is transmitted electronically in a standard format. Printed paper prescriptions and electronic faxes are not considered to be ePrescriptions by CMS rule.

Dispenser—term that the Department of Health and Human Services Centers for Medicare & Medicaid Services uses to specify the pharmacy and pharmacist. It is assumed that this includes in addition to the dispensing of prescription medications that the appropriate verifications and patient education is provided by the dispenser.

NCPDP—National Council for Prescription Drug Programs; an organization that creates and promotes standards for the transfer of data to and from the pharmacy services sector of the healthcare industry. NCPDP is an ANSI-accredited standards development organization that has over 1450 members representing all areas of pharmacy services.[1] NCPDP has developed standards for provider identification and telecommunication standards for pharmacy claims. It has also developed SCRIPT, which consists of multiple standards supporting prescription communication and processing.

PDP—Medicare Prescription Drug Plan (PDP) is the prescription drug plan that was created with the Medicare Prescription Drug, Improvement and Modernization Act of 2003.

Prescriber—the health practitioner who has the legal authority for ordering ambulatory medications.

RXNORM—a clinical drug nomenclature standard produced by the National Library of Medicine. It provides standard names for clinical drugs, strengths and dosage forms. It also provides links between the standard semantic clinical description and the branded representation.

Switch—a company that provides a communication network to support claims adjudication, eligibility checking and electronic prescribing for pharmacies.

Introduction

While there have been many physician-specific articles and books written about ePrescribing, there has been comparatively little pharmacy-specific literature published on this topic. This is because most of the emphasis has been placed on the prescriber, and there is very little pharmacy experience with ePrescribing. The purpose of this chapter is to introduce common ePrescribing terminology, discuss the current state of electronic prescribing (ePrescribing) systems, the impact of ePrescribing on clinical workflows, future directions of electronic prescribing, and the role of the informatics pharmacist in ePrescribing implementation and development. This chapter will provide a pharmacist-centered view of ePrescribing.

The majority of healthcare is delivered in the ambulatory care setting and is increasing. In 2000, Americans made 823 million office visits, 100 million more than 1995.[2] Medication prescribing is the most common therapeutic intervention in ambulatory practice settings. Studies have found 75% of the visits to general practitioners or internists resulted in the continuation or initiation of a medication.[3] Prescription volumes are large and increasing. More than 3 billion prescriptions are written annually in the United States and are estimated to increase to 4 billion in 2007.[4] Prescription meds are used by more than two thirds of U.S. citizens annually.[5] The increasing volumes of prescriptions and the increased costs of prescription drugs has increased the attention to controlling these costs. In addition, prescription drug errors and the management of prescription drug therapy are also costly. Studies estimate that indecipherable or unclear prescriptions result in more than 150 million calls from pharmacists to physicians for clarification.[6] Others estimate the number of prescription-related telephone calls annually at 900 million. Practices report almost 30% of prescriptions required pharmacy callbacks.[7,8] Requesting and receiving approval for refills alone, estimated at nearly 500 million per year, adds to the telephone and fax burdens.[9] These interventions by pharmacists often direct prescribers to less costly therapies and prevent medication errors. It is believed that ePrescribing systems will significantly impact prescribers to select less costly therapy and prevent errors before a prescription is sent to the pharmacy. One study estimates the possible savings from ePrescribing of $27 billion per year in the U.S.[10]

ePrescribing has received a lot of attention in the U.S. over the last several years. The Medicare Prescription Drug, Improvement and Modernization Act of 2003 (MMA) initiated government attention to the current problems with ambulatory prescribing.[11] As part of its direction, the MMA specifically includes the development of ePrescribing standards

The Joint Commission with its identification of National Patient Safety goal #8, "Accurately and completely reconcile medications across the continuum of care," has also increased the interest in ePrescribing systems.[12] This patient safety goal has significantly increased the dialogue in health care organizations on how to capture and maintain ambulatory prescribing information. Many organizations are investigating ePrescribing systems to help meet this goal. The Certification Commission on Healthcare Information Technology (CCHIT) has included ePrescribing as part of their certification requirements. This attention has elevated ePrescribing from a niche application to an important component of an enterprise electronic medical record system. As a result, the implementation and development of ePrescribing has accelerated rapidly and has the gained the attention of the government, health care providers, provider organizations, and patients.

Benefits of ePrescribing

There have been many studies of medication errors with inpatients. Medication errors with outpatients is an important subject with minimal research studies. In a recent study of 661 patients surveyed, 24% experienced adverse drug events. Of these adverse events, 13% were serious, 28% ameliorable, and 11% preventable. The majority of the preventable adverse drug events (ADEs) were due to inappropriate drug choice, wrong dose, and wrong frequency. These results show a higher rate of problems than has been reported in the inpatient environment.[13] Computer checks against allergies, dose, interactions, frequency, and inappropriate drug could have a significant impact on these numbers.

Another study measured the impact of ePrescribing on outpatient medication safety. In this study, 1879 prescriptions for 1202 patients were screened for errors. The rates of errors at ePrescribing sites were not significantly different from paper sites. It was suggested that basic ePrescribing systems may not be adequate to reduce errors. More advanced systems with dose, frequency and other clinical checking are needed to prevent potentially harmful errors.[14]

In addition to the safety provided by automated clinical checks, ePrescribing can reduce errors caused by illegible handwriting, inaccessible medication histories and inaccessibility of drug information. Alerting at the point of prescribing can catch prescribing errors sooner.

In addition to the safety benefits, ePrescribing can also improve operational efficiency. The number of call-backs from pharmacies to physician offices can be impacted by ePrescribing.

Physicians' offices receive 150 million call-backs per year for clarification on indecipherable or unclear handwritten prescriptions and other reasons.[15] It is expected that ePrescribing will reduce the number of call-backs. More studies are needed to identify if call back reductions have occurred with ePrescribing. The findings from the 2006 ePrescribing pilots showed some evidence of cost-shifting where the physician practice settings realized some increased efficiency and decreased efficiency was seen at the dispensing end of the continuum.[16,17]

Increased patient compliance is expected with ePrescribing through better prescription tracking and a more efficient refill process. The new ePrescribing fill status notification will provide the physician with information on prescription fill history. In addition, the electronic prescription communication is expected to better support the convenience of the patient which may increase patient compliance.

Improved communication of formulary information to prescribers is expected to increase the prescriber's formulary adherence. Preliminary pilot data shows that this impact is minimal unless the ePrescribing software has functions to support generic substitution for brand name prescribing.

Components of an ePrescribing System

ePrescribing applications consist of multiple functional components that are integrated into the ePrescribing application. These components consist of registration, new prescription entry, prescription transmission, refill authorization, medication profile management, clinical decision support, and formulary management.

Registration

Registration is the function in the ePrescribing system where the patient information is captured. This registration is commonly interfaced from a medical office registration system. Registration functions are generally handled in a physician's practice by office support staff. Patient clinical information and ePrescribing specific information is often not captured well in registration systems because it is either not entered by clinical staff or not part of the medical office registration system. Such information includes:

1. Pharmacy benefits information
2. Patient height, weight
3. Patient diagnosis or problem
4. Allergies
5. Existing medication therapies
6. Laboratory results

If the above information is not captured in the registration system, it may be necessary to capture it in the ePrescribing system in order to realize many of the safety and cost benefits of ePrescribing. Such benefits include support for checking allergies, doses, drug interactions, therapeutic duplication, formulary verification, and prior authorization with the pharmacy benefits manager.

New Prescription Entry

Prescription entry is often considered the primary function of an ePrescribing system. There are many types of workflows that need to be supported by the new prescription entry function. These workflows will be described later in this chapter.

Prescription Transmission

Prescription transmission includes the transmission of the electronic prescription information to the appropriate places. This information may be codified to meet specific data standards or be non-coded free text information stored in standardized transmission formats. Such transmission will generally go to a prescription hub vendor such as RxHUB which then forwards the electronic prescription to the appropriate pharmacy. ePrescribing systems may also generate a printed prescription for the patient or have the option to fax the prescription information to a pharmacy.

Refill Authorization

Refill authorization can be a complex process. This process and its electronic support in an ePrescribing system can create a tremendous savings of labor and time in the physician's office and the pharmacy. The request for a refill authorization can originate with:

1. A patient call or electronic request to the pharmacy who then requests authorization from the physician's office
2. A patient call to the physician's office clerk.
3. A patient call to the physician
4. During a physician office visit

The pharmacy can electronically initiate a request for refill authorization which is transmitted to the physician's office. The refill authorization response from the physician or office staff is transmitted to the pharmacy electronically, thus avoiding the interruption produced by telephone calls. Many ePrescribing systems have features to allow a physician to remotely authorize refills and enter prescriptions through a PC connected to the internet or via a handheld computer or phone.

Medication Profile Management

Medication profile management is difficult to maintain in an ePrescribing system. ePrescribing systems allow the entry of medications into the profile information only, but this can be very time consuming for the physician or nurse to enter and maintain. Generally, physicians only maintain profile information for those prescriptions originating from their practice. Standards exist for the transmission of prescription activity from the pharmacy benefits manager (PBM) to the ePrescribing system to support a more complete profile. This transmitted information only contains prescriptions covered and processed by the PBM. It often does not include non-covered medications or over-the-counter (OTC) items. Physician practices associated with and under survey of the Joint Commission are identifying processes to meet the requirements for medication reconciliation. This includes comparing a list of the patient's current medications with those ordered as well as passing a complete medication list to the next provider of care when the patient is referred or transferred to another setting.

With ePrescribing, medication profile information originates from many sources. The original prescription information comes from one or more prescribers. The pharmacy and PBM will have more specific information about when and if the prescription was dispensed. Finally, the patient will know specifically what medications they are currently taking which will include OTC items. There is a lot of complexity when combining these multiple sources of medication profile information into a single profile to be reviewed by the ePrescriber. Common profile issues include matching different NDC codes for the same generic drug to identify duplicates, the claims data missing frequency and administration instructions and matching prescription data to the correct patient. There is little experience with this important need to reconcile

medication lists from multiple sources into a meaningful medication profile. Data content standards for coding of medications and sigs will allow for more accurate and usable ePrescribing profiles. Once accurate medication profiles are available, enhanced decision support functionality will shortly follow. The local medication profile consists of medications prescribed and entered directly into the local ePrescribing application. This local information may be enhanced by interfacing profile information from other sources such as a PBM, another affiliated clinic or from one or more pharmacies. It may be difficult to automatically combine an interfaced profile with a local profile because of the difficulty identifying duplicates. For example, a single local ePrescribing entry will match with many pharmacy entries and many PBM entries representing refills of the original ePrescribing entry. Without standard medication prescription coding it may not be possible to match prescription data from multiple sources. For this reason, ePrescribing systems that interface with outside medication profiles normally only support the viewing of the external profile and do not merge and store the external profile with the local profile.

The prescribing of OTC medications is supported by most ePrescribing systems. When an order for an OTC item originates at the physician office it is generally printed to paper for the patient rather than being transmitted to a pharmacy. Most ePrescribing systems allow the physician to document OTC items into the ePrescribing profile. There are generally no good ways to manage OTC items in the ePrescribing profile except via patient interview.

In addition to OTC medications, other medications are often missed in ePrescribing profiles. These include medications taken that were originally prescribed to other family members, prescriptions originating from other prescribers and prescriptions reinitiated by the patient using supplies from previous therapies. Much of this medication information can only be identified by patient interview and manually entered into the ePrescribing system's medication profile.

Clinical Decision Support

ePrescribing systems support the basic clinical decision support functions of drug interactions, therapeutic duplication and dose range checking. The third party adjudicator will often provide clinical decision support rules in the adjudication process to also identify potential problems with the medication being ordered. There is much discussion about how clinical decision support can be improved with ePrescribing systems to reduce the false warnings and to make sure only the valid problems are identified. This functionality is a major justifier for the safety that ePrescribing provides.[18] In addition to automated warning functionality most ePrescribing systems support quick access to drug information electronically. Drug information content providers provide evidence based up-to-date drug information content. The source of this information is considered to be unbiased, though there is concern that biased information and advertising could be inserted into ePrescribing applications. Such bias can be provided by direct advertising or less direct mechanisms such as the sort order of medication selection lists, font selection or continuing education accessible from many ePrescribing systems.

Formulary Management

ePrescribing standards also support the verification of prescribed medications against the formulary of the patient's pharmacy benefit plan. Some systems will even suggest alternates for non-formulary medications. The accessibility of this formulary information is dependent on the management of accurate and up-to-date formulary lists by payers and health systems. In addition, the patient prescription benefit information needs to be captured into the ePrescribing system in order to link to the appropriate formulary for verification. Most formulary listings are available commercially to support ePrescribing systems. Organizations such as self-insured health care organizations and hospitals will often need to maintain these formulary lists manually within their local ePrescribing and pharmacy systems. Such maintenance can require a significant effort that is often not considered when implementing the systems.

Other Integration

In order to provide greater functionality for decision support and better information for the prescriber there is a great need to integrate ePrescribing with other clinical and registration information. The documentation of other clinical information often occurs in systems separate from the ePrescribing system. This documented information is difficult to access in the ePrescribing system. Information that could be integrated with ePrescribing includes:

1. Patient height and weight

2. Problem lists and diagnoses

3. Allergies

4. Laboratory results

5. Other diagnostic test results and findings

6. Pharmacy benefits information and the corresponding formulary.

It is not enough to just interface this information from the originating system. Some of this information may need to be documented or captured during the ePrescribing process itself. Prescribers do not want to access multiple systems to enter this documentation. Therefore it is important that ePrescribing functionality be integrated with other electronic systems in the clinical practice.

Workflows

Workflows are the process steps that people take to accomplish a task. The workflows supported by ePrescribing are complex and vary between physician practice locations and the pharmacies that support them. For example, some pharmacies do not accept electronic prescriptions but do accept faxes. Some accept electronic prescriptions and make full use of the refill authorization functionality of the ePrescribing system interfaces. Within a single physician practice there may be a mixture of physicians where some use the ePrescribing system, some have their clerical staff enter the ePrescriptions and some prescribe only on paper. In order to dispense narcotics most states require a signed paper prescription which forces certain types of prescriptions to print to paper.

The correct matching of ePrescribing system functionality to user workflows results in successful installation of ePrescribing. In some cases the user workflows will need to change to meet a system need. In other cases, the system will need to be adjusted to meet a specific workflow. This process of matching workflows between the physician practice and the ePrescribing system functionality will determine the efficiency, safety, cost effectiveness, and ultimately the success of an ePrescribing implementation. For example, a common problem with ePrescribing is the installation and use of the right type of computer equipment to meet the physician needs. A system that has PCs in every examining room requires the physician to log into the system prior to accessing the prescribing functionality. This login process takes too much time for many physicians and they find that it is easier to handwrite the prescription. Some installations avoid this problem by providing handheld or laptop computers with wireless networking for the physician to carry between examining rooms. The most successful implementations provide full integrated medical record and documentation access from these computers.

Registration and Clerical Staff Workflows

The workflows involving registration and clerical staff normally involve preparation work before a patient encounter and data entry after the encounter. Many offices have workflows that primarily support patient billing needs and therefore the data entry is done after the billing information is captured which is often after the patient visit is complete. Patient registration data needs to be entered in real time in order to support ePrescribing. If this registration information is not available, important ePrescribing functionality cannot be used such as formulary and allergy checking. Many physician offices capture this information on a paper registration form and enter it after the patient visit is complete, which is too late to support ePrescribing. This registration need is often a difficult workflow transition for clinic registration staff since they are used to entering the information into the computer after the paperwork is complete, a workflow common for billing systems. In addition, the physician's registration staff generally do not collect and enter pharmacy benefit member and plan identifiers into their billing system since such information is normally used only by pharmacies. In order for an ePrescribing system to check the PBM formulary, the pharmacy benefit information needs to be captured and entered. In many cases this needs to be entered directly into the ePrescribing application because the clinic registration system does not support it. If this workflow is not incorporated into the registration staff's workflow it is left to the prescriber to enter, or it is not done. Registration information includes: (1) patient demographics, (2) insurance information, (3) patient identifiers, and (4) patient visit information.

Prescription Entry Workflows

The workflows for the entry of ePrescriptions in a physician practice can also vary. In some cases the prescription entry is done totally by physicians but in many cases the entry is done by a combination of physician and clinical support staff (surrogates). The clinical practice workflows of these clinicians consist of constant switching between patients supporting different aspects of the patient's visit. In some cases, the visit will consist of a single encounter between patient and physician but in most cases multiple sub-encounters occur. The first sub-encounter may be a patient interview and data gathering of current medications, height, weight, and patient problems. This initial sub-encounter may end with an order for a test or procedure to be administered during the visit. A second sub-encounter may be the review of the results of the test or procedure and the resulting diagnosis and treatment plan, including one or more prescriptions. A physician may be concurrently handling multiple patients in various stages of their office visit along with telephone and other interruptions.

The ePrescribing application needs to support the ability of the physician to quickly transition from patient to patient and from data gathering to ordering. This workflow is significantly different than what is normally demonstrated when the ePrescribing software is evaluated. These demonstrations normally take a single patient through the ePrescribing process following a specific scenario. To support their workflows, clinicians need to have either portable devices or the ability to quickly log into fixed immobile devices. In addition, they need the ability to quickly select and switch between patients in the ePrescribing application. Errors commonly occur when an ePrescription is accidentally entered for the wrong patient. Finally, prescribers need a system that readily identifies what necessary data gathering has not been completed prior to prescription writing. Such data gathering and entry would include allergies, height, weight, lab results, medication profile reconciliation, and other diagnosis-specific information.

Surrogate Prescribing

Surrogate prescribing is commonplace in physician practices. In these cases physician office staff is involved in the prescribing process. This involvement can include prescription refill authorizations, transcription of handwritten prescription orders into the ePrescribing system, and, in some cases, direct prescribing

Additional workflows may be needed for physician verification if prescriptions are entered by support staff as surrogates. Depending on system functionality and configuration, this verification may occur before or after the prescription is forwarded to the pharmacy. In some cases no verification is done. There may also be multiple ways in which the prescription is communicated by the physician to the support staff prior to the prescription entry. All of these workflow varieties impact the efficiency, safety, and quality of prescribing in the physician practice environment. Research is necessary to understand the safety issues and practice standards necessary for surrogate prescription entry. It may be safer to forward a handwritten prescription to a pharmacist than have a surrogate interpret the handwritten prescription and transcribe it into an ePrescribing system. This is especially true if the ePrescribing system does not have functionality for physicians to verify surrogate prescription entry.

Prescription Transmission and Patient Workflows

Prescription transmission is a new workflow that was created with ePrescribing. This workflow requires the prescribing physician or surrogate to select the destination pharmacy for the ePrescription. With paper prescriptions, the prescriber seldom specifies or needs to specify where the prescription will be filled. With an ePrescription the physician needs to ask the patient and specify where the prescription is to be transmitted. This new requirement for ePrescribing can be a difficult transition for physicians and patients. The ePrescribing system carries a database of pharmacies from which the physician may choose. If the wrong pharmacy is selected, the patient will have difficulty getting the prescription filled, because the pharmacy will need to call the prescriber to make the change. Currently the only way a pharmacy can correct a misdirected prescription is to call the physician's office.

ePrescribing systems generally have a database of pharmacies with each pharmacy's preferred method of communication. The choices are generally paper, fax, or electronic transfer. Signed paper prescriptions will be needed for narcotic prescriptions and when the patient is unable to identify a receiving pharmacy.

The transition from fax-based transmission of prescriptions to NCPDP SCRIPT transactions has been very slow. There has been very little reason, monetarily or otherwise, to upgrade software and hardware to support NCPDP SCRIPT. In order to speed up this transition, CMS is considering the elimination of an exemption that allows prescribers to fax Medicare Part D prescriptions to pharmacies. This rule will have significant impact on pharmacies and prescribers as pharmacies would need to implement ePrescribing interfaces to receive electronic prescriptions.

Pharmacy Prescription Processing Workflows

Once a prescription is entered by a prescriber it is transmitted via the NCPDP SCRIPT standard to an electronic hub company such as RxHUB, who then forwards the message to the appropriate pharmacy's ePrescribing provider, such as SureScripts (see Figure 2-1).

SureScripts connects to the pharmacy's online adjudication switching company, such as eRx or RxLinc, which completes the connection to the pharmacy. Once the prescription is received, the local pharmacy prescription processing software handles the electronic prescription. Due to the lack of standards for most of the data elements of the ePrescription, much of the electronic prescription is manually transcribed into

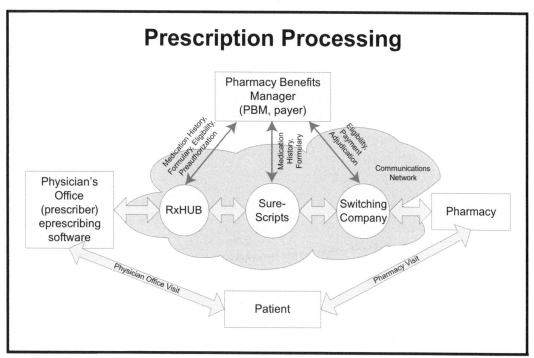

Figure 2-1. Prescription processing.

the pharmacy computer system. Many pharmacy systems print the electronic prescription to paper for re-entering into the pharmacy system. Generally the only systems that are fully integrated between CPOE and ePrescribing are the closed loop organizations, such as Kaiser or the Veteran's Administration, that control the physician's practice, the pharmacy and often the pharmacy benefits manager. Some standards are developing for the content and transmission of this information. These standards are described below.

Prescription Refill Workflows

The ambulatory medication process for prescription refill authorizations has potential for significant improvement with ePrescribing. This workflow is traditionally dependent on telephone calls between the patient and pharmacy, pharmacy and physician, and sometimes the physician and patient. Such a refill authorization normally requires three telephone calls in or out of the pharmacy for each request. ePrescribing software can significantly increase the efficiency of refill requests within a physician practice. In combination with new ePrescribing standards, such efficiency, can also occur within the pharmacy.

ePrescribing Standards

Prior to the implementation of the MMA, the CMS employed the National Center for Health and Vital Statistics (NCVHS) to interview many experts and identify what was needed to best manage prescription costs. It was clearly identified that electronic prescribing and accompanying standards were needed to support efficient and safe management of the prescription benefit. Such standards support safe prescription processing, efficient workflows, formulary management, data quality, patient safety, and management of prescription information at the plan and patient level.

Three types of standards were determined to be necessary for the MMA. Message format standards are needed to support proper communication of data between systems and are needed to communicate transactions that represent specific workflow components in the prescription processing continuum. Terminology standards are needed to assure that the individual data elements are understandable between systems. Terminology standards are equivalent to selecting a standard vocabulary to use when communicating between systems. Unique identifier standards are needed to clearly and safely identify unique components of the prescription process. Such identifier standards include identifiers for drugs, patients, prescribers, and pharmacies.

With the assistance of NCVHS three standards were identified to meet the criteria for "adequate industry experience." These standards are termed "foundational standards" and were adopted as Medicare Part D ePrescribing standards effective January 1, 2006. In addition, six standards were identified as "initial" standards that might, after pilot testing, be adopted as additional ePrescribing standards. Each of these standards is described below.

Foundational Standards

Foundational standards meet the criteria for "adequate industry experience."

1. NCPDP Telecommunication Standard for eligibility verification between retail dispensers and payers. These standards are the communications used by pharmacies to adjudicate prescription claims with payers.

2. Accredited Standards Committee (ASC) X12N 270/271 for eligibility communications between prescribers and payers. This standard supports the verification of insurance eligibility information between healthcare providers and health insurance plans.

3. NCPDP SCRIPT Standard for new prescription, changes, renewals, and cancellation transactions between prescribers and dispensers. This standard provides for the exchange of prescription data

between prescribers and pharmacies supporting basic prescription processes.

Initial Standards

Initial standards are standards "that might, after pilot testing, be adopted as additional ePrescribing standards."

1. Formulary and benefit information. This standard supports the transfer of formulary status, alternative medications, co-pays and other prescription benefit information between the prescription benefit payer and the prescriber. This NCPDP standard is based on the protocol initially developed by RxHub.

2. Exchange of medication history. This NCPDP SCRIPT standard supports the query and display of medication history information from outside sources, normally the pharmacy benefit plan.

3. Fill status notification. This NCPDP SCRIPT standard supports communication from the pharmacy to the prescriber when prescriptions are filled, partially filled, and refilled.

4. Structured and codified SIG. This standard codifies the indication, dose, dose calculation, dose restriction, route, frequency, interval, site, administration time, duration, and stop information for a prescription. This standard is a work in progress and is being developed through cooperative work between NCPDP, HL7, and others.

5. Clinical drug terminology (RxNorm). This standard is a clinical drug nomenclature. It provides standard names for clinical drugs, dosage forms and other related information. It provides links between the clinical drugs, active ingredients, drug components. and most brand names. Originally developed through the Veteran's Administration (VA), RX-NORM is now being further developed through the National Library of Medicine (NLM).

6. Prior authorization messages. This standard supports the communication of relevant information to support prior authorization requests between payer, prescriber, and pharmacy. This standard is being developed by ASC X12N in coordination with HL7.

Future Standards

To date, most of the ePrescribing standards are those supporting the format and transmission of messages supporting specific workflows in the prescribing process. This has focused primarily on messaging standards and communication needs between the prescriber and others. Additional work on vocabulary standards and standard identifiers is needed to eliminate the need to transcribe prescription information into pharmacy systems. Standards are also needed to support specific messaging and workflows not covered by existing standards.

Standards will need to be continually refined in order to support the workflows between pharmacists, prescribers, nurses, payers, and patients. Such workflows will include compliance monitoring, monitoring of other clinical parameters such as lab tests, verifications needed to support pre-authorization, patient and caregiver education, and adjudication and reimbursement communications. Transactions associated with these workflows will be needed to support more efficient pharmacy processes. Experiences from pilot ePrescribing studies have shown a shift of work from the prescriber to the pharmacy. Current efforts have concentrated on the prescriber workflows with less emphasis on downstream needs as the prescription process flows to the pharmacy, the payer, other caregivers and the patient. Future transactions are needed to support these downstream communication needs.

The workflows in the ambulatory medication use process are quite complex. Many individuals need to be integrated into the process and require efficient and accurate communications with each other.

This includes the patient, physician, nurse, pharmacist, physician office registration staff, pharmacy benefits manager, and others. Traditionally, these workflows were dependent on telephones, paper, or information provided by the patient. In order to support these workflows, standard communication methods and data sets are required. For the pharmacist, the most difficult workflows are the communications needs when intervening with the prescriber or payer. These workflows put the pharmacist as the communication conduit between the pharmacy benefit managers, the prescriber, and the patient. These interactions include prior authorization management, generic substitution, and management of rejected online prescription claims. Not only is the use of telephones costly of time and efficiency but they often lead to errors common in verbal communications. There is a great potential for error reduction by using standard ePrescribing transactions to significantly reduce the number of inefficient telephone calls and error-prone communications.

Integration and Medication Reconciliation

In order to provide proper verification and review of new prescriptions, the pharmacist requires an accurate profile of medications currently used by the patient. In the past, this profile consisted of the available prescription history from the dispensing pharmacy's computer system. Such profiles are often incomplete. Prescriptions dispensed from other pharmacies, medications received as samples from the physician's office, and over-the-counter medications are not included in these profiles. Cost reduction efforts through the use of mail order pharmacies often separate the chronic medications from the acute medication profiles in pharmacies. As a result, the ability of the pharmacist to verify prescriptions is compromised by the reduced access to a complete medication profile.

The medication profile needs are the same for all involved in the prescription process. The profile needs to be complete, accurate, accessible, and support the needs of the practitioner. The profile needs to be complete by including all medications actively used by the patient as well as previous medications used. The profile also needs to contain all data elements important to profile review including the frequency, fill history, etc. The profile needs to provide quick access to the information when needed, including quick and accurate selection, matching of the correct patient, and access to prescriber, pharmacy, and pharmacist identification and contact information, if needed. Profile views may differ significantly based on the need at the time of viewing. When reviewing therapies, a profile of prescriptions sorted by therapeutic category may be useful. When looking for a specific drug, an alphabetic sort or search may be useful. When reviewing compliance it may be necessary to view detailed refill history. In some cases, a list of past medication use would be helpful, and in other cases only a list of active medications is needed. These needs can vary based on the practitioner, care location, and specific profile needs at the time.

New Sources of Error

The significant changes in workflows as well as the introduction of new ePrescribing technology is likely to create new sources of error. Known error sources include selection errors from list of choices, mistyped numbers, wrong patient selection, unintended entry or modification of data fields on order screens, inability to identify color highlighting or coding, and errors in the setup of supportive data tables and translation tables. There is likely to be new errors discovered at any time and any part of the ePrescribing process.

The challenges to developers, system managers, prescribers, pharmacists and patients will be to develop processes and workflows the prevent errors and quickly identify and correct errors when they are found. A single error in the ePrescribing system can repeat many times before it is identified and corrected. Such errors can be replicated multiple times within the same physician office or cascade across the whole ePrescribing network. There is some concern that pharmacists, patients, physicians and nurses will be less likely to question an ePrescription that is computer generated even though it may be just as likely to have many of the same type of errors found in handwritten prescriptions. Enhanced decision support can reduce the errors but will never eliminate them.

Pharmacist have always been an important safety and quality component of the prescription process and will continue to be with ePrescribing.

The Pharmacist's Role in ePrescribing

There is some current confusion regarding the pharmacist's role in the ePrescribing process. Much of the current legislation and standards identify the pharmacist as the "dispenser" of medications. This is reflective of the current physician centric focus of ePrescribing. Much of the current direction of ePrescribing standards efforts has not placed very much importance on other clinical practitioners to the ePrescribing process. The pharmacy component of ePrescribing has overshadowed the pharmacist involvement. Further research and evidence is needed to clarify the important role of the pharmacist in ePrescribing. Such importance has already been realized with the inpatient medication use process and inpatient provider order entry.

The increased complexity, costs, and monitoring requirements of medication therapies has increased the importance of the pharmacist as a clinician. There is an increased awareness of the cognitive services provided by pharmacists and the need to reimburse for these services. In order to track and be reimbursed for these cognitive services there is a need for a standard pharmacist identifier. Currently, states

that reimburse for cognitive services assign physician identifiers to these pharmacists. A universal pharmacist identifier is needed to better support the communications between care providers. Such an identifier will support direct communications between specific pharmacists and other providers. Without a universal identifier, such transactions are only identified by the pharmacy of origin rather than a specific pharmacist. The recognition of pharmacists as individual practitioners is important to getting past the current definition of pharmacists as dispensers.

Challenges

The current challenges with ePrescribing are to realize the benefits of quality, efficiency, and reduced costs that the technology is expected to provide. Such challenges involve balancing the business and clinical needs of ePrescribing. The primary goals of ePrescribing include: (1) to support safe and effective therapy, (2) to support cost management for payers, and (3) to support the business needs of physician practices and pharmacies.

An important component that is currently missing from the ePrescribing standards and process development is an organization that oversees the safety and quality of the ePrescribing process. In the inpatient and health systems environment, this quality oversight is provided by the Joint Commission. The Joint Commission has been the driving force to require pharmacist review of medication orders and other requirements to reduce errors.[19] Currently, the Joint Commission only oversees a small number of physician office practices and retail pharmacies. Many physician practices and pharmacies are not reviewed by the Joint Commission. Such oversight is needed in the ePrescribing effort to address the need for profile review, reducing surrogate entry of ePrescriptions without physician review and clarifying the roles of physicians, nurses and pharmacists in the ePrescribing process. As with the Joint Commission, such a quality organization should have oversight over the complete ePrescribing process from the prescriber to the patient administration of the medication. In addition, an error reporting, evaluation, and response process needs to be in place to identify and prevent ePrescribing errors.

There has been much improvement in the functionality and ability for ePrescribing software to support the prescribing workflows. Several challenges exist with the functionalities supported in current ePrescribing software. Increased interest in ePrescribing, standard development and significant efforts to create software that better meets the physician's need has accelerated the need for changes in software.

As ePrescribing use continues to increase, there will be a greater need to develop software that provides similar operation and functionality at all physician practice locations. There will be increased demand to implement and integrate ePrescribing into all ambulatory areas and improve the access to shared medication profiles. Inpatient software will be impacted by the need to access the ambulatory medication profiles upon inpatient admission to support medication reconciliation. Upon inpatient discharge there will be increased need to enter discharge prescriptions as ePrescriptions. Standardization of the computer user interface will occur in order to support physician's use of ePrescribing at multiple practice sites. Such standardization will impact inpatient CPOE systems as discharge prescription functionality is added and standards developed for ePrescribing are adopted in inpatient physician order entry systems.

The visit-based nature of ambulatory computer systems will need to be adjusted to support the continuous prescription support for refills and prescription modifications between office visits. Adoption of standards will force the rewrite of many medication systems as the database structures that create the foundation of these systems change to meet the standards. Adoption of RxNorm medication coding will change the focus of ePrescribing from product selection to therapeutic and problem focused prescribing.

ePrescribing systems will require modifications and additional standards to better support workflows. This will include medication reconciliation, with increased patient access and involvement in maintaining an accurate medication profile.

In order to accomplish this integration of the ePrescribing process it will be necessary for software vendors to understand the complex workflows within and between physicians, nurses, pharmacists, patients, pharmacy benefit managers, payers, and other healthcare providers. Workflow standardization will need to occur in order to develop computer system support of the workflows.

Future Directions

The future direction of ePrescribing systems and software will be determined by the standards currently being developed.

To reduce the errors of transcription and to support profile sharing, all data elements of a prescription requires standardization. This will include completing the standardization of the codified SIGs and drug coding through RxNORM. Standardized patient identifiers will also be needed. Patient identifier standards exist in other countries but are a political hot potato in the U.S. as patient rights organizations have concerns about such standards. Current insurance medication profiles are accessed by requiring exact matches of first name, last name, birth date, gender, and zip code. A national patient identifier would significantly increase the matches that occur with such online profile requests.

Much work is needed to better support a universal medication profile and the reconciliation of this profile. Changes are needed to support the automated combination of profile information from multiple sources.

Additional information such as the originating data source for each prescription entry is needed to identify and combine duplicate prescription entries in the profiles. Additional functionality is needed to support patient involvement in the management and updates to medication profile information. Such updates may include over-the-counter medications, patient problem lists and patient acquired monitoring information such as weight, blood pressure, and blood sugar levels.

Integration of prescribing into other systems and clinician workflows will also occur. One top priority workflow to integrate is currently the medication reconciliation process.

Conclusion

Electronic prescribing has received much attention as the result of the expanded prescription Medicare benefit. The result of this attention has been the development of standards to support better communication of ePrescribing information. The accelerated implementation of ePrescribing software will make ePrescribing the first computerized medication order entry exposure for many physicians. As these standards are further developed and integration continues there will be significant impact on hospital provider order entry and pharmacy computer applications.

ePrescribing Pearls

PHARMACY INFORMATICS PEARLS

- The US government and others have high expectations for ePrescribing to positively impact safety, quality, efficiency and total cost of medications.
- EPrescribing consists of more than just the transmission of new prescriptions to the pharmacy. It also includes two way communication of refill requests, insurance eligibility checking, formulary checking, decision support, pharmacy selection, and the sharing of medication profile information.
- EPrescribing data content and transmission standards are necessary to reduce or eliminate manual transcription of prescription information into retail pharmacy dispensing computer systems. Without these standards there is little pharmacy operational differences between electronic and fax transmitted prescriptions.
- One of the biggest barriers to implementing formulary checking with ePrescribing is the entry of the pharmacy prescription benefit information during ambulatory clinic patient registration.
- It is commonly agreed that stand alone ePrescribing systems are significantly inferior to those developed as components of an ambulatory electronic medical record system.
- Recent research shows that surrogate entry of prescriptions at the ambulatory clinic by non-physician support staff is common. It is currently not known how this impacts the quality and safety of the ePrescribing process.
- Successful implementation of ePrescribing requires careful analysis and design of registration, physician, nursing and patient workflows within the ambulatory clinic.
- EPrescribing system management is needed to prevent the potential for errors and to quickly identify and correct errors when they are found.
- Pharmacists are a very important safety check in the ePrescribing process because they are the last healthcare professional to review the prescription prior to the patient receiving the medication.
- Remember that the patient is the focus for ePrescribing, not the prescriber.

There is a need for increased quality oversight of the ambulatory prescription process. This is one of the biggest differences between the management of inpatient orders and the prescription medication process. Because of the large number of independent physician practices not under Joint Commission oversight, the prescription process does not have a consistent quality. Within the prescription process it is important to understand the difference between the pharmacy as the business entity and the pharmacist as the clinician. In hospital medication processes a nurse administers medications and provides the final clinical check before a medication reaches the patient. In the prescription process the pharmacy is the business entity that dispenses medications and the pharmacist provides the last safety and quality check before the medication reaches the patient. Pharmacists need to step up as the safety and quality advocates for the prescription process. They are the final step in the process before the medication reaches the patient. Ultimately, the patient needs to be the focus for ePrescribing, not the prescriber.

References

1. www.NCPDP.org. Mission statement and organization description. 2007.

2. Cherry DK, Woodwell DA. National Ambulatory Medical Care Survey: 2000 summary. *Adv Data.* 2002;328:1–32.

3. Cypress BW. Drug utilization in office visits to primary care physicians: National Ambulatory Medical Care Survey, 1980. Department of Health and Human Services publication (PHS) 82-1250. Public Health Service, 1982.

4. Estimates. NACDS Economics Department.

5. Kohn LT, Corrigan JM, Donaldson MS, eds. Committee on Quality of Health Care in America, Institute of Medicine. *To Err is Human: Building a Safer Health System.* Washington, DC: National Academy Press; 2000.

6. nstitute for Safe Medicine Practices. A Call to Action: Eliminate Handwritten Prescriptions Within Three Years, 2000.

7. Forrester Research, 2002.

8. Medco Health, 1/29/03, via ePharmaceuticals.

9. NACDS and SureScripts estimates.

10. E-Health Initiative. Electronic Prescribing: Toward Maximum Value and Rapid Adoption. 2004.

11. http://www.cms.hhs.gov/MMAUpdate/, 2007.

12. www.jointcommission.org/PatientSafety/NationalPatientSafetyGoals, 2007.

13. Gandhi TK, Weingart SN, Borus J, Seger AC, Peterson J, Burdick E, et al. Adverse drug events in ambulatory care. *N Engl J Med.* 2003;348(16):1556-1564.

14. Gandhi TK, Weingart SN, Seger AC, Borus J, Burdick E, Poon EG, et al. Outpatient prescribing errors and the impact of computerized prescribing. *J Gen Intern Med.* 2005; 20(9):837–841.

15. Institute for Safe Medication Practices. White Paper: A Call to Action: Eliminate Handwritten Prescriptions Within 3 Years! Electronic Prescribing Can Reduce Medication Errors. 2000.

16. Findings From The Evaluation of E-Prescribing Pilot Sites, AHRQ Publication No. 07-0047-EF, April 2007.

17. Pilot Testing of Initial Electronic Prescribing Standards. CMS Report to Congress, April 2007.

18. Teich JM, Osheroff JA, Pifer EA, Sittig DF, Jenders RA. The CDS Expert Review Panel. Clinical decision support in electronic prescribing: recommendations and an action plan. *J Am Med Inform Assoc.* 2005;12:365–337.

19. *Longo DR, Hewett JE, Ge B, Schubert S.* Hospital patient safety: characteristics of best-performing hospitals. *J Healthc Manage.* 2007;52(3):188–204.

C H A P T E R   3

Clinical Decision Support

Eric Rose and Michael A. Jones

KEY DEFINITIONS

Alert—an urgent notice generated by a computerized clinical decision support system (CDSS). These are usually in the form of a just-in-time, patient-specific message directed to one or more clinicians. It may be a warning regarding a clinician's documented action (or lack thereof) or a documented decision. Or it may be an urgent informational notification of a new clinical condition, circumstance, or change in patient status that requires immediate attention. Some alerts require a response before the clinician can continue.

Alert Fatigue—a state of irritability, exhaustion, or bewilderment triggered in clinicians who have been exposed to too many alerts, or alerts with a perceived history of irrelevance, which cause the user to ignore some or all of the alerts, thereby reducing the safety benefit of the decision support system.[1]

American National Standards Institute (ANSI)—coordinates the development and use of voluntary consensus standards including Health Level Seven's (HL7) Arden Syntax standard. More information is available at the ANSI website: http://www.ansi.org.

Arden Syntax Standard—an HL7 standard designed to allow clinicians to program medical logic into a clinical rule or guideline. The American Society for Testing and Materials first approved the Arden Syntax as a standard in 1992 (E-1460-92). Ownership was transferred to HL7 and ANSI in 1999 with the approval of version 2.0 of the standard. The Arden Syntax is the only approved standard for clinicians to encode medical logic into clinical rules known as medical logic modules (MLM).

Bar Code Medication Administration (BCMA)—an inpatient CDSS to assist nurses with the five-rights of medication administration (right patient, right drug, right dose, right route, and right time). BCMA systems provide warnings if any of the five-rights are violated and most BCMA systems require the nurse to enter an override reason if he or she chooses to proceed. In addition, BCMA systems promote right-documentation (some hospitals call this the sixth right of medication administration).

Centers for Medicare and Medicaid Services (CMS)—the federal healthcare programs for the elderly and indigent. For more information go to: http://www.cms.hhs.gov/

Clinical Decision Support (CDS)—refers broadly to providing clinicians or patients with clinical knowledge and patient-related information, intelligently filtered or presented at appropriate times, to enhance patient care. Clinical knowledge of interest could range from simple facts and relationships to best practices for managing patients with specific disease states, new medical knowledge from clinical research, and other types of information.

Clinical Decision Support System (CDSS)—a system (computer or otherwise) intended to provide CDS to clinicians, caregivers, and healthcare consumers. Automated CDSS are usually just-in-time, point-of-care messages in the form of an alert, reminder, recommendation, or informational notification regarding a patient. Automated CDS systems typically include a knowledge base (which contains stored facts and some method of algorithmic logic), an event monitor (to detect data entry or the storage of data from a laboratory or other system), and a communication system to the end user (unidirectional or bidirectional).[2]

Computerized Provider Order Entry (CPOE)—automated portion of a clinical information system that enables a patient's care provider to enter an order for a medication, clinical laboratory, radiology test, or procedure directly into the computer. The system then transmits the order to the appropriate department, or individuals, so that it can be carried out.

e-Iatrogenesis—patient harm caused at least in part by the application of health information technology.[3]

Health Level Seven (HL7)—an important standards development organization for health information technology (HIT). For detailed information, see the HL7 website: http://www.hl7.org

Healthcare Information Technology (HIT)—any computer system designed to automate and/or enhance a healthcare process or workflow. HIT can be a small apparatus such as an IV infusion pump or a glucometer, a departmental information system such as a pharmacy or laboratory informa-

tion system. It can be an institutional information system such as an admissions, discharge, and transfer (ADT) system, which may interface or interoperate with other departmental systems. HIT can also be a multi-institutional system, such as a regional health information organization (RHIO), or even a national health information network (NHIN).

Information Systems (IS)—(1) Computerized systems for workflow management such as a pharmacy computer system, or an information retrieval system such as a library. The defining characteristic is a database and specialized features and functions for a dedicated purpose. (2) A department of HIT or computer professionals. When designating a department, IS usually stands for Information Services.

Informational Notice—may be a patient-specific automated rule, such as an MLM, to inform of a change in patient status. This type of informational notice may be urgent (e.g., to report a change in renal function) or non-urgent (e.g., to report a hospital admission of a potential study patient). An informational notice may also be product-specific such as a pop-up box during order entry to announce a look-alike, sound-alike (LASA) drug.

Knowledge Base—a collection of stored facts, rules, algorithms, heuristics, and models for problem solving.[2,4] Knowledge base data may be organized in a database or even a simple table in which explicit relationships exist. Familiar examples of commercial knowledge bases that incorporate databases are drug-drug interaction and drug-allergy alerting systems.

Logical Observation Identifiers Names and Codes (LOINC)—a standard to facilitate the exchange of clinical laboratory results. The Regenstrief Institute, Inc. maintains the LOINC database of about 41,000 terms, and its supporting documentation. For more information, see the LOINC website at: http://www.regenstrief.org/medinformatics/loinc/

Look-Alike, Sound-Alike (LASA)—a medication safety designation to prevent confusion between drugs with similar spelling or pronunciation.

Medical Logic Module (MLM)—a rule for an Arden Syntax based clinical rules engine. HL7 defines a MLM as an encoded clinical rule that contains enough logic to make a single clinical decision. MLMs in use today have been developed for many purposes, such as clinical alerts, recommendations, reminders, informational notices, interpretations, diagnosis, quality assurance functions, continuous quality improvement, bio-surveillance, administrative support, and for clinical research.

National Council for Prescription Drug Programs (NCPDP) Script—is a standard for ambulatory prescription messaging between pharmacies and third party payers. The NCPDP standard has been in use for decades. In 2004, HL7 had started its own efforts to develop a standard for institutional prescription messaging, and decided to create a harmonized mapping between NCPDP's script and HL7's RX messages. Their intention is to ensure interoperability of prescription information across the entire healthcare information environment.

Protected Health Information (PHI)—this is information about a person that must remain secure, as defined by Health Insurance Portability and Accountability Act (HIPAA).

Recommendation—an automated rule, such as an MLM, that suggests a course of action. For example, a patient-specific dosage or a suggestion for a laboratory test. Ideally, all recommendations are evidence-based and institutionally approved.

Reminder—an automated rule, such as an MLM, that suggests the clinician has overlooked or forgotten to perform an action such as documenting a decision, event, or finding.

Regional Health Information Organization (RHIO)—proposed definition by the Department of Health and Human Services, BearingPoint, and the National Alliance for Health Information and Technology. A governance entity comprising separate and independent healthcare-related organizations that have come together to improve the quality, safety, and efficiency of healthcare for communities in which it operates and for which it takes responsibility to develop transparent, inclusive processes that enable the interoperable exchange of health information in a manner that protects the confidentiality and security of an individual's information.

Systematized Nomenclature of Medicine Clinical Terms (SNOMED CT)—a comprehensive clinical terminology, originally created by the College of American Pathologists. For more information, see the National Library of Medicine Unified Medical Language System website: http://www.nlm.nih.gov/research/umls/Snomed/snomed_main.html

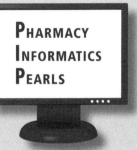

CLINICAL DECISION SUPPORT PEARLS

Vendor-supplied CDS content

- Only as current as the last update, and the accuracy and efficiency of the vendor's editorial staff that creates the CDS content.
- Deactivating CDS alerts to decrease noise may increase the risk of harm.
- Customizing CDS content to improve safety adds a maintenance responsibility.

Medico-legal issues of clinical decision support system

- Legal risk and benefits are largely unknown.
- Are CDS rules and systems under negligence law or product liability law?

Internally developed medical logic modules (MLMs)

- MLMs can cover the gaps in other CDS systems.
- Rule-based surveillance support quality, administrative, cost-containment, regulatory, and research initiatives.
- MLM function is under institutional control.
- Implemented MLMs are the institution's responsibility.

CDS governance committee

- Inventory and evaluate scope of institutional CDS efforts (human and technical) for workflow appropriateness, workload burden, and gaps in coverage.
- Determine clinical group (physician, RPh, RN, etc.) target for each category of CDS. For example, physicians see drug-allergy alerts in CPOE.
- Catalog and ensure appropriate maintenance of CDSS customizations.
- Participate in advising hospital administration of human and technical resource needs for CDSS implementation, customization, and maintenance.

Introduction

Over the past several decades, technology has become an integral part of healthcare delivery. Advances in equipment have improved the efficiency and accuracy of our delivery systems, allowed us to better track our inventory and restrict access to controlled substances, and brought us powerful diagnostic and therapeutic tools. Parallel to these advances in hardware and equipment, computerized clinical decision support (CDS) software solutions have evolved to integrate patient-specific data with an available knowledge base in order to assist the clinician in selecting and delivering the safest and most effective therapies.

There are many types of CDSS. This chapter is not intended as a comprehensive review; instead, it will focus on selected types that the authors felt are currently most relevant to pharmacy practice and pharmacotherapy. Closed-loop systems that automatically regulate therapy without human intervention are beyond the scope of this chapter. In addition, we also avoid those topics addressed in detail elsewhere in this book.

In the early 1970s the first clinical decision support systems became available. These early systems were largely stand-alone diagnostic aids. The clinician would input patient specific parameters, and the CDS system would compare this data to a knowledge base or use it in a set of algorithms to provide an evidence-based differential diagnosis or list of treatment options. Today, prescribers can benefit from CDSS, which provide information to guide diagnosis and recommend evidence-based treatment options, including appropriate medication dosing and information on cost of therapy and institutional formularies.

As pharmacy departments turned more and more to computers to process medication orders and store patient information, systems were developed to assist the pharmacist in screening for allergic reactions and drug interactions by comparing new orders to the patient's medication history and utilizing a commercial knowledge base of known interactions and cross sensitivities. Such systems are only useful if their reference knowledge base is current and complete. Multum and First Databank are two examples of modern vendors who specialize in providing and maintaining detailed drug information knowledge bases that are used as an information source by many CDS systems.

Today, CDSS can still be found as stand-alone systems: POISINDEX, QMR, and DxPlain are some examples. Most often, however, CDSS is found integrated into other technology solutions. For example, bar code technology has been used for years as a tool to track inventory and retail sales patterns. When CDSS are combined with bar code scanning technology, a system is created which can confirm and document that a patient is being given the correct dose of a medication at the correct time and even prompt the administering care provider if recent lab results or new medications may need to be considered before administering an ordered medication. From diagnosis to therapy selection, dispensing, administra-

tion, and monitoring, CDS systems have been incorporated into almost every stage of the medication use process.

HIT Standards

Most pharmacists are not well versed in healthcare information technology (HIT) standards, and they are mentioned in a number of the subsequent sections of this chapter. Standards in general are important to help society function. Two important examples involve automobiles and traffic laws. Most traffic laws are standardized across all 50 states. There was a time in this country when planning a road trip across the U.S. drivers had to research right-of-way laws, etc., because they were different in each state. Today "right-turn on red," traffic signals, and traffic signs are standardized across the country. Another example is the standardization of automobile control devices, which ensures that any licensed driver in this country will understand how to drive different makes of automobiles. We do not have to go to class every time we buy at new make or model of car. By comparison, we are in the early stages concerning mandated HIT standards. The problem is not a lack of HIT standards, but rather too many standards, and currently vender compliance is voluntary. This leads to confusion on the part of HIT developers and users alike.

Imagine if all pharmacy information systems had a familiar look and feel, with consistent functionality. It might not take 6 months to train new pharmacists every time they moved from one hospital to another. Medical residents have a similar problem when they have rotations in multiple hospitals, each with a different computerized provider order entry (CPOE) system.

One of the current federal efforts of the Department of Health and Human Services is to determine which standards should be required for HIT applications. This is no easy task in itself. To compound matters, HIT vendors have been selling their various applications to healthcare organizations for over 20–30 years. When and if the federal government decides to mandate certain HIT standards, that mandate will carry with it a significant price tag that will be passed on to their customers, which in turn will be passed on to our patients (i.e., the rest of us). That is not to say that it should not be done; just that the longer we wait, the more expensive it will be.

Types of Clinical Decision Support Systems

The OpenClinical website (http://www.open-clinical.org/dss.html) defines clinical decision support systems as "active knowledge systems which use two or more items of patient data to generate case-specific advice … are typically designed to integrate a medical knowledge base, patient data and an inference engine to generate case specific advice."[5]

Several expert authors have described clinical decision support systems, including their uses and functions.[1,2,4] Table 3-1 lists some general attributes of clinical decision support systems.

For purposes of this discussion, we subdivide CDS systems into two major categories: patient-specific and non-patient-specific.

Patient-Specific CDSS

1. Commercial drug-interaction alerting systems. These are most common in CPOE and pharmacy information systems and provide alerts for drug-allergy, drug-drug, drug-pregnancy, and other interactions.

   Table 3-2 gives details of the four possible outcomes from this kind of alerting system. These outcomes are true positive, true negative, false positive, and false negative for each drug-interaction check. Modern CDSS allow pharmacy managers to deactivate selected drug-interactions deemed a "nuisance." Most systems allow deactivation by individual drug-interaction or an entire group based on

severity level (e.g., mild, moderate, etc.). Frequently, managers filter out the lower severity alerts to reduce alert fatigue. Although done with the best of intentions, this practice has the potential to increase risk of patient harm by increasing the number of false negatives. As an example of a false-negative causing harm, consider a drug-drug interaction that sometimes causes nausea and vomiting and which has been assigned a "moderate" severity rating by the vendor. Now imagine a patient on total parenteral nutrition (TPN) with orders to discontinue the TPN when she can tolerate oral food. If mild interactions are deactivated in the computer alerting system, the clinician will not be alerted to the interaction that may prolong the TPN therapy. In this case, this so-called moderate drug-drug interaction is significant to this patient.

Remember, false negatives are really true positives.

One limitation of current drug-interaction CDSS design is that severity levels (mild, moderate, etc.) are pre-assigned by the vendor based on the anticipated adverse reaction and cannot be customized based on an individual patient's prescribed dose, age, body size, race, gender, or clinical situation. For example, a drug interaction causing additive sedative effects between anxiolytics and analgesics may be significant in a patient whose neurological status is being closely monitored, but it may be less clinically significant in a hospice patient whose comfort may require the two agents be used together. A solution that we hope will be available in the future is a CDSS that assigns severity ratings at the point-of-care based on patient data and clinical circumstances. Such a system could significantly diminish false positive and false negative outcomes with all of their potentially harmful results. This

TABLE 3-1

General Attributes of Clinical Decision Support Systems

CDSS Attribute	Description

CDS systems are specifically designed for one of three purposes	▪ Augment or improve the quality of clinical decisions (e.g., diagnosis, therapy selection, patient-specific dosing, duplicate lab orders).
	▪ Notify of potential change in patient status (e.g., a change in renal function).
	▪ Prevent errant action at the point-of-care.
	  ● Error of commission (e.g., an attempt to pass medications on the wrong patient).
	  ● Error of omission (e.g., forgetting to give meds post dialysis).

Patient specificity	▪ Information provided applies only to a single patient or healthcare consumer.
Context sensitive	▪ Relates directly to the work at hand ▪ Exception is a CDSS designed to notify of a change in patient status (e.g., a pager alert of a declining serum potassium in patient on digoxin).
Integrated into workflow	▪ Convenient to use. CDSS is a constituent or module of the HIT application.
Intelligently filtered clinical information	▪ The information, advice or warning is relevant and meaningful. ▪ The CDSS uses patient data to infer that the message is actually needed. Ideally, the CDSS does not rely on artificially preset severity rating or on approximated patient information (e.g., proxy-diagnosis). ▪ The CDSS is customizable to clinician preferences (e.g., does not warn an oncologist about a chemotherapy agent causing thrombocytopenia).
Timely	▪ CDSS executes in real time. That is, at the time a clinical decision is made, at the time of a change in patient status, or at the time of an unsafe action.
Pushes information to the clinician, caregiver, or healthcare consumer	▪ The CDSS activity sends unsolicited information before the user recognizes the need for it. ▪ Ideally, the CDSS should employ intelligent filtering to prevent unnecessary or unwanted messages.

new CDSS architecture for drug-interactions requires the implementation of a comprehensive electronic health record (EHR) with codified patient conditions and diagnoses using a standard terminology such as the Systematized Nomenclature of Medicine Clinical Terms (SNOMED CT).

TABLE 3-2

Four Possible Results from an Alerting System

	Positive	Negative
True	■ True positive produces an alert. ■ Example: an allergy warning appears when penicillin is prescribed for a patient with a beta lactam allergy. ■ Alert is relevant to the clinical situation and there is a risk of harm. ■ Clinician needs to see this alert.	■ True negative produces no alert. ■ Example: No alert fires when penicillin is ordered on a patient who has no beta lactam allergies. ■ There is no problem for the clinician to deal with. ■ Clinician do not need to see an alert.
False	■ False positive produces an alert. ■ Example: A duplicate drug warning for a patient appropriately prescribed two antibiotics. ■ There is no check for relevance to the clinical situation and no risk of harm. ■ Clinician considers this alert an inconvenience. ■ Clinician does not need to see this alert.	■ *False negative is really a true positive, but produces no alert.* ■ Example: NO allergy warning appears when penicillin is prescribed for a patient with a beta lactam allergy, because the allergy is undocumented in the computer system. ■ The alert would be relevant to the clinical situation and there is a risk of harm. ■ Frequently caused by blocking low severity alerts so they do not display. ■ Clinicians need to see these alerts, but never gets the chance.

Only the false alerts cause problems. False positive alerts are a nuisance and contribute to alert fatigue. False negative alerts may contribute to harm, because *a false negative is really a true positive* but produces no alert for the clinician to see. These false negatives are frequently caused by turning off the lower severity drug-interaction alerts (e.g., drug-drug and drug-food interactions with a mild or moderate severity rating) in an attempt to reduce alert fatigue.

Two knowledge bases that are possible today, but are still missing from these commercial systems, involve checking for interactions with drug-laboratory tests and drug-disease interactions. Drug-laboratory interactions alerting systems require the use of a standard laboratory coding system such as the Logical Observation Identifiers Names and Codes (LOINC). For drug-disease interaction checking, it is necessary that the patient's problem list and diagnoses use standard terminology such as SNOMED CT.

2. Commercial dose and dose-range checking alerts. Currently, these are rudimen-

tary using few patient data, usually only age. Therefore, these systems only loosely fit the patient-specific category.

3. Commercial clinical rules engine. These allow local development or customization of clinical content (a knowledge base) and programming logic. They include the following:

a. Medical logic modules (MLMs) developed using a rule builder application utilizing the Arden Syntax standard. MLM classes include alerts, reminders, recommendations, and informational notifications about a patient. For more information, see Key Definitions above and the sections below on the Arden Syntax and MLMs.

b. Non-Arden type rules engine. These generally are more difficult to work with and have limited logic relative to the sophistication of the Arden Syntax.

c. Artificial Neural Networks (ANN). These are experimental systems that simulate human reasoning from examples. There is a lot of interest and work in this area, but so far, ANN remains beyond the reach of commercial applications.

Non-Patient-Specific CDSS

These require a clinician to adapt general information to an individual patient and clinical situation.

1. Data mining. Provides population specific relationships and information (see Chapter 11).

2. Informational notice. Usually just-in-time, product-specific information. For example, a pop-up box in a pharmacy system that provides a look-alike, sound-alike (LASA) warning, or other useful information about a drug product, to help the pharmacist with order completion. In CPOE, it might be order-specific information such as the cost of a lab test, or formulary status of a drug, with suggestions for alternatives.[6] It might also be patient-specific, such as informing a RPh that a patient on an expensive, short-stability drug has been transferred to a different nursing unit.

3. Order sets. An organized set of patient care orders that are usually population, procedure or disease specific. It may be evidence-based such as a clinical guideline. Well-designed order sets generally provide plenty of opportunity for clinician customization, which makes it more patient specific in the end.

4. Knowledge retrieval systems (KRS).

a. Primary literature retrieval systems such as Google and PubMed return original articles and expert literature reviews.

b. Secondary KRS are online books (Harrison's Online) or collections of online books (STATRef).

c. Tertiary KRS such as online drug and therapy information are knowledge bases available from several vendors such as ASHP, Lexi-Comp, Thomson Healthcare, and Wolters Kluwer Health. These tertiary KRS and their content are derived from extensive review of the primary literature and expert sources.

Maximizing the Benefit of CDSS

By definition, the value of CDSS lies in its ability to bring together evidence-based best practice information with patient-specific data in order to support clinical decisions. The first step in maximizing the impact of a CDSS is to ensure that the data available for decision-making is as comprehensive as possible. This includes not only complete and accurate patient-specific data such as height, weight, allergies, diagnoses, laboratory values, and medical history, but also access to a current evidence-based knowledge base. Whether this knowledge base is developed and maintained on site, or obtained from a third party, it is vital that the data be current and regularly updated. If a commercial knowledge base is being utilized, the vendor should supply regular updates to the information, and these updates must be installed locally as soon as they become available. To do otherwise is to risk affecting patient outcomes, as clinical decisions are made with outdated information.

The next step is to optimize the method by which the decision support information is delivered to the healthcare provider. Kawamoto et al. conducted an analysis of clinical decision support systems, both computerized and non-computerized, to identify critical success factors.[7] They identified four factors which were most associated with improved clinical practice: automatic provision of decision support as part of clinician workflow, provision of decision support at the time and location of decision-making, provision of a recommendation rather than just an assessment, and computer based generation of decision support. Balas et al. further identified that CDS recommendations based on high-quality published evidence are perceived as being of higher value than recommendations based on locally developed guidelines.[8] Clearly, the greatest impact of CDSS will occur when the decision support is delivered in "real time," provides recommendations for alternative therapy when appropriate, and is based on evidence-based best practice guidelines.

Value of CDSS

The impact of CDS can most easily be described in terms of the various technologies into which it has been incorporated. This discussion will focus on the application of CDSS to medication prescribing, dispensing, administration, and monitoring.

CPOE

Perhaps the most widely studied application of CDSS is within computerized provider order entry systems (CPOE). CDSS in conjunction with CPOE has been shown to reduce medication errors, improve compliance with recommended monitoring or adjunctive therapies, and improve efficiency by reducing the time spent clarifying incomplete orders.[7-11] Essentially all commercially available CPOE systems incorporate some degree of CDSS. CPOE-based CDSS have the ability to screen for a variety of potential risks at the time of order entry, including duplicate therapy, drug-drug, drug-disease, drug–lab value interactions, allergic cross-sensitivities, and appropriate dosing.[9] Ideally, decision support should also provide customized recommendations for special patient populations such as pediatrics, geriatrics, and pregnancy. Such systems should also provide real-time guidance for therapeutic drug monitoring, prompting the prescriber to order laboratory assessments of serum drug concentrations, organ function, coagulation parameters, etc.[9] Mathematical errors can be reduced by automating weight-based and similar dosing calculations. Regulatory compliance can be improved as well, for example, by requiring indication for use of PRN medications. More advanced CDSS systems provide support for dosage adjustments based on renal or hepatic function or actively notify the primary caregiver of critical laboratory values or clinical status changes.

In addition to the active decision support methods described above, more passive methods are also available. Simple measures such as use of tall-man lettering to identify LASA medication names can help avert prescribing errors. Setting default sentences for common orders such as "ceftriaxone 100 mg/kg up to 2000 mg IV Q24H" provide improved convenience and guide the user towards appropriate medication use. Grouping orderable items into procedure- or diagnosis-based order sets can also greatly improve the efficiency of order entry as well as guide best practice. Links to local or web-based drug information resources and evidence-based medicine guidelines also give the prescriber quick access to additional information, if desired.

As a supplement to the real-time CDSS described above, second-tier decision support can enable the pharmacy and other departments to more efficiently monitor patient care. The pharmacy department can identify high-risk medications or diagnoses and the clinical information system may be queried to identify patients who meet these trigger criteria. Pharmacists can then target their clinical activities to focus on those patients most at risk. ADR monitoring and reporting programs can benefit from queries based on common trigger medications. The records of patients who fit selected criteria can be screened to identify those who may benefit from preventative interventions such as vaccines or antiplatelet agents.

Electronic Medication Administration Record

CDSS may also be incorporated into an electronic medication administration record (eMAR). A printed MAR is simply a snapshot of the patient's orders as of the moment it was printed. It then must be manually maintained by the nursing staff in order to stay current with changes in the patient's orders until a new hard-copy MAR can be printed. The eMAR avoids this issue. New orders being placed into the clinical information system are updated to the eMAR in real time, providing all caregivers with an accurate, up to the second record of the patient's medications. CDSS may be incorporated into the eMAR to screen for recent changes in laboratory parameters, vital signs, or allergy status, which may interact with a scheduled medication and alert the nurse prior to administration. For example, a critical potassium level recently returned from the laboratory could cause an alert to display for the nurse which would prompt him or her to confirm with the prescriber before administering the patient's digoxin dose. As with CDSS associated with CPOE systems, an eMAR-based CDSS can only be effective when associated with an up-to-date and comprehensive knowledge base to serve as a source of potential drug–lab value and allergen interactions.

When coupled with bar code labels or radio frequency identification (RFID) technology and bedside scanning, the eMAR-based CDSS can provide real-time confirmation of the "five rights" of medication administration; right medication, right dose, right route, right patient, and right time. Real-time notification or periodic summary reports can also be sent to the pharmacy for missed doses, early/late doses, or doses administered to the wrong patient.

Smart Pumps

In recent years, CDSS technology has been integrated into pumps used for administration of parenteral medications (smart pumps). These systems can provide real time confirmation of the volume, rate and concentration of the solution being administered, or provide alerts when concentration or rate fall outside of established safe ranges. Future generation smart pumps may also promise additional benefits, such as real-time communication back to the eMAR and pharmacy information systems so that all members of the healthcare team can readily identify the current dose of titratable infusion.

Automated Distribution Cabinets

In addition to providing security and documentation of controlled substance access, automated distribution cabinets can incorporate CDSS. Nurses can be notified of a potential hypersensitivity or adverse drug reaction when certain trigger medications are withdrawn for a patient. When synchronized with the pharmacy information system or the eMAR, the automated distribution cabinet (ADC) can also provide alerts when a medication is withdrawn too early or too late based on scheduled administration time. The ADC also presents another opportunity to provide links to additional drug information references. Future systems should also include the ability to display an image of the medication being withdrawn for visual confirmation that the correct product has been dispensed.

CDSS Unintended Consequences

CDSS, above all else, are intended to assist the clinician in providing safe and effective care. However, care must be taken to ensure that the CDSS in place do not hinder efficient patient care in the name of guiding appropriate practice. Some of the common unintended consequences are discussed in Table 3-3.

Alert Fatigue

Just-in-time alerts and warnings are one of the most common and effective methods for delivering clinical decision support information to the clinician. The use of such alerts, however, should be limited to those which present clinically significant, time sensitive information.[10,12-14] Over time, when presented with a deluge of alerts of low perceived value, clinicians begin to reflexively override or ignore an increasing percentage of the alerts. A large number of nuisance alerts and pop-up messages that interrupt workflow will also provide a deterrent to use of the system.

There are several common sources of excessive clinical alerts in CDSS. The commercial knowledge bases used as the backbone of many medication-related CDSS contain a comprehensive and exhaustive list of potential drug interactions and allergic cross-sensitivities rated by severity or potential clinical significance. Criteria should be set to govern what type of interactions should be presented to the clinician as real-time alerts. The number and severity of alerts should also be customized by clinician type and practice setting, if possible. For example, the pharmacy department may desire real-time notification of drug interactions regardless of severity, while the physician practicing in the acute care setting may only wish to see those of moderate or high severity. And the physician in the trauma center may only wish to see those with the highest potential to cause harm.

The knowledge base used to provide interaction and allergy data should also be evaluated for clinical significance and accuracy. Inaccurate warnings or constant alerts for reactions of minimal clinical significance will quickly undermine the credibility of the system and contribute to alert fatigue. If available, alert records should be reviewed closely during implementation of a new system and periodically thereafter. A CDSS governance group should review the most commonly triggered alerts for clinical value and deactivate those that are of low impact. The decision to deactivate any clinical alert should be based on a systematic examination for the clinical significance of the alert and a failure mode effects analysis (FMEA) to determine the potential consequences (e.g., patient harm, liability) associated with not providing the alert to the clinician in real-time.

Alert fatigue may also result when CDS systems constantly provide negative feedback, such as dosage error alerts or non-formulary alerts, without also providing information to guide the correct deci-

---

TABLE 3-3

Unintended Consequences of Clinical Decision Support Systems

Unintended Consequence	Description
Alert fatigue	The tendency for users to become overwhelmed and begin to ignore clinical decision support messages due to a high quantity of alerts or a perception that the alerts have little perceived value.
Delay in care	The risk that interruptions in the workflow caused by clinical decision support alerts or system limitations may lead to a delay in delivery of patient care.
System performance	The risk that processor resources used by the CDSS will cause the hospital information system software to perform slowly.

sion. Whenever possible, any error message should be followed with a concise recommendation. A non-formulary alert, for example, should also provide information on an appropriate alternative and, if possible, a direct link to order the recommended agent, with minimal effort.

Delay in Care

Another potential consequence of CDSS is the risk of delaying patient care. Extensive workflow analysis should be conducted during configuration and implementation of any new CDSS and should continue after implementation in order to ensure that delivery of patient care is not adversely affected. Excessive nuisance alerts, as described above, can be one workflow interruption. Care must also be taken with hard stops or other restrictions in the system which do not allow the user to follow a particular course of action under any circumstances.[15] Two common examples involving medication management are dosage restrictions and formulary enforcement. The practice of medicine is often described as both art and science, and the rate at which new information is generated is staggering. Given the complexity of patient care, it is difficult to predict whether a given medication should "never" be prescribed at a certain dose, or that there will never be an appropriate indication for use of a non-formulary agent. If a clinician is faced with an unusual clinical scenario which requires use of an agent normally considered non-formulary but finds that the electronic system will not allow non-formulary agents to be prescribed, then a delay in care may occur as the prescriber is forced to work around the system to obtain and administer the needed medication. It would be preferable for the system to provide a warning when a non-formulary agent is ordered, and ideally provide the recommended alternative, but still allow the restrictions to be overridden under special circumstances. Such overrides can be monitored and subject to review and follow up by

the pharmacy department without preventing access to care in those cases where it may be appropriate.

Workflow must also be considered in ultra-high acuity settings such as in a trauma center or during a code situation.[15] CDSS guidelines and alerts designed to ensure safe patient care in less acute situations may need to be circumvented or overridden in these scenarios to allow the timely delivery of life-saving interventions.

System Performance

Information technology, especially as related to data capacity and processing speed, is advancing exponentially. The speed and capacity of these systems does however remain finite. In a large healthcare institution with hundreds of patients being cared for by hundreds of providers, the processing resources of even the most advanced systems can be stretched. The development and maintenance of clinical MLMs will be addressed elsewhere in this chapter, but must be approached with impact on system performance in mind. While the system may be able to process any given task in tiny fractions of a second, there may be hundreds of tasks to be attended to at any given moment. A system that is perceived as "slow" by its users will be one that is difficult to adopt and frustrating to use.

A Call for CDSS Research

The goals of automated CDSS are to enhance quality of care and outcomes, reduce cost of care, increase reimbursement, optimize regulatory compliance, align practice with national quality initiatives, and reduce risk and liability (both individual and institutional).[1,2,4] We currently do not know to what extent these goals are met by currently available CDSS.[2] Moreover, we have not fully quantified the effects on clinical outcomes of the unintended consequences, such as alert fatigue. Osheroff et al. describe statistical methods to analyze some aspects of CDSS unintended consequences and CDSS effectiveness.[1] Can the benefits be increased and negative effects decreased with home-grown or extensively customized CDSS? Is it worth the effort and resources to find out?

Commercial CDSS are available from all major HIT system vendors. Maintenance of these systems is relatively easy as vendors routinely provide evidence-based updates. Unfortunately, the design and functionality of the current batch of commercial CDSS have some negative aspects, as discussed in this chapter. The influence of these systems on the goals of CDSS enumerated above still needs much study. The results of these studies could help HIT vendors design the next generation of CDSS.

Home-grown or extensively customized CDSS are resource-intensive, both for initial implementation and ongoing maintenance. Do the advantages of developing to local needs offset the costs? Cost/benefit ratio and return on investment (ROI) are difficult to determine. The benefits part of the equation in most published studies is often too subjective or speculative. Our challenge is to find ways to quantify and define benefits in unambiguous terms so that business cases can more easily justify the expense. Fortunately, CMS and other third-party payers are providing a business case and some evidence for ROI via pay-for-performance and unreimbursed care associated with iatrogenic disease and injury. Whether fortunate or not, these mandates, such as pay-for-performance, do not come with CDSS to drive behavior. Each institution must develop its own processes and CDS tools to help practitioners comply. High-quality CDS and CDSS research is required to find the best CDS methods to assist the institution with these issues.

An import institutional function is to oversee this CDS and CDSS research and also to coordinate institutional CDSS use, customization, and development.[1] These functions should be the responsibility of a multidisciplinary committee focused on CDS governance.

CDS Governance Committee

This may be a new committee for most institutions and should be comprised of CDS stakeholders and champions. It may be piggybacked onto an existing CPOE governance committee, or vice versa, as the two have much in common. Its reporting structure and responsibilities will be determined locally, but its purpose should be reasonably analogous across institutions. That is, to ensure safe, efficient, and effective CDSS; to manage expectations; to handle clinical and satisfaction issues arising from CDSS use; and to otherwise cultivate communications with administration and end-users. Realizing that potentially flawed CDSS content or programming might result in patient harm,[1-4] the committee will have to be adroit at CDSS evaluation as part of the acquisition and deployment strategies, thus underlining the importance of the multidisciplinary nature of this committee. Several professional organizations, such as the American Medical Informatics Association and the Healthcare Information Management Systems Society, have excellent references and books to assist the CDS governance committee with CDSS evaluation, implementation, and ongoing analysis.

Once a CDSS is successfully implemented, maintenance of CDSS must be a top priority. Poorly maintained CDS systems can increase the institution's liability and can adversely affect its budget, especially as the Centers for Medicare and Medicaid Services is increasingly resistant to reimburse for costly preventable adverse outcomes.

In addition, the CDS governance committee should establish that CDSS processes are HIPAA compliant and that exposed protected health information (PHI) is secure from an HIT perspective.

Governance of CDSS: An Opportunity for Pharmacy

Historically, pharmacotherapy CDSS resided within the pharmacy, and a pharmacy manager or management committees informally made decisions regarding CDSS functionality of pharmacy computer systems. Vendors of modern pharmacy information systems are providing increasing control and flexibility for CDS functions. For example, pharmacy departments can make modifications to the knowledge base, change severity levels, and selectively turn on/off individual drug-drug interactions. In addition, some pharmacy systems have facilities for building rules to alert of changes in patient condition, such as increasing serum creatinine. Today, management of all these new CDSS functions are generally still made inside the pharmacy department with little outside influence.

Externally, the medical staff, nursing, and others are usually aware that both human and computerized screening of pharmacotherapy occurs in the pharmacy department, but they are generally unaware of the details or limitations of the various systems (human and electronic). They do not fully understand the burden on the pharmacy workload and consequences to patient care. Alert fatigue as discussed above is a major cause of pharmacist frustration and a serious impediment to quality pharmaceutical care. For example, busy pharmacists often override hundreds of nuisance alerts every day. With this alert burden, it is easy to see how they might miss the significant alerts that they should evaluate more closely. Of the medication errors that have the potential to do harm, only about one third are intercepted, and the cost of each preventable adverse drug event (ADE) is estimated at about $6000 and, as mentioned earlier, this cost may not be reimbursable.[16,17]

A contributing factor to this ADE problem is the lack of a standardized coding system for allergies and drug interactions that would allow this information to move between HIT systems. In 2004 the Institute of Medicine (IOM) published *Patient Safety: Achieving a New Standard for Care,* in which the data standards required for healthcare are identified.[18] It recommends mandating adoption of existing standards already approved by the Department of Health and Human Services, the Veterans Administration, and the Department of Defense. Of these standards recommended by the IOM, the following are of particular importance to pharmacotherapy and associated CDSS: NCPDP script for prescription data; HL7 for clinical data messaging, which includes the RxNorm data standard for clinical drugs and their components; LOINC for laboratory test results; and SNOMED CT for a standard clinical terminology and system of nomenclature. Widespread adoption of the recommended data standards would greatly enhance sharing of information between systems, support patient safety, and encourage private-sector investment in HIT.[18] In addition to providing additional opportunities for medication reconciliation, these standards will also allow development of smarter CDSS that could reduce alert fatigue and have many other benefits.

Meanwhile, as CDSS continue to deploy in advanced point-of-care applications such as CPOE, BCMA, clinical documentation systems, etc., institutions need a way to prevent alert fatigue in physicians, nurses, and other clinicians. The CDS governance committee is born of this need. The notion of an institutional CDS governance committee is a new idea for most hospitals and other healthcare organizations. This committee actually provides an opportunity for pharmacy to ease its alert fatigue burden. One of the possible roles of this committee is to reorganize and distribute alerts to those best suited to make the final decision on them. For example, in most cases, a pharmacist sees an alert and decides whether to contact the physician about it.

If the pharmacist calls the physician, two healthcare providers are interrupted by the alert: the pharmacist and the physician. Since there are many more physicians than pharmacists, one controversial approach is to shift some of the burden to physicians by turning on the "contraindicated" drug-drug interaction alerts, drug-pregnancy interactions (FDA categories C, D, and X), and the drug-allergy alerts in CPOE systems. This allows the physician to deal with these alerts directly and at the most appropriate time (during order entry). For those orders that are not changed, both the physician and the pharmacist see the same alert. However, the historically missing piece (prescriber assessment) is now available during the pharmacist's verification process because most systems allow the pharmacist to see why the prescriber overrode the alert. This should make the pharmacist evaluation easier and reduce the number of calls to prescribers. The CDS governance committee can help legitimize this practice model to prescribing physicians, as it is a multidisciplinary committee with physician leadership.

Structure and Leadership of the CDS Governance Committee

The structure and leadership of this committee is dependent on local resources, needs, politics, etc. It is important that pharmacy leadership ensure that it is well represented on this committee, as a good portion of the CDS issues relate to drug therapy. Some CDS experts perceive pharmacotherapy as low-hanging fruit. There are two reasons for this. First, medications are a well-known source of medical errors.[16,17] Second, CDSS for some other important, error prone domains like diagnosis have proven to be much harder to successfully implement.[2,4]

The chair of the CDS governance committee should be the chief medical information officer (CMIO) or his or her designee, preferably an influential practicing physician who is also a CDS champion.

Membership should comprise CDSS project manager(s); informatics experts from medicine, pharmacy, nursing, etc.; representatives of key medical and institutional committees such as the P&T committee; interested leaders and champions from the medical staff, nursing, pharmacy, information services, quality management, health information management, and risk management; and ad hoc members.

Pharmacy informatics specialists should be active members and be in a position to participate, coordinate, or lead various pharmacotherapy-related CDS projects. Likewise, pharmacy informatics specialists who are involved with CPOE should also be active members of the CDS governance committee.

Functions of the CDS Governance Committee

Here again local circumstances dictate. CDS governance for CDSS selection/development, implementation, deployment, and maintenance has several strategic and associated tactical components that vary by application (CPOE, BCMA, pharmacy information system, etc.) and by vendor. Listed below are some possible activities of a CDS governance committee:

1. Evaluate institutional CDSS needs. This might include:

   a. Research and analyze healthcare-related errors.[18,19] Develop a clear understanding of the nature and sources of errors, and then use this information to guide committee priorities, and educate institutional leadership, clinicians, and other stakeholders.

   b. Create an annual CDSS report to hospital administration that includes a CDSS inventory and an analysis of the scope of institutional CDS efforts (human and technical), focusing on workflow issues, reimbursement issues, workload burden, gaps in CDS coverage, risks for harm; risks for special populations especially pregnant, lactating, neonatal, pediatric, and geriatric; and recommendations.

c. Develop and monitor quality improvement plans for institutional CDSS.

d. Monitor and evaluate quality, performance, and maintenance of CDSS.

e. Consider use of medical logic modules to cover gaps in other CDS systems, and for administrative, research, and quality initiatives. See sections on Medical Logic Modules (MLM), and Figure 3-1 depicting governance of MLM life cycle.

2. Evaluate clinical and CDS issues specific to each HIT system. This might include:

a. Decisions regarding drug-drug interaction severity level for CPOE and the pharmacy information system. For example, physicians see contraindicated drug-drug interactions in CPOE, and pharmacists see all interactions in the pharmacy information system.

b. CPOE order sets with imbedded CDS. Which CDS functions to include in order sets, for example, patient-specific dosing and drug selection rules based on patient factors, indication, antibiogram and formulary; or alerts for duplicate lab tests.

c. Bar code medication administration (BCMA) with CDS reminders. For example, remind the RN to obtain trough serum drug concentration before administering the third IV dose of vancomycin.

d. A point-of-care documentation system with CDS to remind the nurse to document missing pain scores after narcotic administration.

3. Monitor market availability and functions of commercial, state of the art CDSS. It is important to be aware of what other vendors and institutions are doing with these products, and to evaluate this in light of internal CDS issues and efforts. This information is available in the biomedical literature, such as the *American Journal of Health-System Pharmacy* and the *Journal of the American Medical Informatics Association,* and at local and national meetings sponsored by the Healthcare Information and Management Systems Society and professional organizations such as the American Society of Health-System Pharmacists and the American Medical Informatics Association.

4. Stay abreast of CDS national trends, evolving HIT standards, and medico-legal issues. See Table 3-4.

5. Participate in recommending human and technical resource requirements for:

a. CDSS implementation.

b. Development of evidence-based content.

c. Testing.

d. Maintenance.

e. Monitoring various aspects of CDSS.

6. Establish policies and standards for medical logic modules (home-grown or imported) that encompass:

a. Risk/benefit analysis, including the risk/benefit of doing nothing.

b. Development and customization of MLMs.

c. Message development—clinical content, medico-legal, and template formats.

d. Notification and escalation of notification:

i. Notification policy and order of escalation for each MLM.

ii. Mode of notification (pop-up dialog box, pager, email, etc.).

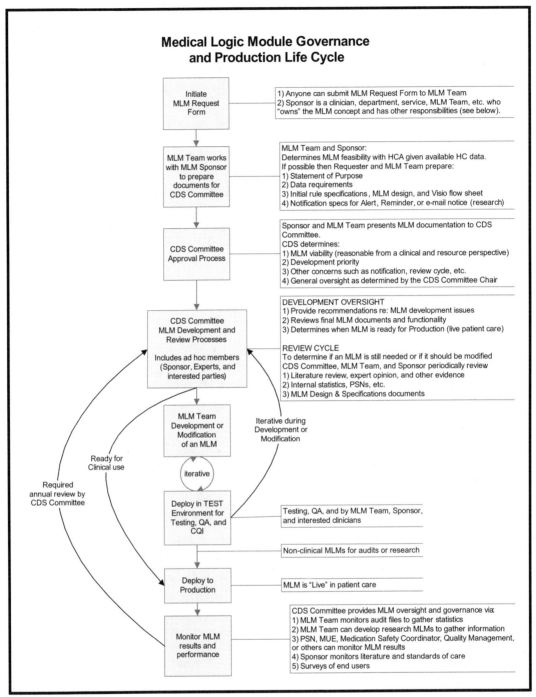

Figure 3-1. CDS governance of MLM life cycle.

e. Audits, audit files, and quality improvement processes.

f. Deployment schedules for new MLMs. The rate of rule deployment (or "rollout") should proceed in an orderly manner as determined by the CDS governance committee. Rule deployment schedule to the live environment should consider the resources of the MLM development team(s),

TABLE 3-4

How to Stay Informed on HIT Issues

Access Point	Opportunity
Professional organizations	ASHP's Section on Pharmacy Informatics and Technology has a taskforce on standards and regulations that monitors evolving HIT standards and regulations, makes recommendations to standards development organizations or government agencies, and informs ASHP membership of its activities and issues of concern. Other healthcare membership organizations have similar committees to monitor HIT standards and regulations. This taskforce is also looking for volunteers as its workload is increasing.
Email list services	■ ASHP, AMIA, HIMSS, and other professional organizations provide email list services to their members focusing on HIT issues. These can be quite valuable for early notification of trends, standards, regulations, and medico-legal issues and to brainstorm and problem-solve HIT issues with colleagues across the country and the world.
	■ Free email news digests such as iHealthBeat and Healthcare IT News report on HIT impact on healthcare, HIT business news, HIT activities of state and federal governments and regulatory bodies, as well as legal issues and legal cases related to HIT.
Academic courses	AMIA 10x10 Program introduces biomedical informatics in a 12-week online course. Their aim is to introduce 10,000 healthcare professionals to biomedical informatics in 10 years.
Active participation in standards organizations	Standards organizations such as Health Level Seven (HL7) are always looking for healthcare professionals to bring new perspectives to their organization. Experience has shown that practicing pharmacists are significantly under-represented. This is a great opportunity to meet and work with accomplished, national figures that are shaping healthcare data standards and consequently shaping the way we all practice our profession.

staff educators to teach end-users about the MLM, impact on clinician workflow, and clinical imperatives to optimize quality care.

g. Maintenance schedules for existing MLMs.

h. Documentation standards for the MLM itself and for the evidence that supports it.

i. Policies for sharing MLMs with other institutions.

Legal Concerns

Liability questions regarding computerized CDS rules and systems have yet to be addressed in the courts.[2,4] Some of the legal questions of interest to the CDS governance committee include:

- Are CDS alerts and reminders legally protected information under risk management and quality initiatives?

- Who is liable for harm caused by a vendor's system (malfunction or otherwise) that is out of direct control of the institution?

- To what extent is an institution liable for harm from a home-grown CDS rule that either causes harm or fails to prevent it?

- Are CDS rules and systems under negligence law or product liability law?[20,21]

- Do institutions incur greater risk with or without CDSS? Would the courts hold an institution liable for harm if it chose not to employ a CDSS that could have prevented or lessened the harm?

Institutions should not delay deployment of CDSS while answers to these and other questions continue to be worked out. The safest approach is for the CDS governance committee to ensure that CDSS are in concert with clinician's needs and are appropriate for clinicians in providing a service. These systems are an adjunct to assist clinicians with their quality and safety efforts and are not intended to replace clinical judgment. The CDS governance committee should vigorously reinforce the notion that the clinician, not the computer, is responsible for its clinical decisions. Realizing that any computerized compilation of data entails the likelihood of some machine errors, omissions, delays, interruptions, and losses of data, for the foreseeable future clinicians must assume full responsibility for ensuring the appropriate use of information provided in computerized messages (alerts, reminders, etc.) in view of the clinical situation.

A separate legal issue that CDS governance committees should follow is the initiatives currently underway to harmonize state and federal laws and regulations. Specifically, the activity regarding HIPAA and interoperability issues that are associated with electronic exchange of healthcare information across networks such as regional health information organization or national health information network. The resulting solutions or mandates may improve or inhibit CDSS functionality in CPOE, e-prescribing, or medication reconciliation.

One last concern is the role of the federal government in regulating CDS systems. Currently the Food and Drug Administration (FDA) sees CDS systems different from medical devices, and favors not regulating CDSS if a licensed healthcare professional uses his or her own judgment to interpret CDSS messages in light of clinical circumstances.[2,4,20-22] However, this FDA policy is controversial, and the CDS governance committee would be wise to follow this issue, as a change in FDA policy could have substantial implications for institutional policies.

As mentioned above, the CDS governance committee may need to bridge a gap in existing CDSS or provide entirely new forms of CDS for quality, administrative, or research initiatives. For these and other CDS efforts, an Arden Syntax–enabled clinical rules engine would provide the flexibility and sophistication to address these interventions and projects. The next section introduces the Arden Syntax standard.

The Arden Syntax Standard

The Arden Syntax is a programming language designed for clinicians to build clinical rules. During a symposium at Columbia University's Arden Homestead in 1989 computer scientists in collaboration with clinicians developed the Arden Syntax. It is a streamlined computer programming language based on Pascal (a computer language designed to teach students good programming style). The Arden Syntax's roots originate from several academic institutions, specifically the LDS Hospital in Salt Lake City (HELP system), Columbia Presbyterian Medical Center in New York, Regenstrief Institute in Indianapolis (CARE system), and others. The American Society for Testing and Materials (ASTM) first approved the Arden Syntax as a standard for encoding medical logic in 1992 (E-1460-92). Ownership transferred to Health Level Seven (HL7) and American National Standards Institute (ANSI) in 1999 with the approval of version 2.0 of the standard. Version 2.7 of the standard was approved by HL7 in 2008. The Arden Syntax is still the only officially approved standard for clinicians to encode medical knowledge into clinical rules. The importance of this standard is that clinical rule developers can move from system to system with relative ease, and clinical rules themselves can be shared with other Arden Syntax–based systems, although some customization will be required. Several major vendors, including Eclipsys, McKesson Provider Technologies, Siemens Medical Solutions, and others have adopted the standard and have developed Arden Syntax clinical rules engines.

The Arden Syntax provides a method to construct clinical rules, such as alerts, reminders and recommendations, known as MLMs. A nice feature of the Arden Syntax is that the MLM developer (usually a clinician) can stay focused on the medical logic. The more technical aspects of program development such as the user interface or data query are not the concern of the MLM developer. The user interface a.k.a. graphical user interface (GUI) is the way a computer program communicates with the person using it. Typically, this is anything displayed on the computer screen, and a person uses the keyboard and mouse, or a touch-screen system, to communicate with the computer program. The computer program automatically handles the user interface. The data queries may be written by the MLM developer but are better managed by database experts in the information systems (IS) department.

The Arden Syntax provides a flexible and clinically sophisticated way to develop MLMs. Most vendors have developed a user-friendly application known as a "tool kit" or "rules builder."

The following are some key features of the Arden Syntax that might be of interest to pharmacy managers:

- HL7 intends MLMs to be sharable between institutions, saving startup time and money in researching the evidence-based rational, and MLM development costs. It is important to realize that MLMs are not "plug and play." This practice of importing MLMs from outside sources always requires clinical and technical validation and local customization. Even so, customizing is usually more economical than developing an MLM from scratch. This savings is in direct proportion to the size and complexity of the MLM. However, implementation and maintenance costs remain the same. There is more information on this topic in the section "CDS Governance and Importing MLMs."

- The Arden Syntax has many built-in conveniences that simplify programming and lessen the burden of development and maintenance. For example:

  - Clinical logic frequently involves temporal reasoning. The Arden Syntax has simplified working with time and durations as compared to traditional programming languages. See Figure 3-2.

  - The clinician developer can focus more time on the medical logic and algorithms. The development environment (rules builder or tool kit) eliminates the need to program the GUI, minimizes the work of building queries to get patient data, and some systems simplify end-user alert notification setup.

  - The Arden Syntax standard promotes extensive documentation of MLMs with several free text slots, as well

Example of If-Then Statement and Temporal Reasoning

The purpose of this IF-THEN statement is to define the safe lower limit of the serum potassium according to the patient's age. In this example, age less than 3 months the lower limit is 4.0 mEq/L, for 3 months to 1 year use 3.5 mEq/L, between 1 and 60 years use 3.6 mEq/L, and for patients older than 60 years use 3.9 mEq/L.

In this example of an IF-THEN statement, the syntax of the IF-THEN statement is highlighted in **bolded text** for clarity. The IF-THEN statement tests the truth of a condition (e.g., age < 3 months) using a "logical" operator (=, <, >, >=, <=, NOT =, etc.). The ELSEIF part of the statement allows multiple conditions to be tested, and ELSE is a catchall if none of the conditions are met. The IF-THEN statement concludes when a condition tests "true," and no subsequent conditions will be tested. Therefore, the sequence of the tests in the IF-THEN statement is very important. The IF-THEN statement concludes with the keyword ENDIF, and all Arden statements end with a semicolon (;).

Temporal reasoning: Notice that the age variable can be tested against any duration. In the first line of the IF-THEN statement, the complier automatically converts the value of age to months; in the subsequent lines, it converts age to years. This is one of Arden's valuable constructs for clinicians. The Arden Syntax knows what units of time are (seconds, minutes, hours, days, weeks, months, and years). It makes encoding this type of logic very easy for clinicians. Unlike other programming languages, the Arden Syntax has many built-in conveniences for clinician developers who are typically not professional programmers.

```
/* Set the safe lower level of serum potassium results according to patient age. */
IF age < 3 months THEN
            K_Lower_Limit := 4.0; /* mEq/L */
      ELSEIF age < 1 year THEN
            K_Lower_Limit := 3.5;
      ELSEIF age < 60 years THEN
            K_Lower_Limit := 3.6;
      ELSE  /* age older than 60 years */
            K_Lower_Limit := 3.9;
   ENDIF;
```

Figure 3-2. Example of the If-Then statement and temporal reasoning.

as the customary comment features found in other programming languages. Well-documented MLMs are very important in reducing maintenance costs. Also, when importing an externally developed MLM, good documentation reduces evaluation and implementation costs.

- The Arden Syntax structure provides the following features:
  - A free text "purpose" slot to briefly describe the objective of the MLM (usually one or two sentences).
  - A free text "explanation" slot to provide in-depth details of the MLM logic.
  - A free text "citations" slot to list references that support the evidence-based rationale for the MLM.
  - The "comment" feature permits the MLM developer to insert comments anywhere in the MLM. This supports liberal documentation throughout the MLM to give details of programming decisions, clarification of methods, and explanations of algorithms. See Figure 3-3 for an example of comment use.

A useful website is the Arden Syntax home page, http://cslxinfmtcs.csmc.edu/hl7/arden/. It was developed and is maintained by Robert A. Jenders, MD, MS, of Enterprise Information Services and Department of Medicine, Cedars-Sinai Medical Center. He is also co-chair of the HL7 CDS Technical Committee that oversees and advances the Arden Syntax standard. This website offers a tutorial on version 1.0 of the Arden Syntax, a library of MLMs contributed mostly from the Columbia Presbyterian Medical Center, a bibliography of Arden Syntax references, and much more information. The HL7 website, http://www.hl7.org, has technical information on the Arden Syntax standards.

CDS Governance and Importing MLM

Editing Imported Rules

The first step after importing a rule that was developed elsewhere, is to carefully review every line of the imported rule to determine what modifications are necessary for safe and effective use at your institution. This includes both technical and clinical validation of MLM content.

Typical modifications include:

- Changing the information in the Maintenance and Library sections to reflect the appropriate use of the rule for your institution should be a high priority of the CDS governance committee. These two sections contain a lot of important information. In the Maintenance section, the local persons or committees who will assume responsibility for the MLM clinical content, customization, and maintenance are identified. The Library section contains the medical evidence base supporting the clinical need for the MLM, and an explanation for the evidence-based logic of the rule.

- Reviewing the clinical content and establishing usage criteria.

- If the rule is a clinical MLM (see next section), then the CDS governance committee must validate the logic and testing of the MLM as part of the approval process for use in a live environment. See Figure 3-1.

- Updating query statements that link MLM to institution data.

- Editing the alert notifications and messages to reflect local style and delivery methods.

Medical Logic Modules

The term *clinical MLM* refers to automated, patient-specific medical logic modules

---

Example of Documenting an MLM with Comment Statements

The syntax for a comments is "/* ... */" and for this example is highlighted in **bolded text** for clarity. Comments provide a way to explain in plain words a portion of the MLM. In this case, it mentions a reference that is listed in the "citation" section of the MLM.

/* Blood volume calculation equations based on the work of Feldschuh & Enson, 1977 */

Deviation := ((weight – LBW)/LBW) * 100; **/* deviation from LBW as % */**
if Deviation is present and Deviation is number then
      if Deviation < –6 then
            cBV := –0.7886 * Deviation + 67.684;
      elseif Deviation < 19 then
            cBV := 69.881 * exp(–0.0072 * Deviation);
      elseif Deviation < 118 then
            cBV := 98.031 * Deviation**(–0.1557);
      elseif Deviation >= 118 then
            cBV := 98.362 * Deviation**(–0.1596);
      endif;
      cBV := cBV * weight / 1000; **/* Blood volume in Liters */**
    endif;

Figure 3-3. Example of documenting an MLM with Comment statements.

that offer a suggestion or warning (alert, recommendation, or reminder) regarding a clinical decision or action, or an informational notice to report a change in a patient's clinical status (e.g., a change in renal function). The target audience of clinical MLMs are clinicians, caregivers, or healthcare consumers.

MLMs are developed within a clinical rules builder (or clinical rules engine) using the Arden Syntax to encode the algorithm. See Figures 3-2 and 3-3 for examples of simple If-Then statements.

MLMs may be either clinical or nonclinical. The main difference is that nonclinical MLMs do not send messages to clinicians engaged in patient care. An example of nonclinical MLM is one that gathers data, such as a patient's serum potassium, for use by a clinical MLM; or one that gathers data for a researcher, manager, or a quality initiative.

The CDS governance committee ensures proper selection, development, deployment and maintenance of clinical MLMs. See Figure 3-1. In this case, the term *development* encompasses both in-house rule development and the pre-deployment evaluation and customization of rules from a vendor or another institution (imported MLM). In selecting which MLMs to deploy, the CDS governance committee will balance factors such as clinical need, financial considerations, potential for e-iatrogenesis, security of PHI, validity of evidence-based content, compliance with internal design standards, and perceived ease of implementation and maintenance. The MLM development team presents MLM proposals to the CDS governance committee. These proposals should be clinically comprehensible. One method is to provide clinically oriented flowcharts. See Figure 3-4a for a textual description of the rule; and Figure 3-4b for a graphical representation of the algorithm flow with an emphasis on the major clinical components. Figure 3-4c shows the other MLMs used in this rule and their relationship to one another. Together these three representations of the rule provide a complete picture that most clinicians can readily understand with only a brief orientation.

Rules for Rules: Planning and Development of Medical Logic Modules

The teams (MLM developers and expert clinicians) and skill sets utilized for implementing imported MLMs are the same teams and skills needed to develop MLMs from scratch. The CDS governance committee may prefer in-house development when suitable MLMs are not available from other sources or when available external MLMs are so complicated or poorly documented that the effort needed to decode and customize them is much greater than starting from scratch.

For in-house development, the CDS governance committee leadership should be aware of certain MLM development principles that will be useful to clinicians aspiring to become MLM developers. The following is a brief, high-level introduction to two of these principles, and other information that might help cultivate the body of knowledge needed for in-house MLM development.

1. Think first, code* later. Henry Ledgard, in *Programming Proverbs* (1975), wrote "The sooner you start coding your program the longer it is going to take." The initial steps to MLM development have nothing to do with computers or programming, but rather gaining an understanding of the problem to be solved. For healthcare professionals, this usually means a clinical problem, or perhaps a gap in the safety net of an HIT application such as CPOE, BCMA, or the like. MLM developers and expert clinicians must take the time to understand the clinical problem and to anticipate the untoward consequences that even a well-designed MLM might introduce, including issues with clinical workflow.[1-4, 23-28]

2. Error trapping: the 80:20 heuristic of MLM development. In well-designed MLMs, approximately 80% of the program logic will be dedicated to "error trapping," and only about 20% of the code is to solve the clinical problem. This strategy grew from a desire to avoid unintended consequences, and naturally it relates directly to the first principle "think first, code later." In general, there are two places for error trapping. These are validation of (1) patient data, and (2) validation of calculated results within the MLM.

In the case of patient data such as a serum potassium result: first make sure it actually exists (not null), is the appropriate data type (number not text), and is within the expected range. For example, a serum potassium result is usually a number in the range of say 2–6 mEq/L. A serum potassium result might also be a non-numeric result that indicates a hemolyzed blood sample. The MLM should be programmed to successfully handle a non-numerical result for serum potassium. This is important so that the MLM does not inadvertently cause an adverse patient event, and that it does not crash the system.

The second form of error trapping is for validating calculated result within the MLM. For example, a calculated volume

---

*The terms *code* and *coding* refer the written program and the act of writing of the computer program. See the If-Then examples in Figures 3-2 and 3-3.

Flowchart MLM Representation

ADE1_Post-Dialysis Meds

(ADE1 = Adverse Drug Event Prevention)

Project Date: 2007-01-04
Last Revised: 2007-05-11

Sponsor:	TBD
Developer:	Michael A. Jones, Pharm.D.
Purpose:	RN Reminder to give post-dialysis medications, only if not given one hour after dialysis.
Use Case:	Triggered by documentation of dialysis completion in Horizon Expert Documentation (HED). One hour after dialysis, the MLM checks the patient's medication profile in AdminRx to determine if the patient has any <u>active</u> medications with a frequency of UDD PRN. If so, it checks the eMAR to determine if these meds have been given after the most recent dialysis. If all meds with a frequency of UDD PRN have been given after most recent dialysis, or if there are no UDD PRN meds, then the MLM sends message to its audit file and ends operation. If there are un-given "UDD PRN" meds then the MLM constructs a message containing a list of these meds and sends a reminder to the RN that these meds MAY be overdue, and it also sends the same message to its audit file.
Comment:	UCH Pharmacy uses this "UDD PRN" frequency for post-dialysis medication orders that do not have a predictable schedule. There are no schedules assigned to the UDD frequency in HMM. UDD (use as directed after dialysis) does not show in AdminRx because there are no associated schedules, and the RN cannot see the medication order in Care Organizer. Therefore, PRN is added so the med order will show in the PRN section of AdminRx.
Trigger event:	Documentation of dialysis completion in HED.
Input:	Required Data: 1. Medication orders and documented times of administration in AdminRx. 2. Patient data from Horizon Clinicals (patient's id, location, and nurse).
Output:	1. Always sends message to audit file for CQI and usage statistics. 2. If criteria are met, a reminder with list of post-dialysis medications will be sent to RN.
Issues:	Monitor usefulness of MLM. 1. Email short user satisfaction survey to RN notified by this MLM (for a limited time only). 2. Query AdminRx data for missed or late doses of post-dialysis medications. 3. Evaluate audit file data for usage and other MLM statistics. 4. Gather pertinent inpatient dialysis statistics for comparison. 5. Monitor inappropriate use of UDD PRN (errors of commission and omission).

Figure 3-4a. Flowchart MLM representation.

of distribution for tobramycin of 1.2 L/kg should not be used for subsequent dosage calculation when the expected value should be something like 0.2–0.5 L/kg.

Body of Knowledge for MLM Developers

There are many excellent introductory books on computer programming that teach

Flowchart MLM Representation

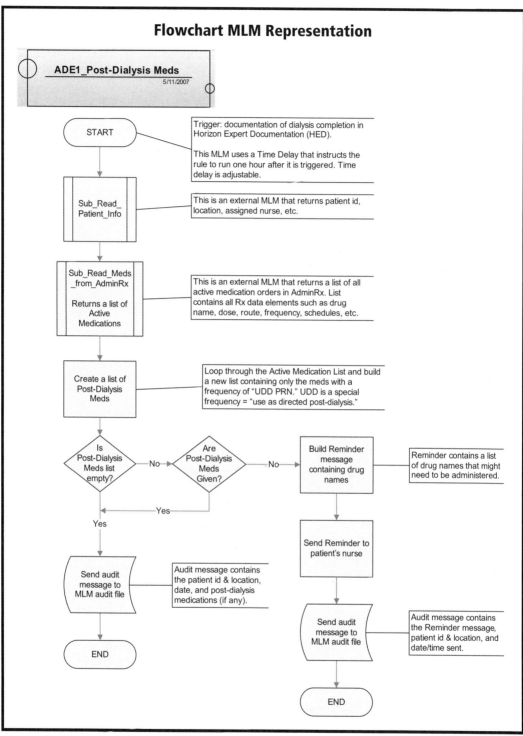

ADE1_Post-Dialysis Meds
5/11/2007

START

Trigger: documentation of dialysis completion in Horizon Expert Documentation (HED).

This MLM uses a Time Delay that instructs the rule to run one hour after it is triggered. Time delay is adjustable.

Sub_Read_Patient_Info

This is an external MLM that returns patient id, location, assigned nurse, etc.

Sub_Read_Meds_from_AdminRx

Returns a list of Active Medications

This is an external MLM that returns a list of all active medication orders in AdminRx. List contains all Rx data elements such as drug name, dose, route, frequency, schedules, etc.

Create a list of Post-Dialysis Meds

Loop through the Active Medication List and build a new list containing only the meds with a frequency of "UDD PRN." UDD is a special frequency = "use as directed post-dialysis."

Is Post-Dialysis Meds list empty? —No→ Are Post-Dialysis Meds Given? —No→ Build Reminder message containing drug names

Reminder contains a list of drug names that might need to be administered.

—Yes—

Yes

Send Reminder to patient's nurse

Send audit message to MLM audit file

Audit message contains the patient id & location, date, and post-dialysis medications (if any).

Send audit message to MLM audit file

Audit message contains the Reminder message, patient id & location, and date/time sent.

END

END

Figure 3-4b. Flowchart MLM representation.

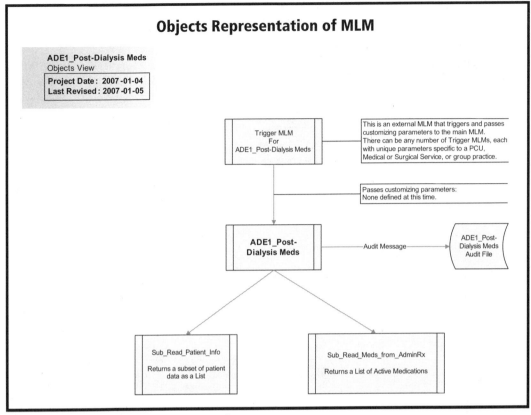

Figure 3-4c. Objects representation of MLM.

general development principles that would be useful. However, few if any are clinically oriented. Although there are no comprehensive textbooks on clinical MLM development with the Arden Syntax, some resources are useful. The Arden Syntax website, http://cslxinfmtcs.csmc.edu/hl7/arden/, has a basic tutorial that is well worth studying. Even though it is for version 1.0 of the Arden Syntax, it provides valuable insight into its features, and has a number of programming examples. Also, an article by George Hripcsak on writing MLMs using the Arden Syntax is useful and informative.[23] Vendors offer classes in the use of their rules builder applications, but these classes focus on the features of the vendor's software and typically do not have time to teach good programming practices. Usually they provide only basic instruction on the Arden Syntax. Ideally, those interested in MLM develop-

ment should train under the guidance of an experienced MLM developer.

The bottom line for managers who see the value of locally customized medical logic modules is to invest in at least one clinician from each of the following departments: pharmacy, nursing, IS, and perhaps medicine to build a cadre of knowledgeable MLM developers. This group of expert MLM developers working through the CDS governance committee will set standards, ensure quality of MLMs, and train others in this very important work.

Future Trends

If we assume inpatient and ambulatory electronic health records (EHRs) will become ubiquitous, and that EHR vendors will adopt the use of standardized medical terminology such as SNOMED CT and Rx-Norm, then interoperability will be possible, allowing easier transfer of health information between EHR systems.

With the implementation of these three indispensable pieces (ambulatory and inpatient EHRs, standardized medical terminology, and interoperability), great advances in the next generation of CDS systems will be possible. Some of the CDS possibilities with these next generation systems include:

- Advanced CDS systems for medication prescribing in CPOE and e-prescribing.

  - Medication reconciliation screening across multiple EHRs. Dentists and ophthalmologists will have access to the patient's complete and current medication history and problem list, and have access to full CDSS screening (see below).

  - CDSS screening or recommendations based on indication, the patient's medication history, problem list, renal and hepatic function, pharmacogenetics, estimated pharmacokinetics and pharmacodynamics, third party payer's formulary, and other conditions and circumstances that optimize pharmacotherapy and other therapies.

- Bio-surveillance for public health issues could automatically notify appropriate internal department(s), the state health department, or the CDC, as appropriate.

- Quality and risk management functions will become more extensive and efficient for infection control and surveillance, antimicrobial stewardship, pay for performance, regulatory compliance, national patient safety goals, and other important quality initiatives and indicators.

- Administrative support and surveillance of all kinds to optimize safety, security, and cost controls, etc., will be possible for the first time with virtually no limitations on available data.

- The promise of continuous quality improvement, total quality management, and Six Sigma will finally be realized as the complete EHR and standard terminology come on line and are easily available for analysis.

Over the last decade, there has been an increase in the political will to proceed with this vision of interoperable EHRs and all of the potential benefits. However, as with any major advance in technology and the inevitable paradigm shifts and resulting transfer of wealth, there are detractors. Namely, those with a substantial stake in the status quo. To achieve this future in the next decade or two, it will take considerable political and social pressure to garner the resources to design, develop, and deploy ambulatory and inpatient EHRs that use standard terminology and are fully interoperable. Such an effort will require a national commitment and funding to secure this future for American healthcare.

References

1. Osheroff JA, Pifer EA, Teich JM, et al. *Improving Outcomes with Clinical Decision Support: An Implementer's Guide.* Chicago, IL: HIMSS; 2005.

2. Berner ES, ed. *Clinical Decision Support Systems: Theory and Practice.* Health Informatics Series. 2nd ed. New York: Springer Science+Business Media, LLC; 2007.

3. Weiner JP, Kfuri T, Chan K, et al. e-Iatrogenesis: The most critical unintended consequence of CPOE and other HIT. *J Am Med Inform Assoc.* 2007;14:387–388.

4. Shortliffe EH, Cimino JJ, eds. *Biomedical Informatics: Computer Applications in Health Care and Biomedicine.* 3rd ed. New York: Springer Science+Business Media, LLC; 2006.

5. Wyatt J, Spiegelhalter D. Field trials of medical decision-aids: potential problems and solutions. *Proc Annu Symp Comput Appl Med Care.* 1991;3–7.

6. Wright L, Grisso AG, Feldott CC, et al. Using computerized provider order entry to implement actions of the pharmacy and therapeutics committee. *Hosp Pharm.* 2007;42(8):763–766.

7. Kawamoto K, Houlihan CA, Balas EA, Lobach DF. Improving clinical practice using clinical

decision support systems: A systematic review of trials to identify features critical to success. *BMJ.* 2005;330(7495):818.

8. Balas EA, Su KC, Solem, JF, Li ZR, Brown G. Upgrading clinical decision support with published evidence: What can make the biggest difference? In: Cesnik B, et al., eds. *MEDINFO 9, Part 2.* Amsterdam: IOS Press; 845–848.

9. Kuperman GJ, Bobb A, Payne TH, Avery AJ, et al. Medication-related clinical decision support in computerized provider order entry systems: A review. *J Am Med Inform Assoc.* 2007;14:29–40. DOI 10.1197/jamia.M2170.

10. Kaushal R, Shojania KG, Bates DW. Effects of computerized physician order entry and clinical decision support systems on medication safety: A systematic review. *Arch Intern Med.* 2003;163:1409–1416.

11. Mekhjian HS, Kumar RR, Keuhn L, Bentley TR, Teater P, et al. Immediate benefits realized following implementation of physician order entry at an academic medical center. *J Am Med Inform Assoc.* 2002;9:529–539.

12. Han YY, Carcillo JA, Venkataraman ST, clark RSB, et al. Unexpected increase in mortality after implementation of a commercially sold computerized physician order entry system. *Pediatrics.* 2005;116:1506–1512.

13. van der Sijs H, Aarts J, Valto A, Berg M. Overriding of drug safety alerts in computerized physician order entry. *J Am Med Inform Assoc.* 2006;13:138–147.

14. Hsieh TC, Kupermn GJ, Jaggi T. Characteristics and consequences of drug allergy alert overrides in a computerized physician order entry system. *J Am Med Inform Assoc.* 2004;11:482–491.

15. Weingart SN, Toth M, Sands DZ, Aronson MD, Davis RB, Phillips RS. Physicians' decisions to override computerized drug alerts in primary care. *Arch Intern Med.* 2003;163(21):2625–2631.

16. Bates D. Preventing medication errors: A summary. *Am J Health-Syst Pharm.* 2007; 64(Suppl 9):S3–9.

17. Institute of Medicine. *Preventing Medication Errors: Quality Chasm Series.* Washington, DC: National Academy Press; 2006.

18. Institute of Medicine. *Patient Safety: Achieving a New Standard for Care.* Washington, DC: National Academy Press; 2004.

19. Guchelaar H, Colen HBB, Kalmeijer MD, et al. Medication errors: hospital pharmacist perspective. *Drugs.* 2005;65(13):1735–1746.

20. Miller R, Schaffner K, and Meisel A. Ethical and legal issues related to the use of computer programs in clinical medicine. *Ann Intern Med.* 1985;102(4):529–537.

21. Miller RA. Legal issues related to medical decision support systems. *Int J Clin Monit Comput.* 1989;6(2):75–80.

22. Young F. Validation of medical software: Present policy of the Food and Drug Administration. *Ann Intern Med.* 1987;106(4):628–629.

23. Hripcsak G. Writing Arden syntax medical logic modules. *Comput Biol Med.* 1994;24(5):331–363.

24. Kendrick DC, Bu D, Pan E, et al. Crossing the evidence chasm: building evidence bridges from process changes to clinical outcomes. *J Am Med Inform Assoc.* 2007;14:329–339.

25. Bates DW, Kuperman GJ, Wang S et al. Ten commandments for effective clinical decision support: making the practice of evidence–based medicine a reality. *J Am Med Inform Assoc.* 2003;10:523–530.

26. Sittig DF, Krall MA, Dykstra RH, et al. Survey of factors affecting clinician acceptance of clinical decision support. *BioMed Central Medical Informatics and Decision Making* 2006;6:6. doi:http://www.biomedcentral.com/1472–6947/6/6

27. Bates BW, Cohen M, Leape LL, et al. Reducing the frequency of errors in medicine using information technology. *J Am Med Inform Assoc.* 2001;8(4):299–308.

28. Musen MA, van der Lei J. Knowledge engineering for clinical consultation programs: modeling the application area. *Methods Inf Med.* 1989;28:28–35.

CHAPTER 4

Pharmacy Information Systems

Chad Hardy

KEY DEFINITIONS

Application—software written to work on a computer and designed to perform a specific task, in this context the PIS. It is what the user sees when he opens the PIS.

Clinical Information System—a group of computers that run databases and software applications to effectively provide a comprehensive repository of patient-specific healthcare information. As a general term, this might be a laboratory, pharmacy, nursing documentation, or ordering system.

Database—a large collection of data organized for rapid search and retrieval by a computer.

Integrated Systems—when information systems that perform different functions share the same database, application space, and often hardware. They are usually provided as a single solution.

Interfaced Systems—when separate information systems (with separate databases) are built to communicate with one another. This requires the development of an interface to normalize information for interpretation by both systems.

Pharmacy Information System (PIS)—a system that provides pharmacy staff the necessary application environment to practice the profession of pharmacy; often includes the ordering, procurement, preparation, dispensing, and monitoring portions of the medication use process.

Server—the heart of a network of computers, providing a centralized and organized location for the PIS, database, and application.

Workstation—the computer in the pharmacy that a staff member uses to interact with the PIS.

Introduction

Pharmacists and managers provide timely, safe, and clinically oriented patient care. In the past few decades, industries such as automobiles, oil, gas, or financial institutions discovered the advantages of storing and retrieving information from computers. This increased productivity, accuracy, and profits for some of the nations leading companies. As a result, information systems were explored as a tool to improve many other industries, including pharmacy practice. These innovative systems grew from printing labels to robust and complex pharmaceutical care applications. Those tools allowed the pharmacist to organize patient demographics, input and store orders, search commonly used information, and screen for potential drug interactions. Today's pharmacy information system builds on these fundamentals while providing features to parallel modern practice.

What is a Pharmacy Information System?

A pharmacy information system (PIS) provides a comprehensive electronic infrastructure to support the provision and management of pharmacy services. Typical systems are designed around pharmacy practice, processes, workflows, and medication use, meeting the needs of the organization. Pharmacy information systems are critical to the efficient and safe operation of any pharmacy business. Not to be confused with a computerized provider order entry (CPOE) system, the PIS is designed for pharmacists and technicians. Consequently, adequate attention should be given to its design, acquisition, implementation, and ongoing maintenance. Many advanced systems require dedicated technical resources for management and configuration.[1] Consequently, the role of the pharmacy informatics specialist is increasingly important to a successful pharmacy team. Focusing on functions, common features can be broken down by practice area, including medication use functions, clinical use functions, and system/business functions.

General Practice Tools

The PIS should meet the general needs of daily pharmacy practice while providing the tools to meet regulatory needs. The guidelines and laws set forth by governing bodies in many ways shape standard pharmacy policy, procedure, and operations. In the pharmacy practice environment, the medication use process is a focal point of pharmacy practice. Prescribing, transcription, dispensing, administration, and monitoring include the critical components of medication use. The process includes a qualified medical provider writing orders (prescribing), the pharmacist or order entry technician interpreting those orders and inputting into the PIS (transcription), dispensing of the product to the caregiver, administration of the product to the patient, and continuous monitoring of the patient's drug therapy. The PIS should provide pharmacy staff the tools necessary to perform these functions safely and productively.

Prescribing and Transcription

Commonly, the PIS addresses the transcription, dispensing, and monitoring of portions of the medication use process. Prescribing features are not typically included in a PIS but can come into play when systems are integrated or interfaced with CPOE. Transcription (or traditional pharmacist order entry) is the process of translating or reducing a provider's order to terms the PIS can understand. These frequently include pertinent fields to support all downstream medication use processes. It is critical to review all of the pieces of information the organization may require throughout the medication use process and to ensure the PIS contains adequate functionality. For instance, the PIS might accept or calculate a rate of administration for an intravenous agent. This rate of administration is used by a nurse administering the drug to the patient or the clinical pharmacist reviewing appropriateness of therapy. In addition, standard administration times, approved abbreviations, and frequencies are commonly communicated between nursing and pharmacy. Some PIS accept patient demographic and admissions data from the hospital business system: social security number, date of birth, ethnicity, insurance, name, sex, admission date, and unique hospital identifiers are commonplace in a system interface. A decision to accept this data is important to the efficiency of the PIS and should be considered carefully. As with any order entry process, the field names and flow of information within the application should be user friendly and aid transcription. Information technology experts use the term *screen fatigue* to describe a system that requires too many prompts or different screens to accomplish a task. The PIS should minimize screen fatigue and allow processing that minimizes mouse clicks or keystrokes. Any relevant clinical information required for order entry should be included in this area of the application, for example labs, allergies, or drug-drug interactions.

Dispensing

In addition to transcription and verification, the PIS should also provide robust tools for medication preparation and dispensing. Some of these tools include automatic calculations (rate, concentrations), ability to customize and print labels in specific locations, and batch processing. Pharmacies distribute thousands of doses to hospitalized patients per day. As a result, they need ways to provide scheduled products by admitted unit or patient type. Batch processing allows the pharmacy to print a group of medication labels for preparation at one time. For instance, the pharmacy may wish to prepare all of the antibiotics for a group of patients on a floor. The PIS can allow all labels to

print, allowing dose preparation prior to administration. This alleviates turnaround times and can improve patient care. A pharmacist focused on clinical activities might use this time to round with providers, create IV to PO switch programs, schedule primary care appointments, or improve pharmacokinetic monitoring services.

Regulatory Considerations

Pharmacy practice is regulated and guided by many groups and organizations. Some of these include the federal government, state boards of pharmacy, the FDA (Food and Drug Administration), DEA (Drug Enforcement Agency), USP (United States Pharmacopeia), ISMP (Institute for Safe Medical Practice), and the Joint Commission. Accommodating changes in system design across multiple states can be challenging. As a result, the manager should pay close attention to the features and configurations of the system to ensure compliance with applicable guidelines. Some examples of regulatory requirements and guidelines related to PIS include labeling requirements (font size, information required), storage of pertinent clinical information (for audit retrieval), and quality assurance tools.

For example, labeling requirements and configuration have seen recent attention by the ISMP with regards to safety.[2] The challenge is designing a label that meets the need of all regulating and accrediting agencies. The PIS should provide the functions and tools that allow the pharmacy to modify labels accordingly. The pharmacy manager should become familiar with local, state, and federal labeling requirements to ensure compliance. In addition, label design should include an interdisciplinary team of pharmacists, nurses, and qualified medical practitioners. This ensures consistency among information provided. For example, pharmacists find a "work label" very useful, providing a breakdown of individual ingredients, concentrations, and preparation quantities. Consequently, nursing has little use for preparation information, concentrating on the amount of medication to administer. Well-designed labels provide features to meet the needs of the healthcare team. If the organization is transitioning to bar-coded medication administration, the pharmacy can ensure the labels print bar codes to support those processes.[11] Some pharmacies have multiple printers with different label sizes to support these preparation types. In the case of intravenous (IV) syringes prepared for neonatal or pediatric patients, smaller labels can help legibility and reduce trimming time by the pharmacist or technician. The pharmacy will also want to pay close attention to where labels print, and ensure the PIS provides capabilities to redirect printing if pharmacies are being covered by another area or do not carry the requested medication.

To meet state and regulatory retrieval requests, data storage capacity is also an important component of the PIS. The pharmacy should ensure that its system can store, catalog, and retrieve all information related to the provision of pharmaceutical care in a timely manner. This author has seen systems run out of memory or computing space, creating challenging situations when asked for an old record by a regulatory agency. As a result, it is important to plan with the information technology (IT) department for the future. Similarly, quality assurance is a critical part of every successful pharmacy operation. The PIS should support reporting, active monitoring, and ready retrieval of information necessary to evaluate quality. The pharmacy manager can evaluate the current QA processes of the organization and ensure that necessary tools are available in the PIS. For example, quantification of order entry or unapproved abbreviations. These are important markers for patient safety and can help justify additional tools to aid the pharmacist. The PIS might provide a monthly report or summary metrics

on errors. More advanced systems would allow some level of analysis as well, without the need to transfer data to an external system.[3] The manager should pay close attention to any experience the vendor of a PIS may have with local, state, and federal regulatory agencies. During a Joint Commission visit, the pharmacy manager will appreciate the time spent evaluating systems for these features.

Clinical Tools and Functions

While general and regulatory considerations require adequate attention, the pharmacy information system is not complete without a comprehensive clinical feature set. These tools revolve around the medication use process, providing the pharmacist with historical, real-time, and future clinical information. In addition, decision support, drug information, and monitoring should be addressed by the system's functionality.

Medication use safety is an important consideration for the pharmacy manager. The PIS should provide the pharmacy specialist with the tools necessary to ensure safe and accurate pharmaceutical care for patients. These tools include drug-drug interaction checking, drug-food interaction checking, drug–disease state contraindication alerts, and allergy screening. Many PIS's accept these types of information and are updated with a drug information repository service, such as First DataBank® or MediSpan®. These services provide a massive amount of drug information that can be uploaded directly into many PIS. Drug Name, NDC (National Drug Code), AHFS (American Hospital Formulary Service) class, default directions, standard strengths, and interactions are example of data elements typically provided. The PIS should provide a way to maintain information such as drug interaction tables, allergy screening methods, and comorbid condition screening if it does not have the ability to accept data from these types of vendors. Maintenance of this information is covered comprehensively in Chapter 8. Ultimately, the PIS should provide accurate, productive features to aid the pharmacist in reviewing relevant interactions, allergies, and clinical alerts. The way this information is communicated to the pharmacist may vary among PIS vendors. It is important to review the way alerts, interactions, and pop-up messages display in the PIS. The goal is to have the information acknowledged and reviewed by the pharmacist each time it is needed. Some systems use so many pop-up messages or screens that many practitioners have become desensitized to their importance. Screen fatigue can have considerable implications on patient care in the hospital and requires careful evaluation. The pharmacy manager should schedule time to test the number of steps it takes for each task in the PIS, to ensure adequate and widespread user acceptance.

Decision support tools play an important role when interacting with or embedded into the PIS. Some of these tools include drug-diagnosis screening, near miss error alerts, or lab alerts for specific drugs. The PIS should provide the ability to create, modify, and maintain this information. As the role of the PIS in the electronic health record continues to evolve, it becomes more important to have multidisciplinary teams involved in reviewing and updating decision support components of information systems. For instance, the pharmacist might provide input on drug monitoring parameters for aminoglycosides and vancomycin. A team of providers, nursing, lab, and pharmacy could decide how to configure the system to alert the ordering provider when a monitoring opportunity arises.

Drug information is a cornerstone of pharmacy practice. To make accurate clinical decisions, pharmacists and technicians should have efficient access to comprehensive tools. This information can be implemented in various ways within a PIS. Some current PIS do little to provide clinically relevant drug information at the right time in the medication use process. For example, drug interactions might show at the end of the order entry process, as opposed to the beginning. In addition, there is great deal of information PIS may not provide. These include IV compatibility and use in specialized patient populations; for example, pediatrics and oncology, to name a few. The pharmacist must rely on external resources for this information. Integration of external electronic drug information databases with the PIS can greatly improve the efficiency and safety of pharmaceutical care. For example, links or look-ups that directly reference online drug information services (e.g., Micromedex, Gold Standard GSM) provided within the PIS allows quicker access to information to streamline the medication use process. These services are typically updated by the vendor, presenting recent and clinically relevant drug information. Additional methods to provide drug information include external programs or the use of textbooks. Both are viable options but someday may follow behind a fully integrated PIS.

Business Tools and Functions

In addition to clinical activities, health-system pharmacies are in the business of taking care of patients. However, this requires that the business generate enough revenue to support the mission of the profession. Although there are varying degrees of dedication to profit and bottom line, operating at a loss, or "in the red," for a prolonged period is detrimental to any operation. The PIS can help automate the charge capture and billing process in pharmacy operations. Pharmacy workflows typically charge on dispense or upon administration of a medication. Charging on administration usually requires some type of bar-coding technology to ensure capture by the caregiver at time of use. Dispense-based charging can occur from an automated dispensing cabinet (ADC) or based on cart fills from the pharmacy. As the system of medication order entry and preparation, the PIS is an ideal medium for configuration of charge capture. Many PIS allow the manager to configure appropriate charge formulas based on many variables (e.g., cost, type of product, dispense units), streamlining any manual necessity for continuous record-keeping. Billing for pharmaceuticals typically involves communication with a secondary system, such as a hospital patient management/accounting system (PMPA). As a result, common identifiers must be used so that both systems can understand what, when, and how much product should be billed. Although there has been recent discussion surrounding discreet NDC-based charge capture,[4,5] many current systems use a charge data master (CDM) or similar identifier to communicate. This number is entered into the PIS for each drug, and paralleled in the PMPA system for patient billing. The actual dollar amount can come from the PIS or be calculated in the PMPA system, although most come from the PIS, as the pharmacy is the department most comfortable with drug costs and is privy to automatic pricing updates from wholesalers or database vendors. Seasoned informatics specialists recognize the challenges of NDC-based billing, which include inadequate system configuration to support NDC specific inventories, inability of wholesalers to provide consistent NDCs in lieu of drug shortages, and ability of the pharmacy to capture the actual NDC administered. Bar-coding provides some solutions to these dilemmas, but challenges with scanning on administration, proper bar code formats, and appropriate scanner hardware at the bedside may need to be overcome to ensure proper charge capture.

In addition to business functions, the pharmacy manager should also understand the underlying hardware and software systems represented by the PIS. At the fundamental IT level, pharmacy information systems consist of hardware and software. While most of the manager's time is spent with the software portions of the PIS, he or she should also understand some aspects of computer hardware. The typical PIS is comprised of servers, workstations, and peripherals. Depending on the size of the PIS, servers can perform split roles. Some servers might run the actual application, while others house the database and all of the patient information. Servers can communicate with one another on the backend via interfaces or take information directly from a shared database. Servers must be very powerful computers, performing multiple task requests from many users at a time. Processing speed, memory, and drive space are fundamental specifications that should be reviewed by the IT group prior to purchase. Most notable to the pharmacy is hard drive space, as this will dictate how much historical information the PIS can house before it must be archived (moved from the primary server) to make room for new pharmacy and patient information. Some PIS vendors recommend a second "history" server or database that is used to minimize the workload on the primary server. Users wishing to run reports or review old data can access the history server without impact to real-time pharmacy operations. Depending on the size of the operation and server configuration, the options for reporting, quality assurance, and monitoring should be considered. It is important to evaluate functions of the PIS in the assessment. Often these create a majority of the processing load on the PIS, slowing the system down. A diagram of typical PIS configuration is provided below in Figure 4-1.

The workstations represent the computers in the pharmacy areas of the operation. Pharmacists and technicians are the users of the workstations. Workstations communicate with the server over the network infrastructure, usually a complex array of cables and network equipment designed to allow data transmission. For this reason,

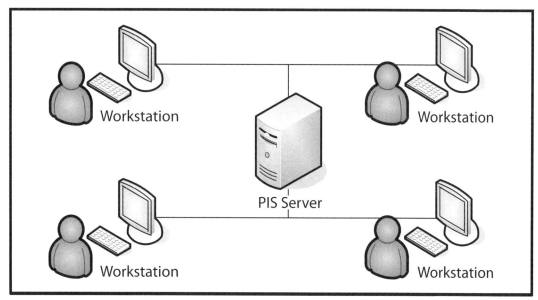

Figure 4-1. Diagram of a pharmacy information system.

when the network is down, the PIS is typically unavailable.

In addition, databases are an equally important system within the PIS, and they are often used to store and retrieve all electronic information contained within the PIS. Knowledge of database terminology and technology can enhance the pharmacy manager's interaction with the IT department. As a result, it is important to understand the basic make-up and functions of a database. Databases store, catalogue, and organize the information in the PIS. Think of the database as the long- and short-term memory of the PIS. Without it, no information could be retrieved or saved. Databases are comprised of fields, tables, and records. An example of a field is a social security number. That field is specifically created to store only this specific number. A group of fields makes up a record. For example, a record might include social security number, last name, first name, date of birth, sex, ethnicity, height, weight, body surface area, and allergies. The record represents the information for a specific patient. Mr. Jones has a record, as does Mrs. Smith. Those records are stored in a table. Tables are used to split information up

in a database, making it easier for the server to retrieve the information. For example, we might store demographics in one table, and medications for the same patient in a second table. Combine all the tables, and we have a database. Figure 4-2 depicts a typical database.

Careful consideration along with collaboration with vendors and the IT department will help pharmacy managers make an informed decision about the current and future needs of the PIS. The pharmacy manager or director often becomes the mediator between the vendor and local IT resources. This presents a unique opportunity to find a solution that meets both operational and business goals.

Goals of Integration with Other Healthcare Information Systems

Many pharmacy managers and directors are faced with an important decision: interface or integrate? Interfaces were the technology of the 1990s, creating new ways for computers to share information and automate processes. Most implementations required tailored creation of each computer system participating in the interface. In many

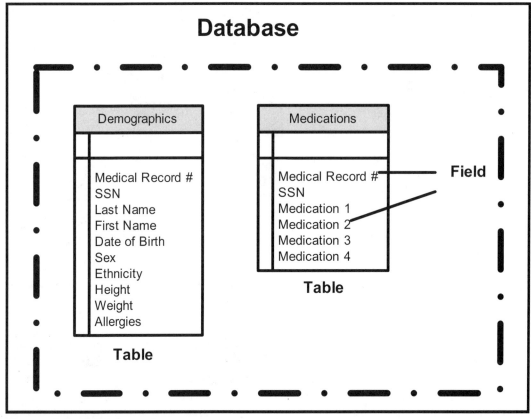

Figure 4-2. A database diagram.

respects, interfaces have brought healthcare IT where it is today. However, due to the difficulty of design and interoperability, many technology experts explore more integrated alternatives. An integrated system often shares the same database, application space, hardware design, and is created by the same vendor. This helps to maintain consistency among system design and ensures that all applications within the health system communicate seamlessly. Most importantly, integrated systems are written by the same vendor and group of developers. Other advantages include support and customization from a single source (Table 4-1). Figure 4-3 displays an interfaced and integrated system.

Communication between pharmacy and CPOE systems require careful design and may present limitations that challenge workflow processes. The type of system-wide clinical information system (CIS) the

organization uses will play an important role regarding the PIS. For instance, many CIS are migrating to CPOE systems, whereby the provider is responsible for keying the medication order into a computer. This often eliminates the need for a PIS to support a robust pharmacy order entry component, focusing the pharmacist's practice on order verification and clinical services. The types of CPOE systems become a key component of an integrated or interfaced PIS. Noteworthy assessment of current practice includes whether CPOE orders should be printed and re-entered by pharmacy into the PIS or electronically transmitted to the PIS for verification. Considerations include efficiency, time required for duplicate entry, and patient safety.[6,7] CPOE orders electronically transmitted to the PIS for pharmacist verification may liberate the pharmacist to provide clinical functions to the healthcare team.

TABLE 4-1

Advantages and Disadvantages of Integrated and Interfaced Systems

	Integrated	Interfaced
Advantages	■ One support contact ■ One database for all information ■ Designed by one group	■ May provide a specific system with more features for an area of health-care (lab, pharmacy, etc.) ■ More competition in market ■ Downtime of other systems may not affect PIS
Disadvantages	■ One database can impact down-time productivity ■ May sacrifice customizability and features for compatibility and interoperability	■ Complicated set-up ■ Extra point of failure and errors ■ Designed by different groups; normalizing data can be difficult

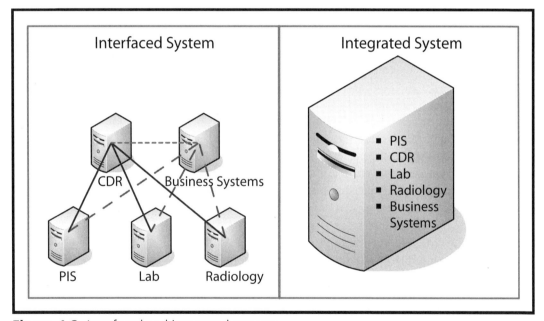

Figure 4-3. Interfaced and integrated systems.

Interfaces are one challenging aspect of communication and implementation of new systems. Hospital and healthcare systems consider technology to streamline their business and clinical processes. Ancillary systems such as pharmacy, lab, and radiology play an important role in providing clinical information to the electronic health record and healthcare team. As a manager, it is important to consider the contributions of pharmacy systems from a global patient perspective. The complexity and variation among interfaces and respective systems warrant careful design, planning, and testing.[8] The pharmacy system may receive lab, demographic, and admitting information from interfaced systems. Similarly, the PIS may send verified order information to electronic health record systems or ADCs. A comprehensive testing plan will minimize the operational impact and emergency fixes required. Some critical areas include drug configuration, ordering, alerts, interfaces, charging, billing, and batch processes. Creating comprehensive workflows for all operational and administration portions of the pharmacy operation will help tease out the needs of both interfaced and integrated solutions.

Future Trends in Pharmacy Information Systems

Pharmacy practice has evolved a great deal in the past two decades. Information technology and automation solutions provide opportunities to streamline operations, and the potential to provide more direct patient care. As a profession, pharmacy has long focused on the preparation and dispensing portions of the medication use process. Technology may threaten our ability to continue this primary method of practice. Automation tools such as automated prescription machines (APMs) are providing medication dispensing in the provider's office. In some situations and settings, it is no longer necessary for a pharmacist to review medications dispensed directly to a patient from an electronic system. As such, the provider's health record and prescribing software provides safety, allergy, interaction, and drug therapy review functions. Consequently, inpatient pharmacy practice is threatened in much the same manner. CPOE systems transition a portion of the inpatient pharmacist's role to the provider. Pre-made and extended shelf life products reduce the need for sterile compounding and product verification within centralized pharmacy operations. So where does the pharmacist fit in? If we don't embrace technology and ensure that we are involved in direct patient care, the question may be answered for us.[9] The PIS provides patient monitoring tools to help pharmacists impact health outcomes and provide more consistent monitoring. For example, verification of orders, therapeutic drug monitoring, pharmacokinetic monitoring, and oncology are specialized areas of pharmacy practice.

Currently, many of these monitoring functions are performed by third-party applications but warrant consideration for inclusion in the PIS. Verification of orders, therapeutic drug monitoring, pharmacokinetic monitoring, and oncology are examples of areas clinical practice. Many PIS are being developed by the same vendor as electronic health record and hospital business systems. This seamless integration provides many opportunities for patient-specific clinical information to show within the PIS. For instance, a pharmacist might be able to see labs related to certain medications from the same window. This minimizes the dependency on additional applications for different types of information (lab, disease state, problem list, and home medications, for example). PIS and automation will become more integrated, driven by regulatory and patient safety goals in healthcare.[10] Certainly the future of the profession is influenced by technologies, and pharmacists possess a unique opportunity to become more involved in patient care.

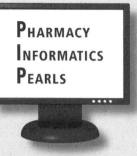

PHARMACY INFORMATICS PEARLS

PHARMACY INFORMATION SYSTEMS

General

- Systems are designed around pharmacy practice, workflows, processes, and medication use.
- Consider dedicated technical resources for management and configuration.
- Should address prescribing, transcription, verification, preparation, dispensing, administration, and monitoring areas in the medication use process.
- Consider the role interfaces play with the PIS and how they impact care.
- Minimize screen fatigue, mouse clicks, and key strokes as much as possible.

Key components

- CPOE orders electronically transmitted to PIS for verification save time and improve access to direct patient care.
- Pay close attention to vendor experience with local state regulatory and legal agencies.
- Involve a multidisciplinary team in the design and decisions of the PIS and electronic health record. The more complex the rule, the more difficult it is to maintain.
- Consider integration of external electronic drug information databases with the PIS to improve productivity.
- NDC billing requires careful planning and consideration but may become a future requirement.
- Don't forget the fundamentals: hardware, software, applications, databases, and interfaces. Consider future hard drive and system memory requirements.
- The database is the long- and short-term memory for all pharmacy related patient information. It is comprised of fields, tables, and records.

Integrating with other systems

- One development group, one support group, one relationship = integrated system.
- Testing, testing, and more testing.
- Creation of comprehensive workflows will help all members of the healthcare team understand pharmacy processes.

Future trends

- If we don't embrace technology and ensure involvement in direct patient care, we may lose part of our profession.

References

1. Mack TA. Decision support considerations in the development and implementation of an electronic medical record. *Pharm Pract Manag Q.* 1998;18(1):21–34.

2. Institute for Safe Medication Practices. "Intravenous Piggyback Medication for Patient Specific, Inpatient Use." (Draft.) Available at: http://www.ismp.org/Tools/guidelines/labelFormats/comments/default.asp. Accessed March 09, 2007.

3. Puckett F. Medication management component of a point of care information system. *Am J Health Syst Pharm.* 1995;52:1305–1309.

4. Centers for Medicare and Medicaid Services. "CMS legislative summary: MMA of 2003. Available at: http://www.cms.hhs.gov/MMAUpdate/downloads/PL108-173summary.pdf. Accessed March 15, 2007.

5. Center for Medicare Services. "Manufacturer average price and the proposed use of ndc based billing for Medicaid affiliated institutions." Available at http://www.cms.hhs.gov/quarterlyproviderupdates/downloads/cms2238p.pdf. Accessed April 15, 2007.

6. Koppel R, Metlay JP, Cohen A, Abaluck B, Localio AR, Kimmel SE, Strom BL. Role of computerized physician order entry systems in facilitating medication errors. *JAMA*. 2005; 293:1197–2003.

7. Kaushal R, Shojania KG, Bates DW. Effects of computerized physician order entry and clinical decision support systems on medication safety. *Arch Intern Med*. 2003;163:1409–1416.

8. Siska MH, Barone LD, Besier JL, et al. ASHP Statement on the pharmacist's role in informatics. *Am J Health-Syst Pharm*. 2007:200–203.

9. Cina J, Gandhi TK, Churchill W, Fanikos J, McCrea M, Mitton P, et al. How many hospital pharmacy medication dispensing errors go undetected? *J Comm J Quality Patient Saf*. 2006;32:73–80.

10. Hartzema AG, Winterstein AG, Johns TE, et al. Planning for pharmacy health information technology in critical access hospitals. *Am J Health-Syst Pharm*. 2007;64:315–321.

11. Food and Drug Administration. FDA Rules Requires Bar Codes on Drugs and Blood to Help Reduce Errors. Available at http://www.fda.gov/oc/initiatives/bar code-sadr/. Accessed April 22, 2007.

CHAPTER 5

Pharmacy Automation Systems

Steve Rough and Joel Melroy

KEY DEFINITIONS

Adverse Drug Event—an injury resulting from a medication or lack of intended medication.

Automated Dispensing Cabinets—secure storage cabinets typically located decentrally on patient care units capable of handling most unit-dose and some bulk (multiple-dose) medications due to storage limitations.

Automation—any technology, machine, or device linked to or controlled by a computer and used to do work. Automation is designed to streamline and improve the accuracy and efficiency of the medication use process.

Carousel Automation—a medication storage cabinet with rotating shelves used to automate dispensing.

Centralized Robotic Dispensing System—centrally located devices designed to automate the entire process of medication dispensing including medication storage, distribution, restocking, and crediting of unit dose medications.

Medication Error—any preventable event that may cause or lead to inappropriate medication use or patient harm while the medication is in the control of the health care professional, patient or consumer.

Supply Chain Management—the management of the pharmaceutical order-to-pay process including management of inventory and distribution of supplies throughout the medication use process.

Technology—anything that is used to replace routine or repetitive tasks previously performed by people, or which extends the capability of people.

Introduction

In today's health care marketplace, payers and patients demand high quality, efficient, and cost-effective service. Through successful implementation of technological advancements, pharmacy departments can play a vital role in providing high quality and efficient service to patients. Efficient use of technology and automation is a prerequisite to the survival of the profession and the advancement of pharmacist patient care services.[1]

The purpose of this chapter is threefold: (1) to provide background on the use of automation in inpatient pharmacy practice, (2) to describe several pharmacy automated dispensing technologies as well as their advantages and disadvantages and intended roles within the medication use process, (3) to identify best practices for maximizing the safe and efficient use of automation, and (4) to provide a predictive model for the impact automation will have on the future of pharmacy practice. On completion of this chapter, the reader should have an understanding of the role of pharmacy-based automation in an integrated health system as well as practical tools for implementing such automation.

Current Trends

The application of automated dispensing systems within the practice of pharmacy began in the early 1960s. However, changes in the health care system and the profession's transition to pharmaceutical care have dramatically increased the demand for incorporation of automation into pharmacy practice over the past 15 years. Corporate and organizational goals of reducing costs, improving operating efficiencies, growing revenues, enhancing safety and quality, integrating and managing data, and providing outstanding customer service are primary drivers of this trend. Pharmacy managers are often expected to improve efficiency by reducing pharmacy staff and nursing workload while increasing quality

through reducing medication delivery time and improving patient safety and clinical programs. All of these important initiatives can be accomplished through appropriate use of automation. As the profession accepts increasing responsibility for improving patient outcomes through implementation of pharmacist patient care services, automation continues to be relied upon to free the pharmacist from technical tasks. Shortages of qualified pharmacists and technicians coupled with shrinking operating budgets are leading managers to explore technologies that can complete less cognitive distributive tasks traditionally performed by pharmacists and technicians.

Strategic partnerships between health systems and pharmaceutical wholesalers are increasing the rate of availability and deployment of new automation and technologies. Wholesalers serve as intermediary businesses that purchase pharmaceuticals from drug manufacturers for resale to pharmacy customers. Rising complexities and costs of day-to-day pharmacy operations, shrinking personnel resources, and limited technology expertise have led pharmacy directors to seek partnerships with vendors possessing a broad line of automated products. Coupled with traditionally strong pharmacy/wholesaler business relationships and declining wholesaling drug distribution business margins, this trend has created incentives for wholesalers to develop more profitable (automation-related) business ventures. Thus, since the mid-1990s wholesalers have acquired pharmacy technology and automation companies at a rapid rate. Mergers between drug wholesalers and medication dispensing automation companies has been a key component to drug wholesaler growth and survival. Traditional automated distribution and information system technologies used by wholesalers to provide services to their pharmacy customers are now being sought after by these same customers to improve pharmacy purchasing and inventory management efficiency. Today's largest pharmaceutical wholesalers (AmerisourceBergen, Cardinal Health, and McKesson) offer similar suites of pharmacy automation dispensing products. See Table 5-1 for a list of technologies and automated devices applied throughout the medication use process.

Medication Errors Versus Adverse Drug Events

Understanding some basic facts from the literature about medication errors and

TABLE 5-1
Technologies and Automated Devices Applied Throughout the Medication Use Process

Prescribing

- Clinical decision support software
- Computerized prescriber order entry

Dispensing

- Carousel technology
- Centralized robotic dispensing technology
- Centralized narcotic dispensing and inventory tracking devices
- Decentralized automated dispensing devices
- Intravenous and total parenteral nutrition compounding devices
- Pneumatic tube delivery systems
- Unit dose medication repacking systems

Administration

- Bar code medication administration technology
- Clinical decision support based infusion pumps

Monitoring

- Electronic clinical documentation systems
- Web-based compliance and disease management tracking systems

preventable adverse drug events is extremely helpful when building a business case to cost-justify the implementation of new pharmacy automation.[2] Some key elements for distinguishing between these terms and important facts related to the implementation of automation may be summarized as follows: Medication errors are preventable, do not always cause patient harm, and may be caused by errors in planning (e.g., prescribing), not just errors in execution (e.g., dispensing the wrong drug for a patient). The majority of medication errors do not result in adverse drug events (ADEs). Reported medication error rates in the literature approach nineteen percent.[3] Reported ADE rates vary in the literature depending on the detection method, ranging from 0.2% using a voluntary self-reporting system to 10% when a system of chart review and computerized screening was used.[4-7] Medication errors resulting in ADEs (preventable ADEs) result in significant consumption of resources in the form of increased lengths of stay, increased cost of care, rework time, malpractice claims, and patient costs (suffering and lost productivity). Prospective, case-control studies estimate that preventable ADEs may result in an additional length of stay of 4.66 days and a $5,857 increase in hospitalization costs. [8,9]

The Medication Use Process

The medication use process encompasses all areas of medication use and is a highly complex, multidisciplinary process. In its simplest form, the medication use process consists of five domains: (1) purchasing/inventory management; (2) prescribing/medication determination; (3) medication preparation, dispensing, and counseling; (4) medication administration; and (5) patient monitoring/assessment. Approaching medication use in terms of a multi-step process or system is critical to understanding and developing strategies for improving medication safety. As Bates et al. described, the majority of preventable ADEs occur in the ordering and administration phases (56% and 34%, respectively) of the medication use process, with only a very small percentage occurring at the transcription and dispensing phases (6% and 4%, respectively).[6] These data suggest that system changes aimed at improving the ordering and administration phases of the medication use process are likely to have the greatest impact on reducing medication errors and preventable ADEs.

Although only a macro-level view of the medication use process has been presented thus far, the medication use system in hospitals is inherently complex, often containing more than 100 steps with multiple hand-offs. Flowcharting the existing medication use process lays the foundation for a system approach for reducing medication errors and preventable ADEs. Flowcharting the process also helps to illustrate weaknesses and unnecessary steps in the existing system and can help identify the multiple points in the system where breakdowns could occur and cause errors. Thus, helping to pinpoint areas where dispensing automation may be implemented to improve the accuracy and efficiency of the process.

Strategies for Automation

A wide array of automation is currently in use in many health systems within all phases of the medication use process. Automated tasks include counting, inventory control (e.g., including maintaining a perpetual inventory), packaging, compounding, labeling, distributing, dispensing and verification of accurate medication administration while electronically documenting all transactions. Goals for incorporating automation include improving patient care, customer services and resource utilization. Automation of the medication use process improves patient safety while significantly impacting the process workflow of nursing and pharmacy personnel.[10] All automation is technology, but the inverse is not necessarily true (e.g.,

information technology software). This section describes several inpatient pharmacy automated dispensing systems and technologies, their advantages and disadvantages, and their intended roles in various aspects of the medication use process. Table 5-2 provides a comprehensive list of technology and automation that can be applied throughout the medication use process. It is important to note that intended benefits are not always actualized within organizations. Pharmacists and pharmacy managers must understand both the positive effects and limitations that automated systems present. Before implementing any new technology, it is important to have realistic expectations of the benefits and limitations of the technology. This chapter will discuss pharmacy supply chain management and automated pharmacy dispensing technology. Technology designed to improve the prescribing, administration and monitoring phases of the medication use process is described in other chapters. Opportunities exist for further development of all technologies discussed in this section.

Drug Purchasing and Supply Chain Management Systems

Pharmacy asset management (order to pay process) can be improved by linking supply re-ordering channels to the medication distribution system.[11,12] Goals include centralizing and automating supply chain management to reduce on-hand drug product inventory or maximize turn rates, improving accuracy and labor efficiency, paying invoices in a timely manner to optimize wholesaler discounts, and reducing product acquisition costs. Supply chain management essentially refers to the distribution of medication supplies throughout the medication use process. For years, pharmacies have used bar-coded product shelf labels and hand-held product reordering devices for physical product inventory and value documentation as well as for reordering pharmaceuticals. Historically, complete and

TABLE 5-2

Guidelines for Safe Use of Decentralized Automated Dispensing Systems

- Assign medications to devices based upon the needs of the patient care unit, patient age, diagnosis, and staff expertise.

- Create an alert system to flag high risk medications stocked in devices (such as a maximum dose prompt).

- Develop an ongoing competency assessment program for all personnel with access to the device. Include direct observations and random restocking accuracy audits; observe dispensing accuracy as part of the assessment.

- Develop a system to locate and remove recalled medications.

- Develop clear, multidisciplinary downtime procedures; included procedures in training and ongoing competency programs.

- Develop systems to account for narcotic waste. Routinely audit controlled substance dispensed quantities against patient orders, medication administration record documentation, and waste documentation.

- Display allergy reminders for specific drugs such as antibiotics, opiates, and NSAIDs on appropriate medication storage pockets or have them automatically appear on the dispensing screen.

- Do not allow nurses to return medications to the original storage pockets/locations; assign a return bin to collect returned medications.

- Establish a preventive maintenance schedule with the vendor that does not disrupt workflow.

- Establish strict security criteria to limit unauthorized access to devices.

- Establish stringent safety criteria for selecting medications that are (and are not) appropriate to store in devices and oversee the process for assigning new drugs to new locations in all care settings.

- Incorporate bar code scanning for restocking and medication retrieval.

- Limit the numbers of medications not available in profile dispense that may be overridden (dispensed without pharmacist review and verification).

- Maximize the use of unit dose medications in ready-to-administer form, with only a few exceptions.

- Only assign medications with minimal harm potential to open access drawers.

- Perform routine expiration date checks, as well as concomitantly verifying inventory quantities.

- Require all personnel to attend formal training and demonstrate competency prior to accessing the devices.

- Require pharmacist medication order review and verification before a medication is accessed for first dose administration (profile dispensing).

- Restrict access to provide single dose (or single drug) availability whenever possible, focus control on high-risk medications and controlled substances (locked lidded pockets).

- Separate sound-alike and look-alike medications; do not stock these medications in the same open-access drawer.

accurate automation of inventory tracking and product reordering has been primarily limited to large chain store pharmacies, which have invested millions of dollars into developing systems to remove human error and labor costs from this process. Many hospital pharmacies continue to experience inefficiencies in this area; however, this gap is closing. Inefficient processes associated with front-end product ordering and inventory procedures can hamper a pharmacist's ability to provide direct patient care. Poor product procurement systems can result in pharmacists spending excessive time locating a product. Several procurement and inventory management software technologies are available from wholesalers and other vendors which can improve the supply chain management process.

In order to develop an efficient supply chain management program, a pharmacy is required to partner with a pharmaceutical wholesaler. Some wholesalers utilize state of the art inventory management technology within their distribution centers which use bar codes and radio frequency signals to track and assure accurate product filling for customers. Since many wholesalers also own automated dispensing technologies and have extensive interface capabilities, they are able to electronically connect with pharmacy automated dispensing software, prescription processing computer systems, and point-of-sale cash register systems. Accomplishing such integration is a major hurdle in accurately and efficiently automating the procurement process for many hospital pharmacies. For example, if a pharmacy's computer order processing system is capable of maintaining an accurate perpetual inventory of products on the shelf while accounting for all dispensing and crediting transactions, that system may be able to electronically communicate real-time inventory levels to the wholesaler's order management system. This functionality would allow the pharmacy to automati-

cally place an order to the wholesaler when inventory levels fall below a predetermined quantity. Such a system works best with robotic dispensing technology which maintains a closed perpetual inventory record of drug products. When products are received in the pharmacy from the wholesaler, the same interface permits new inventory quantities received to be added to the pharmacy computer system's or automated dispensing system's perpetual inventory. Due to dispensing system complexities and multiple drug inventory locations within the hospital, health systems have been relatively slow to implement such systems. Some hospitals have implemented automated procurement systems for a limited supply of medications such as those maintained in a centralized robotic dispensing system or in a pharmacy stockroom, but not for the majority of their inventory. When properly managed, automated inventory management systems have the potential to result in dramatic one-time cost savings by reducing drug inventory (assets) on hand. Long-term savings and efficiency can be achieved by maximizing drug inventory turn rates, avoiding expired inventory, and reducing labor required for the drug procurement process.

Wholesalers are beginning to provide hand-held scanning devices with integrated bar code readers to pharmacies in order to automate the pharmaceutical receiving process at the product (or tote) level. This provides the pharmacy with an automated receiving and invoice reconciliation process, thus automating the labor-intensive and error-prone product check-in process. This process begins with a pharmacy technician scanning a bar code on a delivery tote containing products from the wholesaler, which in turn generates an electronic invoice. Each product bar code is then scanned as it is removed from the tote and the products received are automatically reconciled versus the invoice. The system will automatically credit product invoicing discrepancies, arrange for erroneous picked products to be returned, and update the pharmacy's perpetual inventory for products received. This same scanner may be used to generate orders as well as return requests for damaged or unused products the pharmacy wishes to return to the wholesaler. After products are received, the next step is to generate payment to the wholesaler. Because all necessary information is securely available on the internet, a billing statement can be available immediately following the automated electronic product receiving process. Thus, pharmacies may confirm exactly what products were received on specific invoices as well as the status of paid or outstanding invoices via real-time internet access. The combination of the ordering, receiving, and reconciliation technologies described above may improve efficiency of the pharmacy supply chain management process and dramatically reduce inventory carrying costs.

Drug Distribution and Dispensing Systems

This section briefly describes the advantages, disadvantages, and issues surrounding the use of several existing technologies which, if appropriately implemented, may help improve the safety of the medication use process. The intent is to describe only those technologies thought to have the greatest potential impact on patient safety and is not designed to be all-inclusive. Comprehensive reviews of pharmacy automation are available elsewhere in the literature.[13,14,15,16]

Decentralized Automated Dispensing Devices

Decentralized automated dispensing systems, also referred to as unit-based dispensing cabinets, are secure storage cabinets capable of handling most unit-dose and some bulk (multiple-dose) medications due to storage limitations. These devices are typically installed decentrally in hospitals on patient care units, and are connected

via a real-time interface to the hospital's pharmacy computer system in an attempt to maintain control over drug dispensing. Automated dispensing devices were originally installed in hospitals in the early 1990s with the assertion of providing increased control over controlled substances and floor stock medications in patient care areas. In a national survey conducted by the American Society of Health-System Pharmacists (ASHP) in 2005, over 70% of hospitals in the United States reported incorporating automated dispensing devices for dispensing of medications to inpatients with nearly 90% of these cabinets linked to the pharmacy computer system.[17] In addition to their traditional uses, many hospitals are now using these devices for storing and dispensing nearly all scheduled doses, thereby eliminating the manual medication cart fill and delivery process.

The primary focus of automated dispensing systems is to provide prompt, real time availability of medications for the nurse and patient. They can also help to improve controlled substance accountability, increase productivity, improve charge capture and documentation accuracy, and reduce pharmacy and nursing labor costs. However, the impact of these decentralized automated dispensing systems on medication errors is less clear.[18,19] Decentralized dispensing devices are increasingly incorporating bar code labeling and scanning into the replenishment process, thus improving restocking accuracy and potentially improving medication safety. Also, the use of automated dispensing systems can reduce the time that pharmacists spend on purely distributive tasks such as checking manually filled medication carts and first doses. By decreasing the amount of these distributive tasks, pharmacists can be re-deployed to direct patient care activities including medication therapy management services. New automated dispensing technologies include devices that assist in dispensing prescription medications to outpatients (often located in the Emergency Department) when 24-hour pharmacy services are not available.[20] Due to the novelty and lack of widespread implementation of these devices, the overall impact on medication safety and finances is currently unknown.

Automated dispensing systems may introduce the potential for medication errors. Some systems allow nurses to choose any patient and dispense any drug they choose because the system is not linked to the pharmacy information system to review the patient's profile.[21] Purchasing an insufficient number of cabinets may preclude an institution's ability to maintain a well controlled single-dose access medication dispensing system resulting in a higher potential for product-selection and administration errors. Despite increasing pressure from regulatory agencies, some organizations have yet to link their pharmacy computer systems to automated dispensing devices in such a way that restricts nurses from obtaining medications that are not ordered for patients. These organizations may fail to achieve the potential benefits of automated dispensing devices such as preventing unauthorized medication dispensing and diversion of medications including controlled substances, and ultimately introduce medication administration safety concerns such as the following: (1) nurses having open access to all drugs in a drawer leading to the possibility of incorrect medication retrieval and administration, (2) complacency leading to not verifying drug labels due to a belief that the system is computerized and therefore not as susceptible to errors (or the belief that pharmacy placed the drug there and pharmacy does not make mistakes), (3) drugs stocked in the wrong pocket either because one or more doses inadvertently fell into the wrong slot or due to a pharmacy restocking error, and (4) changing the location of the drug in the cabinet causing an error because the health care professional chooses drugs from particular locations by habit rather than verifying each drug's identity.[22]

Conflicting reports exist in the literature on the impact of automated dispensing devices on medication error rates and provider efficiency.[21-26] Unfortunately, significant capital investments have been made in these systems without full evaluation of the operational changes needed to ensure efficiency without compromising patient safety. Automated dispensing devices may improve nurse efficiency for tasks associated with narcotic record keeping, yet increase nursing time requirements for dispensing non-narcotic doses. In the late 1980s and early 1990s, one could complete a return on investment (ROI) analysis for this technology based on improved charge capture rates. However, in today's environment of prospective reimbursement an ROI based on patient charges is rarely sustainable. Regardless of whether state regulations exist to assure safe use of automated dispensing systems, it is extremely important that every organization develop, enforce, and continuously improve multidisciplinary policies and procedures to ensure patient safety, accuracy, security, and confidentiality. Table 5-3 provides an extensive list of guidelines and considerations for the safe use of decentralized automated dispensing systems. Table 5-4 provides an extensive list of potential advantages and disadvantages of decentralized automated dispensing systems.

Centralized Robotics for Dispensing Medications

Centrally located automated dispensing devices are designed to automate the entire process of medication dispensing including medication storage, dispensing, restocking, and crediting of unit dose medications. Such systems must be interfaced with the pharmacy information system to provide the system access to each patient's medication profile. Requiring bar coding of medication doses for centralized robotics technology to

TABLE 5-3

Potential Advantages and Disadvantages of Decentralized Automated Dispensing Systems

Advantages	Disadvantages
■ Ability to add expansion (auxiliary) cabinets to increase capacity	■ Accurate inventory quantities are difficult to maintain with matrix configurations; results in medication stock outs
■ Ability to only allow access to a single dose of a medication	■ Downtimes may impact patient care
■ Accommodate multiple dosage forms with flexible drawer configurations	■ Duplicate inventory may increase inventory costs and the amount of expired medications
■ Automated controlled substance retrieval, inventory reconciliation and the process to resolve discrepancies	■ If devices are used to replace cart fill, several devices are needed per nursing unit to supply the necessary products and quantities needed to maintain a safe and efficient system
■ Automated medication charges increase the amount of charges captured	■ Inspection and removal of expired medications must be performed manually (devices do not have the software to track expiration dates)
■ Bar code scanning to improve accuracy of restocking	
■ Improve medication distribution response time, thus patients may receive the first dose of a medication faster	■ Multiple dose access still allows for controlled substance diversion and discrepancy follow-up may still be required
■ Improve nursing satisfaction due to fewer missing doses, fewer delays for first doses, and more nursing control over day-to-day medication distribution activities	■ Poor integration with bedside medication storage systems
■ More pharmacy control versus traditional floor stock system	■ Potential cost savings are frequently not realized (labor-neutral for pharmacy technicians)
● stocking the device is time consuming (often because medication dispensing can be centrally controlled by an interfaced pharmacy computerized patient profile	● nursing time saved is difficult to actualize into nursing staff reductions
■ Patient-specific medication profiles to direct and control medication administration (profile dispense)	■ Potential for medication errors and sub-optimal therapy
	● drawers with open access pockets may all product selection errors
■ Provide detailed electronic dispensing and usage reports	● nurses may access a medication before a pharmacist reviews the order
■ Re-deploy pharmacist to perform patient care activities	■ Unable to accommodate all medications (limited by medication size, cabinet size, and risk level for a particular medication to be stocked in a device)
■ Reduce pharmacist time spent towards medication distribution	
■ Save nursing labor	
● eliminate missing or misplaced narcotic drawer keys	
● eliminate narcotic counts at shift change	
● fewer narcotic discrepancies to resolve	
● less narcotic paperwork to handle	

TABLE 5-4

Potential Advantages and Disadvantages
of Centralized Robotic Dispensing Systems

Advantages	Disadvantages
■ Accommodates a very large online inventory	■ Dispensing accuracy is dependent on accurate computer order entry
■ Automates medication restocking and removal of expired medications	■ Dispensing accuracy is dependent on accurate repackaging
■ Automates the credit process for any unused medication doses	■ Does not accommodate refrigerated items
■ Easily integrated with bedside medication storage systems	■ Increased labor requirements for packaging medications because all doses require a bar coded package label
■ Initial platform for point-of-care bar code medication administration and documentation system	■ Lack of standard bar codes in health care

■ Labor saving and improved restocking accuracy by automating and the restocking of the decentralized dispensing systems	■ Nursing acceptance may be mixed
	  ● may not reduce missing doses
	  ● may still experience delays in receiving first doses
	  ● two layers of packaging around most doses

■ Reduces pharmacist time required to verify technician filled medications, allowing a reallocation of time to focus on patient care activities	■ Possible disruption in medication therapy when patients are transferred from one location to another
■ Reduces technician labor required to fill unit dose medication carts and first doses (reductions are easily obtained)	■ Potential to provide more doses than are needed for a single administration time, leading to potential errors

■ Theoretical patient safety improvements
  ● facilitates a pharmacist review of orders before a nurse can administer the first dose of a medication
  ● improved dispensing accuracy
	■ Requires a large amount of space and often physical renovation

properly function allows dispensing accuracy to approach 100%. Thus, as long as a patient-specific computerized medication profile is maintained in an accurate and timely manner, pharmacist time may be re-allocated from tasks such as medication dose checking to more direct patient care activities.

Centralized robotic dispensing systems were traditionally used exclusively to dispense unit dose bar coded medications for scheduled medication cart filling. Through the advancement of these systems, it is now possible to extend the use of this technology to include automation of first dose dispensing whereby the pharmacy information system electronically triggers the robot to dispense the first dose(s) of medication immediately following pharmacist medication order review and approval in the order entry system. This improves first dose medication turnaround time and accuracy, and eliminates much pharmacy technician labor associated with first dose medication dispensing. Another recent expanded use of robotic systems takes advantage of the system's ability to pick medication doses to be restocked in decentralized automated dispensing cabinets. This has the potential to reduce medication administration errors by improving dispensing cabinet restocking accuracy.

Potential advantages of centralized robotics include reducing pharmacy labor costs, restructuring pharmacists' tasks from technical to more clinical activities, and improving medication dispensing accuracy. No published data are available on these advantages, but in one unpublished study a robot decreased the dispensing error rate from 2.9% to 0.6%.[27] However, this improved dispensing accuracy of robotic technology has never been proven to result in improved patient safety since nurses still have open access to all robot-dispensed medications after they are distributed to patient care areas.

Perhaps the greatest advantage of implementing robotic technology is that all doses dispensed by the robot are bar coded, thus facilitating the implementation of BCMA systems. Conversely, this necessity for bar codes on all medications dispensed by the robot has the potential to introduce new error into the medication use system. Although some manufacturers provide bar coded medications, most unit dose medications must be accurately repackaged and bar code labeled by the pharmacy department in order to be read by BCMA scanners. Many manufacturers offer automation and even full service agreements to assist with this labor-intensive packaging requirement. Table 5-5 provides an extensive list of potential advantages and disadvantages of centralized robotic dispensing systems.

Carousel Technology

Carousel automation is a medication storage cabinet with rotating shelves used to automate medication dispensing. Like other centralized robotic systems, the carousel must be interfaced with the pharmacy information system. The carousel utilizes bar code

and pick-to-light technology to improve the efficiency and accuracy of pharmacy technicians who pick and restock medications. Rotating shelves within the carousel bring medications to the technician at one working level, where a light identifies the exact location from which the medication is to be picked. Medications do *not* need to be assigned into the carousel alphabetically to facilitate locating medications; therefore, carousels promote compliance with regulatory requirements standards to reduce errors from sound alike, look alike medications. Properly implemented carousel technology reduces technician travel time, bending, and reaching for medications during the filling process. The rotating shelves allow pharmacies to take advantage of rarely used vertical space to store medications, thereby vacating space for other uses.

Bar code technology implemented for carousels can serve as the foundation for patient bedside bar code medication administration. This functionality can also assist in performing perpetual inventory tracking and tracking expiration dates more effectively. By keeping expirations dates accurate, carousels can improve the efficiency with which expired medications are removed from inventory. Accurate inventory levels with appropriate par levels (i.e., inventory re-order threshold levels) enable a pharmacy to streamline the medication ordering process. Carousels can be integrated with automated dispensing cabinets to increase the efficiency of cabinet restocking eliminating the need for the current paper refill reports and the manual picking process. Comprehensive software within the carousel allows pharmacies to work more efficiently minimizing the number of carousel turns, prioritizing workflow, and processing the most important orders first. Carousel software also allows pharmacies to establish inventory locations outside of a carousel (e.g., on a shelf or in a refrigerator). Using this feature, pharmacies can process orders

TABLE 5-5

Desired Safety Features for Incorporating
Automation Into the Medication Use Process

■ A system must accommodate bar coded unit dose medications and utilize the bar code capability for drug restocking, retrieval, and administering medications.

■ A system should force the user to specify a reason whenever medications are accessed or administered outside of the scheduled administration time or dosage range. All such events are signaled visibly or audibly to the user and are electronically documented and reported daily for follow-up.

■ A unique bar code or user identification code and password are assigned to each user. Audit trials of user actions must be reported in an easily viewed format and should include: identification of the user, the medication, the patient for whom the drug was dispensed, and the time of the transaction.

■ Bar code medication administration systems must be able to identify and document the patient, the medication, and the person administering using the scanning technology function.

■ Devices are interfaced with the pharmacy computer system only allowing the nurse to view and access those medications that are ordered for a specific patient.

■ Devices need electronic reminders to nurses when a medication dose is due (and by a different mechanism when it is past due).

■ Hospital admit/discharge/transfer and medication order entry computer systems are interfaced with automation devices to provide caregivers with warnings about allergies, interactions, duplications, and inappropriate doses at the point of dispensing and/or administration.

■ Patient specific information used in the daily care of patients must be timely, accurate, and easily accessible.

■ Pertinent patient- and medication-specific information and instructions entered into pharmacy and/or hospital information systems are available electronically at the point of care (administration), and the system prompts the nurse to record pertinent information before administration may be documented.

■ Real-time integration or interfaces exist for all steps in the medication use process; starting at the point of prescribing, to order entry and dispensing, and through documentation of medication administration.

through the carousel software to take advantage of the carousel's inventory management for items not physically contained within it. Pharmacies also have the option to arrange checking stations with barcode scanners to facilitate pharmacist checking of medications dispensed outside of the carousel.

An automated medication dispensing system incorporating either centralized robotics or carousel technology will result in improved dispensing accuracy and labor efficiency. However, it is unclear as to the correct configuration of these technologies and

how well they complement or unnecessarily duplicate one another. Research is needed to confirm the theoretical benefits of these technologies when implemented apart from one another as well as when these technologies are synergistically implemented.

Centralized Narcotic Dispensing and Record Keeping Systems

Accounting for every controlled substance dose dispensed and administered is one of the most labor-intensive processes in a central pharmacy. Products exist that can automate this process resulting in improved efficiency and control in the system. Such systems have the capability of recording all doses dispensed from a central pharmacy narcotic room or decentralized automated dispensing devices as well as identifying individuals performing every transaction. In addition, these systems can interface with decentralized automated dispensing devices to verify that every dose dispensed from the pharmacy is stocked into the intended decentralized automated dispensing device. They can also generate bar coded nursing "proof of use" forms for patient care areas without automated dispensing devices. Lastly, the system can suggest reorder quantities based on past usage, provide useful compliance reports for the Drug Enforcement Agency, and facilitate documentation of controlled substance waste.

As discussed in the preceding paragraphs, these systems provide undeniable benefits with regards to tightening control over controlled substance inventory maintenance and identifying potential drug product diversion. Hospitals with one or more dedicated narcotic technicians will likely be able to cost-justify the implementation of centralized narcotic dispensing and record keeping systems by reducing personnel time requirements associated with inventory control and record keeping activities. Thus, it is very common to find hospitals that have reorganized their traditional narcotic vault drug inventory into automated dispensing cabinets linked to narcotic inventory control software as a means to improve narcotic inventory control and dispensing accuracy within the hospital.

Safety Issues Surrounding the Use of Automation

Ensuring System Accuracy and Reducing Errors

Although information technologies and automated medication systems are widely used in health systems and remain integral components of many regulatory and external quality reporting agencies, very little data regarding their appropriate use or impact on patient safety are available.[28] What data are available are limited to computerized prescriber order entry (CPOE) with computerized clinical physician decision support. Other technologies such as robotic technology, bar coding of medications, automated dispensing devices, and BCMA are more widely implemented than CPOE systems, yet their reported impact on reducing medication errors and preventable ADEs is variable. Critical reviews of the safety benefits of various technologies touted to reduce medication errors exist but are limited.[28] Implementing new technology can introduce new sources of error by creating major infrastructure changes. Vendors routinely market their products without sufficient testing or without being able to fully implement the technology as advertised. Nevertheless, all of these systems intuitively show promise in their medication error reduction potential. If properly integrated, all of these systems should ultimately improve patient safety and would likely be incorporated into most medication use systems of the future.

Automation has the potential to reduce medication errors by reducing complexity, simplifying and standardizing processes, avoiding over-reliance on human memory, and improving efficiency. However, technology by itself will rarely prevent medication errors. Effective integration into the existing medication use system coupled with appropriate management is imperative in order to positively impact patient safety. Improper use of technology can prolong a system of errors and introduce dangerous new errors. Implementing technology within a previously sub-optimal manual system will most often yield a sub-optimal automated system. Implementing automation is often a very complicated process that significantly modifies the practice of pharmacy, nursing, and the medical staff. Full implementation can take years to accomplish and often requires dedicated personnel resources. These resources are needed to oversee implementation, manage training and quality assurance and provide ongoing support and maintenance. Without such dedicated oversight, new sources of error will prevail and the automated system may be less safe than the replaced manual system.

Without a comprehensive system to assure that patients receive their correct medications and dosages on time, preventable errors will continue to occur. In preparation of implementing new automation, policies and procedures must be modified to assure the safe and proper infrastructure exists for medication purchasing, ordering, preparation, dispensing, administering, and monitoring. Technology does not preclude the need for all necessary safety checks in the medication use process.

Health systems often possess unrealistic expectations of automation. A false sense of security felt by healthcare professionals can lead to carelessness and errors. For instance, healthcare professionals may neglect to exercise double- and triple-check procedures with medications obtained from automated dispensing devices because of an over-reliance on the technology. To avoid such problems, all personnel must be adequately educated and demonstrate understanding that technology cannot completely substitute for human safety checks. Additionally, managers must make certain that levels of staffing are not overly reduced in response to system automation. Staff must not be forced to work at a pace that precludes the ability to deliver safe and effective health care. With all automation, it absolutely critical that appropriate quality control systems exist to assure the accurate and safe use of automation.

Desired Features for Reducing Errors

Innovative and appropriate use of technology within the medication use process can significantly improve patient safety. Furthermore, the effective merging of information technology and automation can effectively prevent medication errors through different modalities. First, the use of bar coded medications should be maximized throughout the medication use process including the administration and documentation phase of the medication use process. Second, information technologies can be used to analyze and prevent medication errors. For instance, sophisticated pharmacy or CPOE systems may be integrated with patient-specific laboratory and clinical documentation systems to identify ADEs and medication errors when they occur. Potential errors identified by electronic prescribing, BCMA software and "smart" infusion pumps can be analyzed for common characteristics to identify recurring causes of error and facilitate the reduction of potential errors within the organization. Third, automated dispensing systems, especially those incorporating the use of bar code technology, may potentially improve medication dispensing and administration accuracy as well as patient safety. In order to accomplish this task, the system must be properly managed. Fourth, aggressive implementation of computer-generated clinical alert and decision support software will improve patient safety, provided the system is properly designed, implemented and maintained.[30,31] Table 5-6 lists ideal features to assure patient safety throughout the medication use process, regardless of which automated technologies are employed.

Regulatory Issues

In response to a lack of national standards and regulations for the safe use of automated dispensing systems, the National Association of Boards of Pharmacy (NABP) approved a document entitled *Model State Pharmacy Act and Model Rules* in May of 1997. Thanks to the work of some progressive pharmacists, the language in this act is very enabling: the definition of "dispensing"

TABLE 5-6

Automation Selection Criteria

- Can the vendor provide you with established policies and procedures for integrating the system into the pharmacy's daily workflow, clearly defining pharmacist and technician responsibilities, and clearly defining system downtime procedures?

- Cost-benefit analysis: will reduced supply and labor expenses offset the cost of the automation? What is the potential increased revenue as a result of the automation?

- Does the system produce useful statistical and managerial reports, and do they provide a report writing and analysis tool?

- How does the system utilize bar code technology to improve accuracy of transactions?

- How long has the company been in business and how many units do they have in operation?

- How much space will the automation require, and is remodeling required?

- How much time is required for routine maintenance and equipment servicing? Does the company provide full service, routine and emergency software and hardware maintenance? What is the cost of this maintenance and how is it provided? Will routine maintenance disrupt workflow?

- How secure is the system?

- Is training interactive and computer-based? How will new users be trained on the system?

- Is the automation compatible with the organization's strategic goals?

- Is the company willing to guarantee a maximum percent downtime?

- Is the system compatible with existing information systems? Has the company interfaced their system with your pharmacy computer system in another organization? If not, what is the cost for building this interface? Who maintains the interface?

- What do existing customers say about the accuracy and reliability of the system, ease of use, and unscheduled downtime?

- What impact will the automation have on other departments? How are those departments involved in the selection process?

- What impact will the automation have on patient safety?

- What impact will the system have on controlled substance accountability and overall inventory control?

- What sets this company's product apart from their major competitors?

- Will the automation enable the provision of new clinical services?

- Will the vendor adapt the technology to meet your needs, goals, and objectives rather than expect your system to be redesigned to fit their product?

- Will the vendor provide you with a list of all current users?

- Will the vendor's training and implementation support meet your expectations and needs?

includes the use of automated technology. The act provides pharmacists with flexibility in the use of automated devices but appropriately requires such devices be used only in settings where an established program of pharmaceutical care is present that ensures the review of medication orders by a pharmacist in accordance with good pharmacy practice. The act requires policies and systems to be in place to assure safe and secure use of such devices; however, it is not very descriptive or restrictive as to how such quality assurance must be completed. This act is intended to serve as a template for individual states to write (or rewrite) their State Pharmacy Practice Acts.

Despite the model act, some state boards of pharmacy continue to provide a potential barrier to the appropriate and efficient use of automated devices and technologies. Some states may require pharmacists to check every dose prior to that dose being stocked in an automated dispensing device. Other states may allow the pharmacy to develop and document internal quality assurance programs (such as bar coded restocking systems) to assure patient safety. Still other states may require extensive paperwork to be completed which may be interpreted as a barrier to implementing automated devices. Pharmacists must play an active role in assuring their state's pharmacy practice act contains enabling (rather than restrictive) language related to the use of automated dispensing systems and the transfer of electronic medication (prescription) orders. Developing restrictive language will certainly be viewed as "self-serving" to other health care professionals and health systems leading to negative long-term consequences for the profession. Recent automation-related standards developed by the Joint Commission on Accreditation of Healthcare Organizations (JCAHO), particularly those related to the use of automated dispensing devices, are proactive in assuring the safe use of automation. These standards require pharmacist oversight of automated systems as they relate to the medication use process.

Quality Assurance

Regardless of whether state regulations exist to assure safe use of automated dispensing systems, every organization must develop, enforce, and continuously improve policies and procedures to ensure patient safety, accuracy, security, and confidentiality. Specific areas that should be addressed in an organization's policies for safe use of automated dispensing systems and technology include accurate inventory and stocking controls, dispensing procedures, security and breach of security, patient confidentiality, reporting, documentation, training of personnel, initial and ongoing competency assessment, routine quality assurance and safety checks, scheduled (and unscheduled) hardware and software maintenance and support, and contingency plans for maintaining safe systems and service in the event of unscheduled downtime.

Strategic Plan for Selecting Automation Within a Health System

Historically, in order to receive funding, the result of implementing automation had to result in cost reduction, quality improvement, improved service, and/or increased efficiency. While expense continues to be a major barrier to implementing new technologies, various regulatory and external quality reporting groups continue to persuade many organizations to prematurely invest heavily in new technologies that only theoretically improve patient safety. Integrated health systems should not view automation and technology as a complete cure-all; rather, these sophisticated tools should be viewed as instruments to optimize the medication use process. The value achieved by implementing new technology within organizations depends primarily upon three factors: (1) the efficiency of the system being replaced, (2) the level of detail applied to managing and making the most of the system following implementation, and (3) cooperation between departments to assure success of the system.

Within most hospitals, consensus is that automation of the inpatient medication use process should exist, but there is much debate as to the best way to accomplish this task. There is no right or wrong answer. Any of the previously discussed approaches can succeed or fail depending on how well it is managed.[32] Automated systems may either stand alone or be a component of an integrated hospital information system. Suggested characteristics of an ideal system include patient care and safety benefits, responsiveness to customer needs, cost-effectiveness, and ability to leverage the purchase of other technologies. Before purchasing a piece of technology, decision-makers must evaluate the clinical, cost, and safety advantages and disadvantages of competing technologies. To assure successful selection and hospital-wide implementation of automation within the medication use process, it is imperative that pharmacists continuously reiterate the importance of their role in overseeing and coordinating the use of these systems. In the future, pharmacists will be held more accountable for managing and understanding technology interfaces with pharmacy-specific information systems and workflows.[33] Specific technology selection should include a complete analysis of desired system functionality, hardware and software technical requirements, installation and training support, and vendor/system background reference checks. Table 5-7 provides guidelines for pharmacists to use to help guide the automation selection process.

Cost Justification of Automated Systems

Economic Realities in Health Systems

Historically, one could cost-justify the use of new automation if improved medication charge capture offset the cost of the technology. Due to declining hospital reimbursement from government and private payers, this scenario is no longer the case. Directors of Pharmacy often feel as though they must pass through bureaucratic red tape to gain administrative and financial support for new services and new technologies. Despite even the best cost- and quality-justifications and organization-wide support, health systems may simply not have the available financial resources to purchase new technologies. Many vendors now offer lease options to address this problem. Regardless of an organization's financial situation, a solid ROI analysis demonstrating the positive financial effects of a particular technology is a great way to gain administrative approval for financing that piece of automated technology. System costs vary dramatically depending on institution size, infrastructure needs, and the number and type of hardware purchased. Initial capital costs dramatically vary—training and other hidden expenses often double these costs. Pharmacy involvement in the cost-justification of automated technologies is essential.

Return on Investment Analysis

With the rising costs of healthcare, providing hospital administration with evidence of a technology's ability to positively impact the organization financially is becoming increasingly more important. Many drivers for automation exist including improvements in patient safety, customer service, operational efficiency, revenues, regulatory compliance, overall quality of care, and reduced costs. Whether or not automation saves money is a function of how well the system is managed, the efficiency (or inefficiency) of the manual system being replaced, and the extent to which different disciplines cooperate to maximize the system's capabilities. The goal of an ROI analysis is to compare the total costs of implementation to the financial benefit resulting from implementation of

TABLE 5-7

Future Roles of Pharmacy Personnel
As a Result of Automation and Technology

- Attend patient care rounds assuring the appropriate use of medication.
- Collaborative drug therapy management (with physicians) for medications and diseases which require specialized monitoring, patient assessment and education.
- Coordinate and oversee the entire medication use system.
- Coordinate services to maximize patient medication therapy compliance including medication administration teaching, medication counseling, and automated prescription refill reminder and incentive programs.
- Develop, implement, and oversee medication error and adverse drug reaction prevention and reporting programs.
- Develop, implement, and oversee programs that promote and assure cost-effective use of medication therapy.
  - Case management and medication use algorithms for high cost and/or high risk diseases and medication therapies.
  - Guidelines for the use of high cost and/or high risk medications.
  - Medication formulary and medication use policy strategies.
  - Medication use evaluation programs (MUE).
  - Monitoring and assuring compliance with established guidelines of care.
- Develop decision support capabilities (e.g., rules, alerts, order sets, treatment guidelines, etc) to be incorporated into electronic prescribing systems.
- Facilitate efficient information exchange and continuity of care for patients' medication regimens.
- Maximize timely transitions from intravenous to oral therapy.
- Medication reconciliation activities (medication admission histories, discharge medication order reconciliation, and patient teaching).
- Participate on multidisciplinary patient care teams.
- Pharmacokinetic dose adjustments.
- Review and verify all physician entered orders to make sure they are appropriate for a given patient.

automation. If a positive ROI is demonstrated (i.e., the total financial benefits outweigh the costs), the decision should be made to support the automation.

An ROI analysis is often separated into three distinct sections: capital purchase, ongoing operating expenses, and ongoing savings. For ongoing savings, two components include "hard" and "soft" dollar savings. Hard dollar savings are directly attributable to a reduction in FTEs or the elimination of a direct expense. Hard benefits are directly related to an increase in revenue and an increase in reimbursement. Soft benefits include customer service improvements, reduced wait times, reallocating staff to another activity, regulatory compliance enhancement and cost-avoidance. Depending on the institution, soft savings may or may not be included in the ROI analysis. The decision on whether to lease or purchase a technology impacts the placement of those dollars into the ROI analysis. For automation that is purchased, the expense will often be capitalized and appear in year-zero. For leased automation, the annual lease expense will usually appear as an ongoing operating expense. See Figure 5-1 for a model ROI analysis template for cost-justifying a centralized robotic dispensing system. This ROI template has been kept very simple for the purposes of illustration and individual organizations may require alternative formats and approaches, including the calculation of net present value, internal rate of return and payback period, all of which are not included in this template. Pharmacists are highly encouraged to work with their finance department on such detailed calculations if they are necessary.

Every organization will have a slightly different format for presenting financial business plans; however, several pieces of information are crucial for financially evaluating automation, regardless of the format. First, clearly state all capital, lease, maintenance, and supply (hardware and software) expenses as a result of implementing the new technology. Second, obtain a quote from your information technology department for projected computer system interface expenses. Third, incorporate fixed labor costs (salary, benefits, vacation, sick leave) of any new support activities the automation will require. If the automation to be implemented is a means for providing a new service (which is often the case in ambulatory settings), be sure to calculate added personnel expense which will be incurred if the automation is not approved. Fourth, evaluate undeniable minimum expenses which will be eliminated from the budget as a result of the new technology. Examples include fixed tech-

nician and pharmacist labor costs associated with activities the automation will replace, supply costs, and labor cost savings which can be achieved in other departments (e.g., nursing). Fifth, factor in additional savings the department can commit to as a direct result of implementing the automation. For example, pharmacist time saved as a result of the new technology may be re-deployed to a more direct patient care role ensuring the appropriate use of medications. Department medication expense reports and clinical literature can assist in determining a projected dollar savings for expenses to be reduced as a result of new clinical pharmacy services and target drug programs.

At this stage of the analysis, many organizations will only allow those cost savings which will be eliminated from the organization's budget to be factored into the ROI equation. However, in recent years, literature targeted towards health system administrators has been filled with reports of the value of clinical pharmacy services on patient care, safety, and reducing total health care costs. Depending on the organization, it may be possible to factor less tangible but real organization-wide cost savings for medication error avoidance into the ROI analysis. Most administrators have probably heard about cost increases in the range of several thousand dollars for every preventable adverse drug event. Since the release of the IOM Report in 1999, patient safety has risen to the top of many organizations' priority list allowing directors of pharmacy to more effectively sell the benefits of error reduction to a higher level. Many insurance companies and employer payers are beginning to select health care facilities based on safety records. If acceptable to an organization's top-level administration, this will make the cost-justification of most dispensing technologies a simpler process. Less tangible cost savings due to re-deployment of pharmacists' time include ordering of fewer laboratory tests, reduced lengths of

Fictitious Centralized Robot Dispensing System Return on Investment (ROI) Analysis

	Capital Expense	1	2	3	4	5	6	7
Capital Purchase								
Purchase Price of Robot	$950,000							
Vendor Implementation	$50,000							
Total Capital Expenses	**$1,000,000**							
Ongoing Operating Expenses								
Supplies [a]		$25,000	$26,250	$27,563	$28,941	$30,388	$31,907	$33,502
Robot Service and Maintenance Costs [b]		$55,000	$55,000	$55,000	$55,000	$55,000	$55,000	$55,000
Total Operating Expenses		**$80,000**	**$81,250**	**$82,563**	**$83,941**	**$85,388**	**$86,907**	**$88,502**
Ongoing Savings (Costs avoided)								
5 FTE technician labor savings [c]		$162,240	$168,730	$175,479	$182,498	$189,798	$197,390	$205,285
1 FTE pharmacist labor savings [d]		$123,500	$128,440	$133,578	$138,921	$144,478	$150,257	$156,267
Preventable ADE cost avoidance [e]		$117,500	$117,500	$117,500	$117,500	$117,500	$117,500	$117,500
Total Savings Potential (Costs avoided)		**$403,240**	**$414,670**	**$426,556**	**$438,919**	**$451,775**	**$465,146**	**$479,052**
Total Net Savings (Loss)	($1,000,000)	$323,240	$333,420	$343,994	$354,978	$366,388	$378,239	$390,550
Cumulative Net Savings (Loss)	($1,000,000)	($676,760)	($343,340)	$653	$355,631	$722,019	$1,100,259	$1,490,808

(a) Envelopes and bar code labels $20,000/year, other supplies $5,000/year. Assume 5% annual cost increase.
(b) Service and Maintenance Costs are fixed for 7 years.
(c) Technician labor savings (5 FTE) is projected to increase at a rate of 4% each year for the seven year analysis. $12/hr + 30% benefits.
(d) Pharmacist Labor savings (1 FTE) is projected at a rate of 4% each year for the seven year analysis. Average salary of $95,000/year + 30% benefits.
(e) ADE cost-avoidance calculations are as follows:
1. Avoids 25,000 dispensing errors per year via improving dispensing accuracy from 98.9% after pharmacist double-check to 99.9%.
2. Assumption is that 1 in 1,000 dispensing errors results in a preventable ADE.
3. System implementation will avoid 25 preventable ADEs per year.
4. Cost of a preventable ADE to the hospital is $4,700.
5. Annual cost-avoidance to the hospital is $117,500.

Figure 5-1. ROI spreadsheet.

stay, reduced emergency room visits, and fewer re-hospitalizations. An organization's likelihood of successfully incorporating such findings into an ROI analysis depends on the extent to which pharmacy cognitive services have been marketed to local physicians and administrators. Sixth, projected increased revenues as a result of improved charge capture should be incorporated into the analysis. Most hospital administrators will have a fair understanding of the increased income for the organization due to improved charge capture. Organizations may have a higher capture rate for ambulatory services; therefore, increased charge capture should be broken down by inpatient and outpatient areas. Lastly, a solid ROI analysis will include a payback period (how long it will take to pay the organization back for their initial investment) and internal rate of return (how much the money spent on the automation will earn the hospital back) in the analysis. The hospital's finance or fiscal department is often a valuable resource in helping to perform ROI calculations for new technologies, and they must be involved in the analysis from the start to ensure that all contributing factors are addressed. This not only helps to maximize finance department understanding of and buy-in into the project, it also prevents rework on the part of the person completing the ROI analysis calculations.

Many health system pharmacy departments have been successful in cost-justifying advanced automation and technology through the elimination of technical positions and the redeployment of pharmacist time to clinical activities. Technology vendors should be able to provide contacts in other organizations that have already completed a similar ROI analysis.

Automation Impact on Pharmacy Manpower

Pharmacists are often concerned that the implementation of automated dispensing systems will decrease the number of necessary pharmacist positions and consequently

the demand for pharmacists. Theoretically, automation (as well as expanded use of pharmacy technicians) increases the amount of work that can be accomplished by the existing work force. In the early and mid 1990s, pharmacy thought leaders predicted that increased use of automation coupled with a dramatic increase in the use of prescription mail order service would result in a reduced demand for pharmacists. Fortunately, increased organizational recognition of the high financial and quality impact of the clinical pharmacist role, the growing population of older Americans who take more and more medications, the soaring number and complexity of medications, and unrecognized theoretical time savings within departments following implementation of automated systems have resulted in quite the opposite trend. However, as automated dispensing and patient monitoring technologies advance, it is reasonable to predict a reduction in the number of pharmacist and technician positions in which preparing and dispensing pharmaceuticals is the principle work activity.

Within health systems, cost-justification of new technologies will likely require a reduction in the number of full-time pharmacy technician positions (and possibly pharmacist and nurse positions). Technicians will increasingly be expected to oversee automated dispensing systems and even possibly "smart" IV pump and BCMA systems. These new tasks may create new patient care technician roles that are expanded to provide support activities across all phases of the medication use process. The pharmacist's traditional distributive roles of preparing and distributing medications will most certainly be challenged as technicians and technology become increasingly responsible for dispensing activities. Many pharmacy departments have been successful in re-deploying pharmacists' time from distributive to clinical roles. As technology continues to provide pharmacists with opportunities to be more involved with direct patient care, the impact on pharmacist manpower needs will be mostly determined by pharmacists themselves. If pharmacists and pharmacy directors are successful at demonstrating the quality and economic value of pharmacists' patient care services, it is reasonable to predict an increase in the number of available health system pharmacist positions. However, if the patient care role of the pharmacist does not continue to grow and demonstrate overall value, pharmacists may increasingly be displaced by technology. Automation is currently forcing the issue of pharmacist professional role redevelopment in health systems.

Given that continued automation of the dispensing process is inevitable, future work activities of pharmacists depend primarily on four issues: (1) the breadth of tasks that a pharmacy technician is legally allowed to perform (and/or allowed to perform by an employer); (2) the extent to which pharmacists are reimbursed for medication therapy management services; (3) the level of productivity which can be achieved through automated systems; and (4) the extent to which pharmacists are able to demonstrate improved quality and overall lower cost of patient care as a result of their role on the patient care team. Existing dispensing automation clearly creates the potential for pharmacists to focus more time on direct patient care activities instead of product preparation.

Future Roles of Pharmacy Personnel as a Result of Automation

The transformation of the pharmacist role from distributor of drugs to cognitive provider of care has largely resulted from pharmacists' access to patient-specific information about diagnosis, laboratory results, treatment progress, and the patient's entire drug therapy regimen. Integrated delivery systems and automation will continue to provide pharmacists with opportunities to work more closely with physicians, other healthcare providers, and patients to assure appropriate drug therapy decisions and outcomes. Towards this end, pharmacists must continue to assume increased accountability for understanding patient drug-related needs, identifying, solving and preventing drug-related problems, designing and initiating drug therapy plans, and continuing drug therapy plans once they are initiated. Pharmacists have an important responsibility in creating systems to improve the quality and safety of drug distribution and administration. Pharmacists must possess good time management and problem solving skills while being able to focus the majority of their time on issues related to high-risk drugs and high-cost diseases. In the future, clinical pharmacists may have three primary responsibilities: to assess (1) patient compliance and medication-related outcomes, (2) drug and disease education, and (3) intervention. The optimization of such roles is essential in both inpatient and ambulatory environments to avoid the displacement of pharmacists by automation. Additionally, pharmacists in all practice settings must continue to capitalize on the advances of dispensing technologies in order to maximize their potential to provide patient care services that improve outcomes and safety.

Conclusion

Automation is not a panacea. There is no perfect technology, and all systems must be well managed in order to achieve desired results. No existing automated system fully supports the profession's transition to pharmacist patient care services. To be successful in the future, pharmacists must view automation-induced productivity and efficiency as desired goals, not as threats to their work. Optimized use of automation to perform distributive functions currently performed by pharmacists and technicians is essential to provide pharmacists the opportunity to use their clinical knowledge and skills to

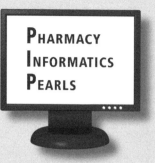

PHARMACY AUTOMATION SYSTEMS

Current Trends

- Changes in the healthcare system have increased the demand for integrated automation systems
- Automation is increasingly relied upon to help minimize the amount of time pharmacists spend on drug distribution activities, thus maximizing their time available for the provision of direct patient care services

The Medication Use Process

- The medication use process encompasses all areas of medication use and is a highly complex multidisciplinary process
- Integrating functional and well-managed automation into the ordering and administration phases of the medication use process are likely to have the greatest impact on reducing medication errors and preventable ADEs

Strategies for Automation

- Automation can be introduced in to any phase of the medication use process
- Goals for incorporating automation include improving patient care, customer service, and resource utilization
- While automation can assist in decreasing medication errors and preventable ADEs, unintended consequences of automation may lead to more error-prone systems if implementation is not managed properly

Drug Purchasing and Supply Chain Management Systems

- Goals for implementation include centralizing and automating supply chain management to reduce on-hand drug product inventory (maximize turn rates), improve accuracy and labor efficiency, pay invoices in a timely manner, and reduce product acquisition costs
- Completely integrated systems that incorporate wholesalers have been slow to catch on due to multi-system complexities and multiple drug locations throughout the health system

Drug Distribution and Dispensing Systems

- Decentralized automated dispensing devices can be implemented to provide prompt, real time availability of medications to the nurse and patient, yet conflicting reports exist on the impact on medication rates and provider efficiency
- Properly managed centralized robotics and carousel systems can result in increased rates of dispensing accuracy, yet only case reports exist on the true advantages of these systems
- Centralized robotics require all unit dose medications to be bar coded—this is an important step before implementing BCMA

Safety Issues Surrounding the Use of Automation

- Critical reviews of the safety benefits for various technologies touted to reduce medication errors exist but are limited; however, implementing new technology can introduce new sources of error by creating major infrastructure changes

- Bar coding medications should be maximized throughout the medication use process to ensure safe medication use

Strategic Plan for Selecting Automation Within a Health System

- Integrated health systems should view automation as a sophisticated tool to optimize the safety and efficiency of the medication use process rather than a panacea
- Characteristics of an ideal system include patient care and safety benefits, responsiveness to customer needs, cost-effectiveness, and the ability to leverage the purchase of other technologies

Cost Justification of Automated Systems

- A comprehensive return on investment (ROI) analysis demonstrating the positive financial effects of a particular technology is essential to gain administrative approval for financing that piece of technology
- Drivers for automation to be highlighted in an ROI include improvements in patient safety, customer service, operational efficiency, revenues, regulatory compliance, overall quality of care, and reduced costs

Automation Impact on Pharmacy Manpower

- Integrated delivery systems and automation will continue to provide pharmacists with opportunities to work more collaboratively with physicians and other healthcare providers to assure appropriate drug therapy decisions while positively impacting patient care

provide medication management therapy to patients. Every change must be implemented with an understanding of human factors engineering and safety science since unexpected consequences can result from unexpected new hazards. The capabilities of pharmacy automation will continue to increase at a rapid rate over time. Efficient electronic physician prescribing systems, fully automated dispensing systems, and virtual patient monitoring systems will be commonplace in the medication use process of the future. Pharmacists have a choice to make such systems successful or to resist change. Embracing automation, providing leadership within organizations to assure that automation is implemented safely and efficiently, and continuing to find innovative ways to incorporate automation into pharmacy practice is vital.

References

1. Rough S, Temple J. Automation in practice. In: Brown TR, ed. *Handbook of Institutional Pharmacy Practice.* Bethesda, MD: American Society of Health-System Pharmacists; 2005:329–352.

2. Kohn LT, Corrigan JM, Donaldson MS, ed. *To Err Is Human: Building a Safer Health System.* Washington DC: National Academy Press; 1999.

3. Barker KN, Flynn EA, Pepper GA et al. Medication errors observed in 36 health care facilities. *Arch Intern Med.* 2002; 162(16):1897–1903.

4. Cullen DJ, Bates DW, Small SD, Cooper JB, Nemeskal AR, Leape LL. The incident reporting system does not detect adverse drug events: a problem for quality improvement. *Jt Comm J Qual Improv.* 1995;10:541–548.

5. Classen DC, Pestotnik SL, Evans RS, Burke JP. Computerized surveillance of adverse drug events in hospitalized patients. *JAMA.* 1991;366:2847–2851.

6. Bates DW, Cullen DJ, Laird N, Petersen LA, Small SD, Servi D, et al. Incidence of adverse drug events and potential adverse drug events. *JAMA.* 1995;274:29–34.

7. Jha AK, Kuperman GJ, Teich JM, Leape L, Shea B, Rittenberg E, et al. Identifying adverse drug events: development of a computer-based monitor and comparison with chart review and stimulated voluntary report. *JAMIA*. 1998;5:305–314.

8. Classen DC, Pestotnik SL, Evans RS, Lloyd JF, Burke JP. Adverse drug events in hospitalized patients: excess length of stay, extra costs, and attributable mortality. *JAMA*. 1997;277:301–306.

9. Bates DW, Spell N, Cullen DJ, Burdick E, Laird N, Petersen LA. The costs of adverse drug events in hospitalized patients. *JAMA*. 1997;277:307–311.

10. Smaling J, Holt M. Integration and automation transform medication administration safety: successful eMARs mandate a multifold integration strategy that includes people, process, applications and technology. *Health Manag Technol*. 2005;26:16–19.

11. Louie C, Brethauer B, Cong D, Rudomin M. Use of a drug wholesaler to process refills for automated medication dispensing machines. *Hosp Pharm*. 1997;32:367–375.

12. Carroll NV. Changes in channels of distribution: wholesalers and pharmacies in organized healthcare settings. *Hosp Pharm Report*. 1997;Feb:48–57.

13. Barker KN, Felkey BG, Flynn EA, Carper JL. White paper on automation in pharmacy. *Consult Pharm*. 1998;13:256–293.

14. Vermeulen LC, Stiltner RS, Swearingen LL. Technology report revision: automated medication management in departments of pharmacy. Oakbrook, IL: University Hospital Consortiium, 1996.

15. Thielke TS. Automation support of patient-focused care. *Top Hosp Pharm Manage*. 1994;14:54–59.

16. Perini VJ, Vermeulen LC. Comparison of automated medication-management systems. *Am J Hosp Pharm*. 1994;51:1883–1891.

17. Pederson CA, Schneider PJ, Scheckelhoff DJ. ASHP national survey of pharmacy practice in hospital settings: Dispensing and administration–2005. *Am J Health-Syst Pharm*. 2006;63:327–345.

18. Ray MD, Aldrich LT, Lew PJ. Experience with an automated point-of-use unit-dose drug distribution system. *Hosp Pharm*. 1995;30:18–30.

19. Lee LW, Wellman GS, Birdwell SW, Sherrin TP. Use of an automated medication storage and distribution system. *Am J Hosp Pharm*. 1992;49:851–855.

20. Gordon J, Hadsall R, Schommer J. Automated medication-dispensing system in two hospital emergency departments. *Am J Hosp Pharm*. 2005;62:1917–1923.

21. Paparella S. Automated medication dispensing systems: not error free. *J Emerg Nurs*. 2006;32:71–74.

22. Barker KN. Ensuring safety in the use of automated medication dispensing systems. *Am J Health-Syst Pharm*. 1995;52:2445–2247.

23. Sutter TL, Wellman GS, Mott DA, Schommer JC, Sherrin TP. Discrepancies with automated drug storage and distribution cabinets. *Am J Health-Syst Pharm*. 1998;55:1924–1926.

24. Borel JM, Rascati KL. Effect of an automated, nursing unit-based drug-dispensing device on medication errors. *Am J Health-System Pharm*. 1995;52:1875–1879.

25. Guerrero RW, Nickman NA, Jorgenson JA. Work activities before and after implementation of an automated dispensing system. *Am J Health-Syst Pharm*. 1996;53:548–554.

26. McIntosh S, Petropoulos J. Using data from automated dispensing units to identify adverse drug reactions. *Am J Health-Syst Pharm*. 2005;62:2397–2400.

27. Weaver PE, Perini VJ, Pierce D. Random sampling process for quality assurance of the Rxobot dispensing system. ASHP Midyear Clinical Meeting. 1998;33:289E.

28. Oren E, Shaffer ER, Guglielmo BJ. Impact of emerging technologies on medication errors and adverse drug events. *Am J Health-Syst Pharm*. 2003;60:1447–1458.

29. Garg AX, Adhikari NK, McDonald H, Rosas-Arellano MP, Devereaux PJ et al. Effects of computerized clinical decision support systems on practitioner performance and patient outcomes – a systematic review. *JAMA*. 2005;293(10):1223–1238.

30. Degnan D, Merryfeld D, Hultgren S. Reaching out to clinicians: implementation of a computerized alert system. *J Healthc Qual*. 26(6):26–30,2004 Nov-Dec.

31. ASHP Automation and IT Policy Positions. Available at: http://www.ashp.org/s_ashp/cat1c.asp?CID=518&DID=560. Accessed 04/01/07.

32. Darby AL. Considering a hybrid system for automated drug distribution. *Am J Health-Syst Pharm*. 1996;53:1128, 1134, 1137.

33. Rough S. The pharmacist-technology interface: current and future implications for the practice of pharmacy. *The Pharmacotherapy Self-Assessment Program*. 4th ed. PSAP Book 2. Kansas City, MO: ACCP,2001:85–116.

C H A P T E R   6

Bar Code Medication Scanning at the Point of Care

Kevin C. Borcher

KEY DEFINITIONS

Bar Code—a series of vertical lines and spaces of varying widths that encode data to be scanned and decoded through a computer.

Bar Code Medication Administration (BCMA)—an inpatient clinical decision support system to assist caregivers with the five rights of medication administration (right patient, right drug, right dose, right route, and right time). BCMA systems provide warnings if any of the five rights are compromised, and many BCMA systems require the nurse to enter an override reason if he/she chooses to proceed. In addition, BCMA systems promote right documentation (some hospitals call this the sixth right of medication administration).

Bar-coding at the Point of Care (BPOC)—a process in which the patient and various patient therapies are documented with a bar code scanner at the bedside.

eMAR—electronic medication administration record.

Imager—an electronic device similar to a scanner that analyzes an image, including linear and two-dimensional bar codes, and digitally converts it into data.

Linear Symbology—a one-dimensional bar code consisting of vertical lines and spaces.

Radio Frequency Identification (RFID)—a computerized chip or tag with an antenna capable of storing data in conjunction with a receiving module for purposes of product identification or tracking.

Scanner—an electronic device that analyzes an object, such as a linear bar code, and digitally converts it into data.

Symbology—the pattern represented in a bar code that encode data and allow it to be converted into information with the use of a scanner or imager. A symbology is similar to a computer language.

Two-dimensional (2D) Symbology—a bar code that may use dots or lines arranged on the vertical and horizontal axes that can contain up to several thousand characters.

Introduction

Medical and medication errors have been a focus of healthcare facilities for years. Many organizations, including the Institute of Medicine (IOM), the Institute for Safe Medication Practices (ISMP), and the Federal Food and Drug Administration (FDA), are advocating various forms of technology for the benefit of patient safety. One of the most promising methods of technology used to prevent medication errors is the bar code scanning of medications at the bedside. A bar code is a symbol, often containing a series of lines and spaces of varying widths that contains data that is read by a scanning device and decoded through a computer which can be used with many applications. Bar code technology was developed over 50 years ago. It has been widely used in the commercial retail industry for more than 30 years. In healthcare, bar code technology is used to assist in the administration of medications to patients. This process is commonly referred to as bar-coding at the point of care (BPOC), bedside scanning, or bar code medication administration (BCMA). The term BPOC is more encompassing than BCMA, since BCMA refers specifically to the scanning of medications. BPOC includes the bar-coding and scanning of other applications. Some of these additional applications include the patient scanning and documentation of vital signs, blood products, and laboratory specimens.

The benefits of BCMA include the reduction of medication errors for patient safety. Studies (Leape, Bates) have demonstrated that over one third of preventable adverse drug events occur at the point of administration.[1] Yet, only 2% of these errors are caught at this point.[2] Medication administration is the last opportunity for a medication error to be prevented. Thus, BCMA provides a significant opportunity to capture and prevent medication errors.

There are additional benefits to BCMA besides medication error prevention. BCMA systems have been in place in hospitals since 1993, when the Department of Veterans Affairs introduced a bar code scanning system. BCMA has slowly increased in utilization over the last several years. Liability may be reduced by ensuring complete and accurate documentation, since the patient wristband and medication are scanned at the actual time of administration and not at the end of the nursing shift or later in the day, when the nurse may become distracted and inadvertently forget to document.

There is a potential for greater charge capture through the use of BCMA. Traditionally, medications are either charged on dispense from the pharmacy or an automated distribution machine or charged on charting by the nurse. The former method requires the pharmacy staff to take responsibility for patient charges, regardless of whether the medication was documented. This requires persistence on the part of the pharmacy department to charge and credit medications that have been administered or returned to the pharmacy, respectively. With systems in which charges are contingent on charting on the electronic medication administration record (eMAR), if the medication is not charted, the medication will not be charged. This process is dependent on the nurse charting the medication. If the nurse is distracted and does not chart at the time the medication is administered, the medical record will not be complete and revenue will be lost. With accurate documentation and charging based on the scanning of the medication, the facility would be in greater compliance with billing processes and may have a lower chance of issues if a patient record is audited by internal or external billing departments.

As technology has improved, so has the implementation rate of bar-coding systems. In 2002, only 1.5% of hospitals surveyed had reported the use of bar code technology at the bedside. In 2005, the number increased to 9.4%.[3,4]

Bar Code Symbology

Before investing in expensive packaging and scanning equipment, a basic understanding of bar code symbologies is needed. Familiarity with different symbologies is important in order to determine which to place on products when needing to package. As per the FDA mandate that took effect April 26, 2004, each unit of a product must contain the NDC in a linear bar code format by April, 2006. The Global Standard 1 US (GS1 US), formerly known as the European Article Numbering Uniform Code Council (EAN.UCC), is the United States member of the international organization which supports the identification and standardization of bar codes, among other electronic information used in e-commerce. Two of the most commonly employed symbologies include linear and two-dimensional formats. See Table 6-1.

The linear symbology is a one-dimensional format. Linear bar codes contain a series of black and white lines and spaces of

TABLE 6-1

Types of Bar Codes

Linear Symbology	Example	2-Dimensional Symbology	Example
UPC	N3 3 64455-993-94 3	Data matrix	
Code 39 (3 of 9)	*12345678902*	Aztec	
Code 128	6258474611	Pdf 417	
GS1-128	(01) 1 030409 471302 8		
GS1 Databar		Pharmacode	
GS1 Databar-Stacked	(01) 00311098508058		

varying thickness and distance between the lines. Scanners read the contrast or reflectance of the lines and spaces in decoding the information. Some symbologies can contain letters and numbers, whereas others contain numbers only. One of the first linear symbologies to be used commercially, and which is used routinely in the grocery industry, is the universal product code (UPC). This format begins with a prefix digit. The prefix number 3 is reserved for pharmaceuticals. The next series of numbers contains the NDC for medications, and ends with a check digit. The check digit is used to validate that the number represented in the bar code, such as the NDC, is correct. Code 39 is a common symbology used in healthcare. It can contain alpha and numeric characters. This code requires an asterisk (*) at the beginning and end of the code to be interpreted correctly. Because each character is a combination of nine black or white bars and spaces of varying widths, this symbology may be rather long and therefore difficult to use on small packages. A type of code that is used more frequently is Code 128. This symbology compresses the data more than Code 39 by using fewer and more compact bars and white spaces and, thus, may be more advantageously placed on smaller medication packages.

GS1-128, formerly referred to as UCC/EAN-128, is a variant of Code 128. GS1-128 is found on products that may be packaged or shipped in different units, such as intravenous fluids, which have individual bags shipped in a case of six or twelve units. On February 27, 2007, the GS1 organization officially changed the name of reduced space symbology (RSS) to GS1 DataBar. This format is being widely used by manufacturers. Because of the small size, this linear symbology is often used on small packages, including ampules and vials. A variation of GS1 DataBar is known as GS1 DataBar Stacked. This type can encode additional information, such as lot number and expiration date, in a second row. An often confusing code seen on some injectable products is known as the pharmacode, or pharmaceutical binary code. This is a small series of lines used as a package printing control to ensure the printing on the package is correct and free from defects. The pharmacode is not able to be scanned by traditional scanners. This becomes confusing when the nurse attempts to scan this code and believes that there is not a scannable bar code. See Table 6-1.

A newer symbology format that is becoming more popular is known as two dimensional, or 2D. These symbologies encode significant amounts of data, up to 3,000 alpha-numeric characters, in a very small space. Instead of lines and spaces, 2D uses small dots or lines arranged in an order using the horizontal and vertical axes. Two of the most common forms of 2D codes used in healthcare are data matrix and Aztec. Two-dimensional codes can be very small, enabling them to be placed on medication packages in a variety of places. They are omni-directional, meaning they can be positioned and scanned in any orientation. PDF417 is a two-dimensional symbology made up of several one-dimensional codes. It is a series of one-dimensional lines and spaces that can contain a considerable amount of information. Aztec has some advantages over data matrix. Data matrix is identified by two perpendicular anchor lines on the border. Aztec contains a square located in the center of the code. The scanner reads the Aztec symbology from the inner square, so that if part of the code is damaged or torn the bar code can often be accurately scanned. By contrast, if the outer lines of a data matrix code are damaged, the bar code will be difficult to read. Many symbologies require an area surrounding the bar code with no markings that could interfere with reading the code. This area around the bar code is called the white space, or quiet space. Aztec offers an advantage over other symbologies because the Aztec codes can be directly adjacent to one another without requiring white space. See Figure 6-1.

Whichever symbology is selected, the NDC is the common number used for many systems to read. The NDC is a 10-digit code used by the FDA representing a unique product identifier. The NDC is broken into three segments. The first segment may be four or five digits and represents the manufacturer or labeler of the product. The second segment identifies the product (drug name, strength, dose formulation) and is three or four digits. The third segment is one or two digits and identifies the package size and type. The 10-digit code may need to be changed to an 11-digit NDC for HIPAA and billing purposes, in which case a zero is placed in the appropriate segment of the 10-digit NDC. Although the FDA requires the manufacturer's bar code to include the NDC, the code often includes more than the 10-digit NDC. This number is referred to as the scan code or scan ID. One of the problems encountered with small packages is that symbologies, such as GS1 DataBar, can be printed too small to be reliably scanned except with some of the newer or more advanced imagers with high density optics.

Medication Distribution Models

When the assessment has been made to move forward with BCMA, there are several decisions to make. One of the first steps is to establish the medication distribution model. This decision will drive many other steps regarding the type of equipment used to package, store, and distribute medications. The most common medication distribution methods include a centralized, a decentralized, and a hybrid model.

The centralized method is commonly used to perform a traditional cart fill. The pharmacy prepares a supply of medications for each patient for a time period, often 24 hours. The medications are delivered to the nursing units for distribution from a medication cart or a nurse server (servidor) in or near the patient's room. The decentralized model typically allows for most or all of the patient's medications to be obtained from an automated distribution machine (ADM). Some of the vendors of these systems include AutoMed, McKesson, OmniCell, and Pyxis. Medication profiles may be maintained on the ADM, which can be more current than with the cart fill, allowing for a greater benefit in terms of patient safety and medication availability turnaround time. The hybrid model incorporates methods or functions from both the centralized and decentralized approaches. A cart fill for a time period may be performed by the pharmacy, with the ADM used to obtain controlled substances, PRN medications, and some first dose or stat medications.

Figure 6-1. Spacing between data matrix and Aztec symbologies.

Once the distribution model is defined, the most appropriate bar code packaging equipment for the organization's needs should be determined. A robot (e.g., McKesson, Swisslog) is able to package medications for patients to be placed in a medication cart and may work better for a centralized distribution system. Doses may be packaged ahead of time based on usage. The robot can then perform much of the cart fill process, including the bar code packaging of topical and injectable products. Robotic systems are often very large machines, requiring a significant amount of space within the pharmacy.

Space planning and selection of the style and size of the robot to make the best use of available pharmacy area will accommodate placement of the equipment into the pharmacy. Walls and doorways may need to be removed and rebuilt due to the size of the individual pieces. These systems may also have special electrical, ventilation, and humidity needs. This could become an expensive endeavor and should be well thought out prior to signing any contracts or agreements. Robotic systems are not inexpensive. They vary in price depending on the size and features and may range from $250,000 to over $1 million.

A bar code packaging system (AutoMed, McKesson, Talyst, others) can be used to package individual doses for patients, or for ADM replenishment or refills. These systems can vary greatly in price, depending on size, speed, degree of automation, features, and design. Packaging machines can be priced at approximately $5000 for an entry level machine that can package oral solid doses with or without a bar code. These often require an individual to place each tablet or capsule on a "platter" or in a chute for the machine to package the dose. The next levels of systems have calibrated containers that use bar code technology to verify that the correct product is placed in the correct canister for packaging. Systems

of this type range from $50,000 to $250,000. These may be able to interface to the ADM or pharmacy information system to perform patient-specific or ADM-specific refills.

The pharmacy department must work closely with nursing and the information technology departments when developing the medication distribution model. Involvement from the information technology, biomedical, plant maintenance, and construction teams needs to recognized in the early stages of equipment evaluation as well. The size of the equipment needs to be considered in this phase. Prepare a cardboard cut-out, if needed, to determine if the largest single piece can fit through doorways and other openings from the dock to the final point of placement. Some equipment may be too large to fit through doorways, creating an additional expense. Construction costs should include any work to remove and replace walls and doorways. If the movement of the equipment requires the use of an elevator, involve the necessary departments to help facilitate this phase. Determine interface development costs, electrical, and humidity requirements during contract negotiations and before contract signing.

Specific functionality and timelines of deliverables with penalties need to be clearly defined in the contract. Also, support and service agreements are integral components of the contract. The equipment will require preventative maintenance and occasionally repair. Such complicated pieces of equipment will require staff to be available to keep it in working condition. If the bar code is an integral part of the daily function, then having a contingency plan is crucial. That may include having a two- or three-day supply of medications prepackaged, or purchasing a backup machine that can meet the organization's needs for the downtime, or having spare parts readily available.

Bar code packagers are a means of providing valuable benefits in terms of medication error reduction and patient safety. In addition, a financial benefit can be realized with the use of packagers. There may be a cost savings by purchasing medications in bulk instead of the manufacturer's unit dose packages, and also by buying in larger sizes (e.g., bottles of 500 count or larger vs. 100 count). The cost of repackaging bulk products into unit dose will cost between $0.005 and $0.03 per package or more and should be a factor of the annual budget. In addition, the cost of waste and expired products must be taken into consideration. Manufacturer unit dose packages often have expiration dating of 2 years or greater. When repackaging, the expiration is immediately shortened, based on United States Pharmacopeia (USP) standards. For products with low use, this could increase waste. This can be minimized by packaging a portion of the bottle instead of the entire contents.

Atypical Product Packaging

Since the FDA mandate went into effect on April 26, 2004, manufacturers have either placed a bar code on their unit dose packaging or have opted to no longer produce some products in unit dose form. Those institutions which have adopted BCMA over the last several years have realized the necessity of packaging doses internally. Those who are serious about future implementation will need to be evaluating bar code packaging devices. Bar code packaging systems are designed for oral solid dosage forms. They do not address the handling of oral liquid packages. Liquid packagers exist that can bar code label oral liquids in unit dose cups or in oral syringes. If obtaining such a system is not possible for the pharmacy, the department will have to manually prepare and label syringes.

There are several third party software programs available that are inexpensive and easy to use to assist in the labeling of products. These programs are often very flexible and can design any size label with

multiple bar code formats. They can also be used to design labels for placement on other products, such as ampules, vials, suppositories, and topical items. For products that do not have space for a large label, a label with a tail, often referred to as rat tail, tadpole, or flag label (see Figure 6-2) can be used and wrapped around the neck of the product or affixed to allow the bar code to be scanned. The manually produced labels should include, at a minimum, drug description and NDC or scan ID. The pharmacy needs to have a process in place that can ensure that the label does not get inadvertently placed on the incorrect product. The material used for packaging or repackaging products should conform to USP standards to allow for sufficient stability, dating, and moisture impermeability. Another consideration is user acceptance. Some types of packaging material are easier than others for the nurse to open to remove the medication. Paper or foil may be easier to open than plastic.

Wristbands

Once the hardware and software solutions have been determined, the BCMA process should be outlined. The first step in this process involves the ability to scan the wristband. If the nurse is unable to identify the patient by scanning the band, his or her trust in the system is compromised. It only takes one unsuccessful attempt to create a perception that the entire system is problematic, and the perception of success or

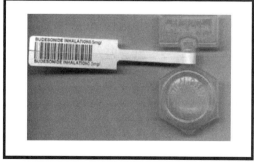

Figure 6-2. Flag or rat tail label.

failure becomes reality in the minds of those using the system. Patients are fascinated by the use of scanning technology and are willing participants in their treatment. There are a variety of factors to consider when developing functional wristbands. Choosing the appropriate material and size is essential. Paper with plastic covers may obscure the bar code with condensation or may smear the print on the band. The band should not contain metal pieces, which could interfere with magnetic resonance imaging systems. Material that is too glossy or uses colored paper or plastic may not be able to be read by the scanner if there is not enough contrast and reflectance when scanning. As an additional form of identification, the facility may opt to use a wristband large enough to allow placement of the patient's photograph.

Placement and size of the bar code on the wristband are important in developing a band that will be reliably scanned. If the bar code runs parallel to the length of the wristband, it may wrap around the patient's wrist, creating a difficult scan. This may be more of an issue with pediatric and geriatric patients with smaller wrists. Placement of the bar code perpendicular to the length of the wristband can reduce difficulty in scanning. If the patient identifier is a long number, or if the bar code is too large, it may be difficult to read. Manipulation of the band and turning the patient's wrist to access the bar code can be frustrating to both staff and patient. A successful method is to place several 2D bar codes all the way around the band. See Figure 6-3. Either data matrix or Aztec symbology can be used, but Aztec has an advantage over other 2D symbologies. Aztec doesn't require white space or quiet space around the bar code, so more copies of the bar code can be place directly adjacent to one another.

Before implementing the wristbands, the samples should be tested in different conditions with several staff for comfort and ease of scanning. Conditions should include scanning in dark rooms and direct sunlight. Test the bands after they have been twisted, folded, and crinkled, since patients who are bored or confused, or pediatric patients may manipulate the bands. The bands should be submerged in water and then scanned, since many patients do take showers in the hospital, which may affect the scan reliability. If there are sharp edges on the band the patient may complain and become dissatisfied. This is of particular importance to neonatal patients who have fragile skin.

A process should be developed to limit work-arounds of the scanning practices. Limiting wristband printing access will reduce the chance of finding wristbands attached to patient charts, doorways, or bed rails instead of the patient. If a label is used on the patient chart or physician order sheets and progress notes, one method is to code the wristband bar code with a prefix or suffix which is different than that on the patient chart labels. This bar code should not be recognized by the scanner as a patient identifier.

Devices and Equipment

The determination of the hardware to be used needs to be a multidisciplinary process and should be well thought out. There are many different devices to consider, depending on the type of BCMA system used. A stationary bedside computer offers the patient an opportunity to use the internet and other programs. The patient is entertained as well as more involved in his or her treatment. A disadvantage exists in that the healthcare member needs to sign in and out of the PC at each patient's bedside. This leads to frustration and complaints of delays

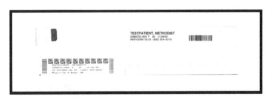

Figure 6-3. Linear vs. 2D bar-coded wristbands.

with logging in and out each time a patient is seen by the physician or medication needs to be scanned and administered.

A popular device is the mobile computer, often referred to as a computer on wheels (COW). The use of this acronym has caused some confusion and complaints at times on the nursing units, with patients mistaking the mobile computer device with an inference to the patient's weight. Because of this, some facilities may opt to use the term wireless on wheels (WOW). These devices are comprised of a desktop computer (CPU), monitor, mouse, keyboard, and scanner on a specially-designed cart on wheels. In order to supply power to the system, a portable battery is attached to the unit. The hospital must invest in a wireless network if the decision is made to use these devices. The wireless network must be tested not only in all hallways but also inside patient rooms to ensure connectivity is maintained. See Table 6-2. These systems can be expensive. The battery life is limited, so the unit must be plugged in to recharge throughout the day. Staff may be reluctant to use the carts because of the bulky nature. These carts may be very heavy, weighing in excess of 150 lb. Depending on the weight and wheel size, these may be difficult to push on carpeted floors or over door thresholds in and out of patient rooms. Because of size, these carts

may be difficult to maneuver in the patient rooms, particularly if the rooms are small, non-private, or have many IV poles and other equipment. The facility needs to involve other departments, including hospital safety and plant operations, to locate areas to store and charge the devices. Fire codes may restrict the placement of the devices in the hallways. Electrical outlets need to be of sufficient quantity to handle recharging of the devices.

An apparatus similar to a COW is a smaller, lighter device which uses a laptop computer on a smaller cart. The wheel size and base of the unit should be tested on actual patient care areas to ensure that it rolls easy and is not prone to tipping. These devices may weigh 50 lb or less. Some nurses may prefer a full-size COW because the screen size on a desktop PC can be much larger than a laptop. Depending on the number of USB or serial ports on the PC, there may not be enough ports for all ancillary devices (scanner, extra battery, mouse). Some staff may not be comfortable using a touchpad or other built-in pointing device. In addition, the battery life on a laptop may only last 2–4 hours. As with their larger cousins (COWs), these devices will need to be charged throughout a typical shift. Another option is to attach an external battery to the laptop, which can increase the

---

TABLE 6-2

Mobile Device Characteristics

	Computer on Wheels	Laptop, Tablet	Hand-held Personal Digital Assistant	PC Wired in Patient Room
Mobility	+	++	+++	-
Size/weight	-	+	+++	n/a
Screen size	+++	++	+	+++
Battery life	+	++	++	n/a
Cost	+++	++	+	++
Wireless connectivity	+++	+++	+++	n/a

battery life up to 8–12 hours. Depending on the type of battery (Ni-Cad, NiMH, Lithium ion), recharging cycles and battery life may decrease faster than expected. It may be preferable to have an extra set of batteries for each system so the staff is minimizing their time dealing with these issues or adding a new task to their already busy day. Replacement batteries need to be calculated in the budget and exchanged as their life cycle runs out. See Table 6-3.

Another point to consider is the high amount of use and abuse portable devices go through. Unlike the typical computer that is used only a few hours each day, these devices may be used continuously, particularly if an eMAR is used. The information technology department should have a plan in place to handle calls of broken or damaged devices through all hours of the day. Replacement parts or backup equipment needs to be available so as not to interfere with the performance of the staff. The hospital should determine the number of devices per floor. Not only will the nurses be using the devices, but physicians and other departments will need to access patient information and perform documentation in the computer.

Some health systems use a handheld device. Somewhat larger than a PDA, these devices are useful for charting medications when minimal patient information is needed. Some BPOC systems use a handheld device as the sole means of scanning and documentation, whereas other vendors have developed systems to incorporate the use of multiple devices. The size of the screen on these devices limits the amount of information which can be seen without scrolling. These devices work well for patients in isolation rooms. If a COW with a tethered (corded) scanner is used, the entire device may need to be wiped down with a disinfectant after it has been in the room. Handheld devices are evolving. Battery life, screen size, weight, size, and comfort are improving. These devices are becoming more popular as the manufacturers modify and develop these for use in healthcare. Some of these devices operate through a wireless network, whereas others may need to be synchronized in a cradle to update scanning information. Hand-held devices can be a very useful complementary method for systems that can use multiple devices. It may be advantageous for the facility to utilize two or more types of devices, since there may not be one solution to fit all needs. When evaluating device selection, the staff needs to participate in the decision. Demonstrate several different devices and let the staff trial them, evaluating for ease of use and mobility on a patient care area.

Scanners

Another important decision involves the devices that scan the patient wristband and medications. Scanning devices were initially designed for the retail industry. Applications

---

TABLE 6-3

Budgetary Considerations

Mobile computers or laptops, carts, spare batteries	Bar code packager
Scanners/imagers	Bar code label software and printer
Wireless network infrastructure	Construction and remodeling for any robotics or bar code packaging equipment
Printers for wristbands	Wristband material

in healthcare, such as BCMA, are relatively new. Manufacturers are receiving feedback from users and are designing or redesigning equipment for specific uses in hospitals. Linear scanner technology has been around since the 1960s and was first used in commercial retail applications in 1974. Significant improvements in imaging optics have emerged in recent years. These scanners typically produce a thin beam that projects onto the bar code and reads the reflection of contrast of the width of lines and spaces. Linear scanners are able to interpret one-dimensional symbologies.

A newer technology, similar to that of digital cameras, has been developed. The design and evolution of 2D imagers have paralleled that of digital cameras. These devices take a picture of the image, interpret the image using search algorithms, and decode the data. The 2D imagers can read both linear and two-dimensional symbologies. Bar codes can be scanned from a distance of up to 12 inches, depending on the optimal focal length of the imager lens. Although most codes can be read without difficulty, an imager that is designed to read very small codes may have difficulty with focusing on very large codes, such as those on IV bags. On the other hand, imagers designed to read large codes may not be able to readily interpret very small codes. Imagers are the preferred technology for hospitals, as they can read a greater variety of bar code formats and are suited for future uses, such as incorporating lot number and expiration date into the bar code.

Whether scanning or imaging technology is used, the next step is to determine if the devices will be tethered or cordless. Corded (tethered) scanners may attach to the PC via a USB or serial connection. One of the challenges with a corded scanner is that when the nurse scans the medication, he or she may pull the cord out of the port. Tethered scanners also draw power from the COW, which might already have lim-

ited battery life. Cordless scanners have the advantage of not having to be physically connected to the PC. Typically there is a cradle that the scanner needs to synchronize with. Bluetooth technology is also developing as an alternative to tethered devices. An external power supply is required for cordless scanners, therefore, an electrical outlet needs to be available to charge cordless scanners. Rechargeable battery packs are an alternative to external power supplies. Cordless scanners have an advantage for the nurse in that only the scanner would need to be cleaned if it were taken into an isolation room. However, the nurse may miss a warning or alert if the computer is not close enough, defeating the patient safety benefits. If the PC is outside of the room, the nurse will need to go between the patient and the PC multiple times during the medication administration, producing distractions and increasing the risk of medication errors. A hand-held device offers the advantages of displaying pertinent information directly on the PDA-type screen. This device may also offer the nurse the advantage of not necessarily having to disturb the patient during the night if an IV needs to be hung, providing the hospital's policy allows for the scanning as a means of identification. The facility may be using isolation rooms more frequently during certain times of the year, so planning for a sufficient number of devices to handle such situations is of critical importance.

Printers

Printers are another piece of equipment that requires understanding of the various types of devices and technology. The type of printer used will make an impact on the ability of the bar codes to be scanned. Dot matrix and ink jet printers are not able to produce a reliable print job and are not recommended. Laser printers may also have difficulty, depending on the dpi resolution and the material used to print on. A commonly-used type of printer for bar-coding is a thermal printer, a compact and inexpensive means of printing high quality bar code labels. They are extremely flexible, printing almost any type of bar code symbology in various sizes. There are two types of thermal printers: thermal transfer and direct thermal printers. Thermal transfer printers use a ribbon, similar to that of a dot-matrix printer. Direct thermal printers avoid the costs of ribbons by allowing the print heads to imprint the image onto a specially treated label material. Direct thermal printers do not need a ribbon, which saves cost and time involved with purchasing and changing ribbons, and potential HIPAA issues with disposal of the ribbon. Because of the special label stock required for direct thermal printers, the labels may have an increased cost compared with off-the-shelf labels. In addition, the imprint on the labels may not last as long as traditional labels, which do not require the special treated label material.

Implementation

Once all of the equipment is installed and processes are determined, the preparation for implementation can begin. Determine which departments will be using scanning for purposes other than medications. Areas may include respiratory therapy for treatments, phlebotomy for blood draws, dietary for food delivery, and nursing assistants for vital sign documentation. Ensure that there are devices available for the staff to perform their jobs and that these areas have been incorporated into the training plan.

The go-live of the system can take months of preparation. To ensure that all bar codes can be reliably scanned into the system, pharmacy staff will need to test every line item used and identify those products that need to be corrected or labeled. In addition to validating the medication scans in the pharmacy, sufficient time and resources need to be made available so that all medications and IV fluids stored on the patient care areas as floor stock and in the

automated distribution machines can be verified for successful scans. The pharmacy purchasing department and other areas that supply medications and IV fluids should work to identify products that need to be bar code packaged or labeled. If using a robot or automated bar code packaging system, canisters may be calibrated to a specific NDC and, therefore, cannot be interchanged with like products from different manufacturers. This can be a challenge if the specific manufacturer's product is out of stock or discontinued by the wholesaler or manufacturer.

A key software component to a successful BCMA system is the translation table. This reference table or crosswalk is used in many BCMA systems to convert the bar code on the package (scan ID) to the product identifier within the BCMA system. The scan ID in the bar code on the manufacturer packages often includes other digits, such as a prefix or check digit. The software may be able to read the bar code but may not be able to determine the NDC from the scan ID. A translation table allows the pharmacy to enter the bar code on the package into the database within the BCMA software and reference it with the drug product. Because the pharmacy may stock the same product from different manufacturers, these items may need to be added to the translation table. Also, new products should go through a quality assurance process that includes validating the bar code and adding it to the translation table if needed prior to being released from the pharmacy.

A continuous post-implementation evaluation should be in place to ensure the efficacy of the system. Reports should be used on a regular basis to identify drugs that are not scanned, to determine if the product is difficult to scan, or to determine whether the BCMA process is being followed. A helpful method is to create a simple troubleshooting form with basic information, including patient name, the drug in question, the time that the drug was scanned, and the error message or result of the failed scan. The staff need to have a mechanism in place to contact the appropriate department for rapid resolution to a problem, whether the problem is related to hardware, software, or product. If issues are addressed and resolved in an expeditious fashion, the system will be more reliable and effective.

Staff training should involve the understanding of the system and the reasons why it is being implemented to increase the acceptance and use of the system from the beginning. Nurses may perceive the system as taking additional steps and time with little or no benefit. Taking the time to educate the staff on the benefits will help with the understanding. Also, providing examples of published reports of unfortunate incidents in which bar code scanning would or should have been used may help the staff to realize the importance of scanning and the consequences of not scanning. Training on the proper use of the scanner, including how to achieve optimal scans, will decrease some of the early frustration. The staff also needs to be instructed in how to identify issues with product bar codes and to report them in a timely manner so that problems can be rectified expeditiously and scanning compliance can be adhered to. This training program must be mandatory for all staff who administer medications, with no exceptions. Training of the pharmacy staff is also necessary, as questions are often referred to those working in the pharmacy.

Not only do the pharmacy staff need to understand how the system works for nursing, but they must know how to ensure that all products leaving the pharmacy have a valid bar code, and how to troubleshoot basic issues. To reinforce the benefits, obtain testimonials from the hospital nursing staff that have experienced the near-miss observations and publish them within the institution. Using a pilot unit for a short period of time may be beneficial in identifying any processes or issues that need to be adjusted or resolved. Some practices may be different on weekends that need to be accounted for, such as wristband printing and resolving medications with bar code issues. Weekend staffing is often reduced on weekends, evenings, and holidays. Staff need to know who to contact during these times to answer questions and resolve issues. Printing wristbands may be limited to registration staff or house supervisors instead of secretaries during the weekday shifts. Only certain individuals may have the access to add new medications or bar codes to the BCMA translation table, so a process should be in place to accommodate these off-hour occurrences.

Reports and Monitoring

To maintain an ongoing, successful system reports are needed from the system to ensure compliance and to identify those individuals who are not adhering to the policies and practices of the institution. Reports should produce a summary to identify the overall success but also produce detailed information to identify individuals who are struggling with compliance or to find medications which are not routinely scanned. Beneficial data elements include the date and time of the administration event, patient identifier, drug, and the user. A report incorporating the alerts of the five rights (right patient, right drug, right dose, right route, right time) is a powerful testimonial to the effectiveness in relation to patient safety (see Figure 6-4). Reports can also be useful in determining if a particular medication is repeatedly identified as not scanning, which could be a result of a lack of a bar code or one that is not readable. Reports can also bring to light areas or situations that the staff believes are or should be exempt from the scanning process. These situations should be evaluated and corrected wherever possible.

It is most beneficial to identify causes of the failure to scan based on system issues

Nurse Unit: IMC   Point of Care Audit Alert Numbers

Legend (MAE = administered Med Admin Events, AA = where Audit Alert, Pt = Patient, MM = Mismatch, Inc = Incompatible)

User	Total # of MAE	# of MAE AA fired	% of MAE AA fired	Pt MM	Over Dose	Under Dose	Inc Drug Form	Inc Drug Form Route	Task Not Found	Expired Med	Early/ Late
Patient A	1	0	0	0	0	0	0	0	0	0	0
Patient B	3	1	33	0	18	0	0	0	0	0	0
Patient C	3	0	0	0	0	0	0	0	0	0	0
Patient D	1	0	0	0	0	0	0	0	0	0	0
Patient E	1	0	0	0	0	0	0	0	0	0	0
Patient F	0	0	0	0	0	0	0	0	0	0	0
Total	9	1	11	0	18	0	0	0	0	0	0

***** End of Report *****

Figure 6-4. Example of report demonstrating verification of Five Rights.

rather than user issues. Attempt to rule out issues that are not in the nurse's control. The scanner may have lost firmware settings from a power loss and may need to be re-initialized. The bar code on the patient wristband or the medication package may have been damaged or is unable to be scanned. If the computer system had downtime, the nurse will be unable to scan after the fact. After identifying individuals who have difficulty in complying after system issues, discuss the reasons why they are not adhering to established policies. Publicize the near-misses or good-catches and testimonials from the users throughout the hospital. Leadership support is crucial to the success of the process. Management must routinely monitor the compliance of the staff and take corrective action to produce adherence. The power of peer pressure is also a strong method to increase scanning compliance. A subtle method to encourage compliance is to post scan compliance reports with staff names in the staff lounge. Patients pay attention to their treatment and are aware of those who are scanning and may question why their wristband or medications are not being scanned, especially if they understand that it is done for their safety.

Downtime

Downtime policies and procedures must be in place to handle such situations. BCMA systems may be inoperable for a variety of reasons. Electrical or network failures, equipment failures, system upgrades, or system crashes can all contribute to the BCMA not functioning. These interruptions will impact reporting and BCMA metrics and should be taken into account. It is not reasonable to withhold medications and wait until the BCMA system is functioning. Rather, the nurse needs to realize that the safety checks are not in place and should implement additional manual checks to ensure safe and accurate medication administration. Documentation of the medication will often need to be completed through the electronic MAR or by utilizing a paper MAR that is later used to enter into the eMAR or as part of the permanent patient record. Supervisors should be aware of when these downtimes and not hold users at fault during these periods.

Future Trends

With the improvement of technology, BCMA systems will continue to evolve. Hand-held scanning devices will be lighter, have larger screens, and be more ergonomic for the users. Although the FDA requires manufactures to place a linear bar code on products, there may be an additional 2D bar code that can hold much more data, including lot number and expiration date. Radio frequency identification (RFID) tags have an intriguing potential in the future. They

PHARMACY INFORMATICS PEARLS

BAR CODE MEDICATION ADMINISTRATION

Medication distribution models

- Determine the model (centralized, decentralized) prior to obtaining bar code packaging equipment

Packaging equipment

- Be aware of equipment size, electrical, and special construction requirements
- Ensure that package size and bar code will fit in and work with automated distribution cabinet pockets

Bar code devices

- Select devices that are ergonomic, lightweight, and easy to use
- Purchase enough devices for all users that will need them, including physicians and ancillary departments
- Devices need to be able to handle both current and future symbologies

Symbology

- Consider symbology type, size, and placement of manual bar code labels on products
- Scan all products, enter them into the "translation table," then test in an environment to ensure that the scan IDs can be read in the BCMA system

Future trends

- 2D symbologies can hold much more data than linear bar codes, including information such as lot number and expiration date
- RFID technology shows great promise in the ability to track and identify medications

are miniature computer chips with antennas that can be programmed for storage and retrieval of various data, including NDC, lot number, expiration date, and distributor. Devices can read the information from a short distance. Some retailers use RFID technology commercially to track products and pricing information. Some manufacturers are using RFID for tracking and tracing medications in the distribution process. RFID use is expected to increase as the cost of the technology decreases.

Summary

As the benefits of medication error reduction are publicized and the cost of imple-

mentation decreases, more healthcare institutions will be moving toward BCMA systems. The planning phase is cumbersome and must involve multiple departments for its success. Computers, scanners, bar code packaging equipment, and wristband material are some of the pieces to evaluate. As the technology improves, more facilities will implement BCMA. In addition, technologies such as radio frequency identification (RFID) may be used. Understanding how these relate to the bar code symbologies and the software used will ease the execution of the project. With well-trained staff and supportive leadership, the compliance will remain high and patient safety will be realized.

References

1. Bates DW, Cullen DJ, Laird N, et al. Incidence of adverse drug events and potential adverse drug events. Implications for prevention. ADE Prevention Study Group. *JAMA*. 1995;Jul 5(274):29–34.

2. Leape LL, Bates DW, Cullen DJ, Cooper J, Demonaco HJ, Gallivan T, Hallisey R, Ives J, Laird N, Laffel G, et al. Systems analysis of adverse drug events. ADE Prevention Study Group. *JAMA*. 1995;Jul 5(274):35–43.

3. Pedersen CA, Schneider PJ, Scheckelhoff DJ. ASHP national survey of pharmacy practice in hospital settings: dispensing and administration—2002. *Am J Health-Syst Pharm*. 2003;60:52–68.

4. Pedersen CA, Schneider PJ, Scheckelhoff DJ. ASHP national survey of pharmacy practice in hospital settings: dispensing and administration—2005. *Am J Health-Syst Pharm*. 2005;62:378–390.

CHAPTER 7
Smart Pump Technology

Helen T. Giannopoulos

KEY DEFINITIONS

Adverse Drug Event—any injury due to medication.[1]

Clinical Advisory—a decision-making tool that is identified for a specific medication. Nursing guidelines are often created as an advisory. An example would be a suggestion by the pump to the user to use a 0.22-micron filter when administering a medication.

Dataset—the recommended parameters for each medication programmed into the smart pump software such as dose, dosing unit, rate, or concentration.

Drug Library—list of medications programmed in the smart pump software. The library includes properties such as name, dose, and concentration for each medication listed.

Hard limit—a dose that serves as the absolute limit (high or low) for drug administration by the pump. Once this hard limit is reached, the dose cannot be overridden, serving as a warning to the pump user that the dose needs to be verified prior to drug administration.

Infusion Pump—a device that administers drugs or nutrition to a patient through intravenous, subcutaneous, intramuscular, intrathecal, epidural, or intra-arterial routes. Infusion pumps can administer fluids in very controlled amounts.

IOM—the Institute of Medicine.

Profile—unique set of options and best practice guidelines for a specific patient population.

Smart Pump—a computerized infusion device that can be programmed to include a specific set of data.

Soft Limit—similar to hard limits but can be overridden and a dose can be programmed for delivery.

Introduction

In its 1999 report "To Err is Human," the Institute of Medicine (IOM) estimated that between 44,000 and 98,000 deaths per year result from adverse events in hospitals. In comparison, approximately 45,000 deaths annually are caused by automobile accidents. In the 2006 publication "Preventing Medication Errors," the IOM reported that medication errors occur in all stages of the medication use process but most frequently at the prescribing and administration stages. The IOM estimated that at least 1.5 million preventable adverse drug events (ADEs) occur each year in the United States. As a result, they have developed an action agenda for health care organizations to address this issue. The agenda includes adoption of new technologies such as computerized provider order entry (CPOE) and smart pumps.

This chapter will describe smart pump technology and discuss the implementation process associated with smart pumps in health care systems.

What is a Smart Pump?

A smart pump is in very simple terms a computerized infusion pump. Infusion pumps are devices that administer drugs or nutrition to a patient through intravenous, subcutaneous, intramuscular, intrathecal, epidural, or intra-arterial routes. Infusion pumps can administer fluids in very controlled amounts. There are two basic classes of pumps. Large volume pumps can pump nutrient solutions large enough to support a patient. Small-volume pumps infuse hormones, such as insulin, or other medicines, such as opiates.

While traditional infusion pumps are manually programmed by individual clinicians, smart pumps are programmed to include a very specific set of data created by the hospital staff. Part of this data is the drug library. A drug library is a list of medications programmed in the smart pump software. The library includes proper-

ties such as name, dose, and concentration for each medication listed. Smart pump software is customized to "alert you if a programmed infusion is outside of a particular medication's recommended parameters (or dataset), such as dose, dosing unit, rate or concentration."[2] In other words, smart pumps are designed to facilitate medication administration and prevent medication errors that have been associated with more traditional infusion pumps.

There are several manufacturers of smart pumps. B. Braun Medical, Cardinal Health, Hospira, Inc., Smith Medical, and Sigma International all manufacture smart pumps and have developed proprietary smart pump technology. Each system must be evaluated by hospital staff before a decision to acquire the technology is made (see Figure 7-1).

Steps to Implementing Smart Pump Technology

Establishing a Multidisciplinary Team

The pharmacist's role in this new technology is to be part of a multidisciplinary team that will plan, evaluate, and implement the software and procedures for use. During the smart pump implementation process, multiple teams are assembled to support a successful system go-live. The three teams consist of the core team, clinical team, and implementation team.

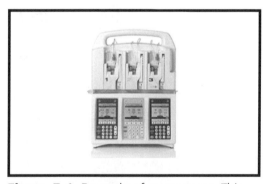

Figure 7-1. Example of smart pump. This product allows for programming of soft and hard dose and rate limits.

Core Team

A core team needs to be established at the inception of smart pump implementation. The core team's primary role is to assist the organization in selecting a smart pump vendor. The core team consists of representatives from senior leadership, bioengineering, nursing, pharmacy, information technology, and supply chain management. The senior leader's role is to assist with solidifying the organization's financial commitment to the project as well as the resulting culture of change associated with implementation. Bioengineering will provide expertise in the mechanics of the smart pump and evaluation of the safety and specific functions of the pump. The nurse team member evaluates the efficiency and usability of the pump as the primary user. The pharmacy representative will be in charge of evaluating the software's programming capabilities.

For example, the software should allow for multiple patient populations to be programmed into the pump, specifically both pediatric and adult patients. A medication safety officer would be an ideal pharmacist to be involved in this implementation. It is the responsibility of a medication safety officer to be a leader in the hospital's medication error reporting program. If the institution does not have a medication safety pharmacist then a pharmacist with clinical experience who works closely with the nursing department could serve in this role. Finally, a representative from supply chain management will assist with negotiations of contracts with the vendor. The supply chain representative will work with the bioengineering representative to define maintenance packages and technical assistance to be provided by the vendor.

Clinical Team

The clinical team consists of nurse educators, staff nurses, pharmacists, members of the quality assurance (QA) department, and a representative from the vendor. The clinical team will work closely to develop a dataset for the infusion pump system which includes drug name, dose, infusion time, standard concentrations, and clinical advisories. The pharmacist plays a key role in this stage of the process. The team also discusses programming issues and provides solutions for the implementation of the new infusion pump. As an example, safety measures need to be established with programming parenteral nutrition since it is considered a high-alert medication. In this case, the clinical team may decide to create dosing parameters such as the grams of protein per kilogram ordered per day.

Implementation Team

The implementation team will be responsible for downloading the dataset to the new infusion pumps and distributing them to all areas of the healthcare system. This team consists of representatives from bioengineering and nursing as well as the vendor and the pharmacist who created the dataset. Bioengineering will work with the vendor representative to download the dataset to each infusion pump or potentially use wireless technology to deliver the drugs to the pumps. A clinical nurse (i.e., staff nurse) will assist in exchanging active infusion pumps with the new infusion pumps. The pharmacist should be available to answer specific questions nurses may have about locating medications or programming the new infusion pumps. Development of educational materials is also key at this point. Nursing-focused and pharmacist-focused education should be developed in various formats, including PowerPoint, video, and writing. The educational process can be live or loaded onto the institution's website for viewing.

Conducting a Failure Mode Effect Analysis (FMEA)

Prior to the development of the dataset, a member from the QA department will assist with conducting a failure mode effect analysis (FMEA). A FMEA is a process improvement tool used to identify risk points with a product prior to implementation. The steps in a particular process, in this case the process is the implementation and use of smart pumps, are evaluated for potential risks and failures. These potential risks or failures are prioritized based on potential for harm to the patient, frequency of occurrence and the ultimate effects of the failure. The result of the FMEA is to develop an action plan to eliminate or reduce failures, starting with the highest priority.

The clinical team should assist with this process. The members of the clinical team that should be represented at the FMEA include frontline nurses from all the units the pumps will be implemented with special emphasis on specific patient populations such as transplant, critical care, pediatric units (NICU, PICU, general), hematology/oncology, cardiovascular, and others. A member from the QA department should lead the FMEA, as they are considered process experts. It is essential to have the pumps on site for the practitioners to experiment with using various real-life scenarios. This activity uncovers potential failure modes.

There have been several articles published in AJHP specific to FMEA and smart pump implementation.[2,3] Wetterneck et al. discussed their experience with the FMEA process, including programming process for new intravenous pumps, hazard scores comparing the old pump with the new pump, and what the recommended actions were recorded. The article discussed problems that appeared after the implementation of the smart pump and what actions were taken.[3] A FMEA was conducted to analyze the intravenous drug administration process. Their experience with the FMEA process steps identified potential failure modes. They focused on IV pump programming errors since that was identified as a hazard. Two main interventions were performed from their FMEA results: updated pre-printed order sets and implementing smart pump technology. Consistent risk points

identified by multiple institutions are (1) bypassing the safety software, (2) selecting the wrong medication concentration, and (3) not reading or verifying override warnings causing a patient to receive an inappropriate dose of medication. There are many process improvement tools that can be used to assess the implementation of smart pump technology. It may be helpful to contact the quality department to determine the process specific to your institution.

Designing and Building the Dataset

Often hospitals that have merged to become one health system use various concentrations specific to their campus. If the smart pumps are accidentally transferred to other campuses, an error could easily occur. Newer pumps include the capability of wireless transfer of information. This means that a pump update conducted by wireless transfer will affect the pumps at each site in the system. Standardization in the preparation and dispensing of medications must occur throughout the healthcare system in order to provide a safe environment for the patient. Standardizing concentrations, volumes to be dispensed, and placement of pharmacy labels on syringes are just some steps that will assist in the preparation of designing the dataset. In standardizing concentrations, the minimum volume delivered by the pump should be taken into consideration to ensure that the appropriate dose can be delivered to the patient.

Another important step in preparing to design the dataset includes gathering all resources to identify medication name display, dosing range, length of infusion, and administration guide (clinical advisories).

Often the infusion pump manufacturer will provide training for the pharmacist who will be developing the dataset. First the pharmacist should review the pharmacy computer system and evaluate how the medication name appears on the product label and medication administration record

(MAR) to create the list of medications that will be programmed into the pump. For instance, if the pharmacy computer system displays dopamine as DOPAmine, then the dataset should display the medication in the same manner. Doing this allows for consistency and aids in the programming of the pump in a systematic method. Multiple concentrations of a drug should also be included in the dataset.

Tools used by licensed healthcare professionals to order medications for patient administration should be gathered. These tools may include, but are not limited to, pre-printed orders, hospital pathways, and protocols. All doses listed in each tool should be evaluated to determine the dosage range for each medication. Once the range has been established, a soft limit (a dose that is out of range but can still be programmed for administration) and hard limit (a dose that is exceedingly out of range that cannot be programmed for administration) should be defined. In doing so, the pharmacist can ensure the dosing safety alerts set will not cause unnecessary warnings for the nurses.

It is important to have an infusion time range identified for each medication prior to building the dataset, otherwise the pump software may not allow the medication information to be programmed. The pharmacy computer system should provide the first resource to determine infusion times for medications. If the infusion times are not already defined, then alternate resources such as *Physician's Drug Reference* (PDR), package inserts, and any dosing handbook that includes nursing administration guidelines should be reviewed.

The administration guide or clinical advisory is a note that displays on the pump as the nurse programs the medication. Its purpose is to assist in the appropriate administration of medications by providing clinical information. Clinical advisories may be driven by healthcare system policy (i.e., high-alert medications necessitate two

nurses to verify dosing information), or by medication administration guidelines (i.e., 0.22-micron filter required for administration). In determining which clinical advisories should be included in the dataset, it is important to understand that the pump will alert the nurse each time the medication is programmed; therefore, the advisories should be limited to pertinent administration guidelines so as not to desensitize nurses to important alerts. It is also important to understand that a clinical advisory is not necessary for each medication that is included in the dataset.

Once the preparation process has been completed, the next step is to begin building the dataset. The pharmacist responsible for building the dataset should coordinate with the clinical team to determine which profiles will be designed in the dataset. A profile is a unique set of options and best practice guidelines for a specific population. The name of the profile should be determined next. Some institutions determine the profile name according to a specific patient care area (i.e., the intensive care unit may be labeled "ICU"). Other institutions, such as pediatric hospitals, may label the profile by area and weight range (i.e., PICU 2–10 kg). Once the nomenclature of the profiles has been decided, the clinical team will determine the medications included in the library for each profile. The library should consist of medications that are used in the specific population defined by the profile. The components of a library consist of medication name, infusion type, infusion units, standard concentrations, dosing parameters, and clinical advisories (see Table 7-1). The medication name will be displayed as it is in the pharmacy computer system. The infusion type may be listed by dose per time, dose per weight per time, or volume per time (see Table 7-2). The infusion type will determine which dosing elements are options for that infusion type. The infusion unit is defined as the dosing unit for the medication.

TABLE 7-1

List of Library Components

Drug Program Properties

General

(Drug Name)	dopamine
Display Text	DOPamine
Infusion Type	dose/kg/min
Syringe Model	(none)
Syringe Size	(none)

Infusion Units

Concentration Units	micrograms (mcg)
Delivery Units	ICRP grams (mcg)

Main

Concentration Maximum	(none) mcg/mL
Concentration High	(none) mcg/mL
	1600 mcg/mL
Concentration Low	(none) mcg/mL
Concentration Minimum	(none) mcg/mL
Dose Maximum	(none) mcg/mL
Dose High	(none) mcg/mL
Dose	(none) mcg/mL
Dose Low	(none) mcg/mL
Dose Minimum	(none) mcg/mL
Patient Weight	(none) mcg/mL

Options

Loading	Disabled
Loading Dose Maximum	(none) mcg/kg
Loading Dose High	(none) mcg/kg
Loading Dose	(none) mcg/kg
Loading Dose Low	(none) mcg/kg
Loading Dose Minimum	(none) mcg/kg
Loading Time	(none) MM:SS
Loading Time Limit	(none)
Bolus	Disabled
Bolus Dose Maximum	(none) mcg/kg
Bolus Dose High	(none) mcg/kg

Concentration

Enter the drug concentration

TABLE 7-2

Examples of Types of Infusions

Basic infusion	mL/ hour
	Volume over time
	Intermittent volume over time
Dose per time	Dose/min
	Dose/hour
	Dose/time
	Dose/day
Dose per weight (kg) and time	Dose/kg/min
	Dose/kg/hour
	Dose/kg/time
	Dose/kg/day
Dose per weight (m²) and time	Dose/m^2/min
	Dose/m^2/hour
	Dose/m^2/time
	Dose/m^2/day

In order to ensure appropriate programming of the pump, a nurse may verify the medication label with the medication order. In turn, the units displayed on the pump should match the units on the medication label. The standard concentrations, dosing parameters, and clinical advisories defined during the preparation process will be incorporated into the dataset.

Quality Assurance Check

Once the dataset has been designed and created, the clinical team should perform a quality assurance check. The dataset should be downloaded into the pumps so that actual doses can be programmed. By programming a dose, the team can evaluate the types of overrides a nurse will encounter once the pump is implemented on the floors. The team can then determine if the defined dose ranges are appropriate. Nursing should be

involved in reviewing the drug library to ensure that most medications used in their patient care areas are available for programming under the appropriate profile. A staff pharmacist or clinical pharmacist should be involved in checking and confirming the appropriate drug name spelling, dose, concentration, and length of infusion. Any changes required to the dataset should be communicated to the pharmacist developing the dataset. Once the quality assurance step has been completed by the clinical team, some manufacturers may provide a final check of the dataset prior to the date the pumps are implemented for use in patient care areas (go-live day).

Staff Training

While smart pumps have the potential to significantly reduce medication errors, it is inherent in new technologies that there is a learning curve for the staff. As with any new technology, some research shows that these pumps may not result in fewer errors if the behaviors and work patterns of the staff using and programming the pumps is not taken into consideration. Training is critical.

As discussed earlier, the pharmacist can receive training from the pump manufacturer in the creation of the dataset. The nursing staff may be trained by a clinical nurse who has participated in training by the manufacturer. The manufacturer may provide a representative to assist the clinical nurse in training the staff nurses in the use of the pump. The training sessions should, at minimum, involve identification of profiles, location of medications, and set-up and programming of the pump. The length of the session should not exceed 1 hour, so as not to disrupt patient care. Training sessions should be conducted during all shifts to ensure participation of all nursing staff. A computer-based training program may be an option to assist in educating the nursing staff. In large integrated health systems, there will need to be creative solutions for

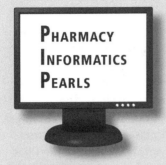

PHARMACY
INFORMATICS
PEARLS

PEARLS

Establishing a multidisciplinary team

■ It is imperative that there is a nursing representative from each area of the hospital where the pump will be implemented. This allows for a voice for the end user and allows for the nursing representative to communicate the change in a workflow process prior to the week of implementation. By doing this, the late adopters to change can prepare for the change and decrease staff resistance to this new product.

Conducting a failure mode effect analysis (FMEA)

■ Identify potential risk points prior to implementing the new product to the healthcare system.
■ A representative from each nursing unit is needed to provide valuable input of the potential risk points.
■ Minimize the actual meeting time by sending out emails to the team members involved in the FMEA to brainstorm and bring ideas of risk points to the meeting.

Preparing to design the dataset

■ Make sure all pathways, protocols, and guidelines have been collected, especially in high-risk areas such as critical care units and radiology.

Designing the dataset

■ Involve the clinical team from the very beginning. Ultimately, the end users of the pump will be nurses. By doing this it will assist with nursing staff acceptance of the new product.
■ The goal is to limit the number of concentrations for a specific medication in a profile to decrease the risk of a nurse selecting the wrong concentration when programming the pump.
■ When creating dosing parameters make sure to look at the pump key pad to determine how the numbers appear. For example, when creating a dosing parameter with a max being 25, if the numbers 2 and 5 are next to each other you may want to use the number 6. By using 26 as the dosing parameter it may assist in identifying or preventing a miskey or key bounce errors. ISMP has reported several programming errors due to those programming problems.

Quality assurance

■ Make sure the clinical team members review and evaluate the medications created in each profile. This provides them an opportunity to determine if any changes need to be made to the dataset prior to go-live.
■ Actually pull medication labels and program them into the pump to determine what alerts the nurse may see as they program medications. If multiple alerts are fired then the dosing parameters created for that medication may need to be re-evaluated.
■ Make sure the clinical pharmacists in the respective areas review the medications and dosing parameters for their respective areas. They may identify a dosing parameter that needs to be changed specific to their area and a medication that should be added to the profile.

educating large numbers of full-time, casual, and on-call staff who work days, evenings, and night shifts.

Future Trends

Informatics is in essence the integration of compatible technologies into a business environment to improve performance and quality. In the healthcare community, informatics is being embraced to reduce errors and improve patient care and safety. Smart pump technology is only part of the solution. The future of the smart pump is as part of a facility-wide system that also includes CPOE, and bar-code medication administration (BCMA) as well as other automated delivery and record keeping systems. When all components work together, the benefits to the patient increase dramatically.

Smart pump technology continues to evolve rapidly and the debate continues over which type or brand of pump is best suited for certain clinical settings.

References

1. Bates DW, Cullen DJ, Laid N, Petersen LA, et al. Incidence of adverse drug events and potential adverse drug events. Implications for prevention. ADE Prevention Study Group. *J Am Med Assoc.* 1995;274:29–34.

2. Beattie s. Technology today: Smart IV pumps. Available at: http://rnweb.com/rnweb/article/articleDetail.jsp?id=254828 (Accessed June 13, 2008.)

3. Wetterneck TB, Skibinski KA, Roberts TL, et al. Using failure mode and effects analysis to plan implementation of smart i.v. pump technology. *Am J Health Syst Pharm.* 2006;63:1538–1538.

Bibliography

Adachie W, Lodolce, AE. Use of Failure mode and effects analysis in improving the safety of i.v. drug administration. *Am J Health Syst Pharm.* 2005;62:917–920.

Institute of Medicine. Preventing Medication Errors. 2006.

Institute of Safe Medication Practice. Safety Issues with Patient-Controlled Analgesia. Part I. How Errors Occur. July 10, 2003. Vol. 8 (14).

Ibid. Part II. How to Prevent Errors. July 24, 2003. Vol. 8 (15).

Ibid. Misprogram a PCA pump? It's easy! July 29, 2004. Vol. 9 (15).

Ibid. Hazard Alert Key Bounce and Keying Errors. October 19, 2006. Vol. 11 (21).

Ibid. Example of a Health Care Failure Mode and Effects Analysis for IV Patient-Controlled Analgesia. 2005.

Smaling J, Holt, MA. Integration and automation transform medication administration safety. *Health Manage Technol.* April 2005. Available at: http://www.healthmgttech.com/archives/0405/0405integration_automation.htm

System Maintenance

Doina Dumitru

KEY DEFINITIONS

Electronic Health Record Systems—software programs designed for use by clinicians to electronically store clinical information related to patients.

Formulary—a health system's specific list of medications approved for use by its clinicians.

Maintenance—work that must be done to a software program to ensure that the system is updated and accurate.

Medication Masterfile—compilation of records that individually contain data elements that compose the medication information presented for use in an EHR system.

Order Set—compilation of medication and procedure orders that can be accessed and ordered from a single source in the EHR. These are analogous to paper pre-printed order forms.

What Needs To Be Maintained?

When the excitement of implementation is over and the electronic health record system (EHR) is being used by clinicians, the issues related to system maintenance begin to take center stage in the information technology (IT) department. One of the earliest questions IT project managers must ask is: what type of maintenance needs to be done? Because we work in the medical field where the knowledge base is constantly changing, our IT support systems must change as well to reflect updates and new trends in the discipline. In an EHR system, the pharmacy IT support team will focus its maintenance activities on updating medication masterfiles, formularies, clinical decision support tools, and clinical order sets (Table 8-1).

TABLE 8-1

Types of Maintenance Required

Maintenance Type	Example(s) of Required Maintenance Activities	Key Points
Medication masterfile	■ NDC changed by drug company ■ Drug discontinued from the market ■ New drug approved by FDA	■ Frequency of database updates ■ Post-update data validation/testing required ■ System availability to end users during updates ■ Plan for data elements being deleted or inactivated ■ Impact of data changes on existing interfaces ■ Post-update build
Formulary and related drug information maintenance	■ Drug addition to the formulary ■ Drug deletion from the formulary ■ Links to drug information sources updated or changed	■ Timeliness of formulary updates ■ Setting clinician expectations for delivery of updates ■ IT support must work with inventory personnel ■ Commercial vs. home-grown drug information sources
Clinical decision support	■ Dose alerts added to the system ■ New allergy cross-reactivities added to the system ■ New laboratory triggers added to a drug	■ Complexity of CDS ■ Commercial vs. home-grown CDS rules ■ Frequency of updates
Order sets	■ Changes in clinical practice require medications to be added or removed ■ Medication masterfile changes	■ Quantity of order sets needing updates ■ Manual vs. automated update process

Medication Masterfile Maintenance

Many EHR systems use masterfiles as the building blocks of the data that comprises the system. Masterfile type examples include frequency files, medication files, and system user files. While much effort is often first directed on accurately setting up these files, post-implementation support of the data is equally important. Support activities can include building new frequencies, adding new medications to the system, and setting up access for new users. The types of support activities will vary greatly at each organization and will often be determined by how frequently end users require (or in some cases demand) updated information. The amount of support required will often depend on how much customization was done in the system. The greater the amount of customization, the greater the amount of system maintenance required. Because of the importance of the file in an EHR system, this section will focus on discussing medication masterfile support issues.

The medication masterfile is one of the key building blocks of an EHR system. The masterfile must contain accurate and up-to-date information on all medications that may be used in the patients of a given institution. Additions to the masterfile done after the initial installation process must be consistent with principles used to set up the file. Any changes made to the initial data load must be thoroughly tested to ensure that new information is valid, without error, and is consistent with other medications built into the system. Finally, existing data must be revalidated following any upgrades made to the software system.

While the initial process of setting-up and loading a medication masterfile into an EHR is time-consuming, the maintenance of the file also requires significant time investments to ensure that the data is accurate and up to date. If the computer-assisted provider order entry (CPOE) system component does not have the latest FDA drug approvals available for ordering, clinicians may lose their faith in the system and revert to workarounds such as medication ordering done on paper. To that end, the first step in medication masterfile maintenance revolves around selection of the drug database used to supply basic drug information to the EHR. Institutions have the option of using drug database vendors such as First DataBank or Medispan or using custom databases developed by an internal IT department. Drug information such as drug names, dosage forms, NDCs, and package sizes are examples of information that a database would provide. There are several key questions that project team managers must consider when deciding how much support will be required for the medication masterfile:

1. How often will the drug database be updated: daily, biweekly, monthly, or quarterly?

2. What type of post-update data validation or testing must be done to ensure that no errors occurred during the update process?

3. How will update activities affect the availability of the system? Do updates require scheduled computer down-time periods?

4. What happens to existing data in the system if drugs or NDCs are removed from the database by an update?

5. If NDCs are used for interfacing with various types of automation (e.g., automated dispensing systems), how will NDC changes as a result of an update affect the ability of the interface to function?

6. How much post-update build is required to set up new data loaded into the system?

The frequency of medication masterfile updates is an important consideration in EHR projects. Systems which rely on commercially available databases can be updated by data loads provided from the database vendor. The healthcare organization must decide how frequently this will occur. This decision is made by considering many factors, including:

■ Clinician expectations. For example, when will new drugs be available for use in the system, e.g., the day after the FDA approval or one month after the approval? When will drugs removed from the market be inactivated in the system?

■ Resources required to install an update. Can one person load the software or are multiple resources needed to complete all of the steps in the process?

■ System downtime required. Must the system be made unavailable while an update takes place? Or can clinicians continue to use the system as new data is loaded?

Table 8-2 outlines the advantages and disadvantages related to various update frequencies.

Once the masterfile information has been updated, the data in the system must be validated and tested to ensure that the integrity of the data has been maintained. Validation activities may involve testing CPOE with new drugs added to the system. For example, does the new drug behave like existing drugs in the system when ordered via CPOE? Other testing and validation activities include: ensuring that all needed dosage forms are available, testing clinical rules such as dose alerts for newly added or deleted medications, that system defaults are applied to the new data, and that existing data has not been altered. The last consideration is especially important. In some systems, data loads make changes to end user screens instantly. For example, while a physician is entering an order into the CPOE system, the medication name changes slightly as the new data is loaded into the system. In this case, the drug database vendor has made a change to the drug record name which is then loaded into the system by the masterfile update process. Such situations could lead to end users doubting the integrity of the system and the data within it. It is imperative that clinicians trust the information if they are to use the system effectively and consistently.

System availability to end users is another important consideration in medication masterfile maintenance. If the maintenance required to keep the file up to date also mandates frequent system downtime, clinicians will be resistant to supporting the technology's use. However, if clinicians can write prescriptions and document medication histories during the update process, the maintenance will appear seamless to the end user. Conversely, some systems may not require scheduled downtime for an update. However, the EHR system may be slowed by the update process. In this case, if the EHR has many users logged into the system, the data load could lead to excessive system slowness and clinician frustration with the software.

During the masterfile update process, medication records and related informa-

---

TABLE 8-2

Advantages and Disadvantages of Various Medication Masterfile Update Frequencies

	More Frequently	Less Frequently
Advantages	■ Latest FDA approvals available ■ Drug withdrawals from the market not available to clinicians	■ Post-update data validation and testing done less frequently ■ Less system down-time required
Disadvantages	■ In custom-built databases, greater number of resources needed to keep up with frequency of updates ■ Post-update data validation and testing must be done more frequently ■ System may be unavailable more frequently	■ Latest FDA drug approvals not immediately available for use by clinicians ■ Drugs withdrawn from the market still available in the system

tion may be inactivated or deleted. In many systems, NDC data is frequently modified in response to manufacturer changes. If the EHR relies heavily on the NDC to identify discrete drug products, frequent changes can create a maintenance quagmire. In such cases, processes must be developed to allow IT support staff to quickly identify: which NDCs have changed or been deleted, what data was tied to the NDC, what is the new NDC, and how will the new NDC be tied to the data? Sophisticated processes involve software system utilities which find and re-place NDCs throughout the system with the ability to track what was changed and when it was changed. More rudimentary processes involve running reports to identify affected NDCs followed by manual replacement of individual NDCs by IT support personnel. If manual processes are used, many more resources would be required to keep pace with medication masterfile updates.

One important consequence of medi-cation masterfile updates is the effect that is had on systems interfaced to the EHR. Systems commonly interfaced include automated dispensing systems (ADS), inventory management systems, medica-tion compounding machines, and pharmacy information systems. While each of these systems may be significantly affected follow-ing an update to the medication masterfile, interfaces to ADS and pharmacy informa-tion systems are most often affected by such updates with results affecting both phar-macy and nursing personnel. In the case of the ADS, if a drug's NDC was deleted from the EHR database and the ADS uses NDCs to communicate with the EHR, the link between the two systems is now broken and must be rebuilt. When pharmacy informa-tion systems are not integrated into the EHR but are interfaced, changes made in the EHR database must be mirrored in the pharmacy system to ensure that orders entered in the EHR will cross the interface and produce the same information in the pharmacy system.

In such cases, interface testing must be done to ensure that medications ordered in the CPOE system are sent to the ADS (where they can be retrieved by a clinician on the nursing unit), and in the pharmacy system where pharmacy personnel can accurately use medication lists and other information retrieved from the EHR.

A final consideration is the amount of post-update build required to newly added or deleted drug information. For example, if the update process added a new FDA drug approval to the EHR, the drug record must be set up to match existing medications in the systems. Build principles initially used to set up the system must be applied to the new medication added to the database. Examples of post-build activities include: specifying dose defaults, indicating frequency defaults, and identifying dosage forms and sizes to be used within the system.

Formulary and Related Drug Information Maintenance

In many EHR systems, maintenance of the formulary is closely related to that of the medication masterfile, as the data used by the formulary is dependent on the accuracy and relevance of its component medica-tion records. Stated differently, the medica-tion masterfile is the building block of the formulary in a clinical information system. Formulary related issues include implemen-tation of pharmacy and therapeutics (P&T) committee decisions in the system and up-dating drug information links in the EHR.

Ensuring that formulary changes made by an institution's P&T committee are reflected in the EHR in a timely manner is crucial. If a non-formulary medication was approved by the committee for use on February 26, clinicians expect to be able to order the medication that same day. How-ever, setting clinician expectations for such updates is a key factor in acceptance of CPOE processes. If clinicians are consistent-ly told that the EHR will be updated within two days of a P&T committee meeting, therapeutic plans may be adjusted to reflect these expectations. Setting realistic expectations is also key, as different types of input are required to ensure a successful formulary update. Pharmacy IT support teams must coordinate such updates with inventory personnel as medications that can be ordered via CPOE must also be available in the pharmacy for dispensing. This illustrates the importance of both clinical and IT staff input into building formulary changes into the system.

Drug information links are related to formulary updates as some EHR systems provide internet hyperlinks to drug information sources. Examples of such information include links from a specific medication record ordered in the CPOE system to the dosing section of a drug monograph from a database. As databases are updated, associated links must also be changed to reflect new information. Commercial drug information systems, similar to commercial medication drug databases, may be easily updated using software tools provided by a vendor. Home-grown drug information sources, however, may require significantly more maintenance. If system utilities are not developed to make information changes simple to implement, changes may need to be made one a time, drug record by drug record.

Clinical Decision Support Maintenance

EHR systems vary in their use of clinical decision support (CDS) tools. Some systems may employ simple CDS such as allergy and drug interaction checking while other systems use sophisticated rules engines to selectively display laboratory values, diagnoses, and radiological alerts based on data stored in the patient's medical record. As the complexity of the CDS grows, the amount of maintenance grows proportionately. Factors that affect the amount of mainte-

nance required include: complexity of CDS, commercial vs home-grown CDS rules, and frequency of updates.[1-3]

Clinical decision support available in EHR systems varies widely in complexity.[4,5] Simple forms of CDS such as allergy checking, when purchased from commercial database vendors, usually require little maintenance. Once an update is available from the vendor, the new data is loaded into the system and is available for use by the end user soon after the update occurs. In more complex CDS alerts, such as selectively displayed laboratory alerts, rules engines may require a programming change in order to update the information used to generate the alerts. In such cases, the maintenance needed for the system may require specialized IT support to accomplish the change.

A second consideration in the maintenance of CDS systems is the source of the data. Commercially available CDS is often updated via data loads done at regular intervals. These updates are fairly simple to accomplish as they involve loading the data from a compact disk (CD) into the EHR. If CDS is custom-designed by an organization, then the maintenance required is often extensive. In such cases, decision rules must be individually revised by the IT support team to achieve the desired update. Depending on the software type, this may require specialized programming knowledge which in turn limits the resources that can be used to update the CDS system. Regardless of source, both commercial and home-grown CDS systems must undergo post-update testing and validation, similar to the medication masterfile, to ensure that the data is accurate and the software behaves as expected.

Finally, the frequency of CDS updates is also an important factor in determining the extent of maintenance required. Alerts and rules updated weekly instead of monthly or quarterly require more time and resources to accomplish.

Order Set Maintenance

Order sets are powerful tools that can be used to expedite order entry and minimize medication errors during the ordering process.[6,7] Although many electronic order sets often allow order entry of both medications and procedures, only applicability to medications is discussed below. Creating order sets and protocols in EHR systems is often most time-consuming during the build and implementation phase. After go-live, these tools can usually be used for quite some time before changes are required. Needed modifications can result from changes in practice or prescribing habits that must be implemented or in maintenance resulting from medication records that must be added or removed from the order sets. Regardless of the reason that generates the request for change, the steps needed to accomplish the update are the same.

Changes made to the medication masterfile often impact order sets in the CPOE system and will likely occur more frequently than those required by changes in clinical practice. Examples of such medication masterfile changes include: naming convention is changed for a medication by the database vendor, dosage form is removed from the database due to being discontinued by the manufacturer, and new medication strength is added to the database. If an existing order set contains a medication that is changed by an update to the medication masterfile, then the order set must be reviewed and the drug record on the set updated to ensure that clinicians are able to order the medication. For example: an institution's monthly database update is loaded into the system, resulting in the removal of the 10-mg tablet size of medication ABC. Because ABC 10 mg is on several order sets in the CPOE system, the IT support team must remove this strength from the order sets on which it is located. In some systems, this step is accomplished automatically by utilities provided by the CPOE system vendor. In other systems, this must be done manually by support personnel. If changes must be made manually to order sets, maintenance may become very time consuming.

Future Trends

Regardless of system type used by an organization, maintenance requires much time and many resources. In many institutions, the amount of maintenance is often proportionally related to the number of different systems used throughout the organization: the greater the number of systems, the greater the amount of maintenance required. Further, if the systems are interfaced to each other, information translation across that interface becomes an issue. Because data transfer between systems is often imperfect, system changes or updates must be made in multiple systems simultaneously. This results in duplication of work by the pharmacy IT support team and may pose a risk for the health system. For example, in organizations where the EHR is supplied by Vendor A and the pharmacy system is supplied by Vendor B, updates to the medication masterfile must be made in both systems separately. If the support team makes an error in the update to the EHR, risk is introduced by having information that is wrong in one system but correct in the other. As a result, information translation across the interface to the pharmacy system could introduce error in a patient's medication profile.

In 2004, the president of the United States installed a National Coordinator for Health IT. Since that time, the federal government has supported a movement to achieve interoperable health IT systems throughout the country. In response, various efforts have begun to improve the communication between disparate clinical systems. Of great significance is the focus on developing standardized clinical vocabularies that can be understood by various systems, regardless of vendor. Examples of such vocabularies include SNOMED for diagnosis codes and RxNorm for medications. For pharmacy IT support teams, uniform terminology translates into fewer maintenance hours required and more importantly, consistent medication data being supplied to the EHR system.[8]

RxNorm has the potential to significantly impact how clinical information systems work with medication records in masterfiles. Maintenance activities will also be affected

as the need to maintain records in multiple systems disappears as different systems use the same language to transfer medication data. However, adoption of RxNorm is dependent on the willingness of EHR software vendors to incorporate the data into their programs. Such efforts will require vendor personnel and financial resources to rework existing programming or to write new programs which incorporate the medica-

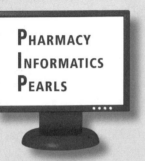

PHARMACY INFORMATICS PEARLS

SYSTEM MAINTENANCE

Medication masterfile

- Customize a system at your own risk: more customization equals more maintenance.
- Be consistent: additions made after go-live must reflect the same principles used to set up the file initially.
- Test every time: all changes should be tested and validated before they go live.
- Minimize downtime: clinicians don't trust systems that are frequently not functioning.

Formulary and related drug information maintenance

- Coordinate: IT support and pharmacy inventory personnel must work together to ensure that both the system and the pharmacy has medications available for ordering.
- Set realistic expectations: let clinicians know when additions or deletions to the formulary will be available.
- Drug information links: great tools, but must be kept up to date. Commercial sources of information are easier to update than home-grown versions.

Clinical decision support

- The more complex the rule, the more difficult it is to maintain.
- Commercial CDS is easier to maintain but the information may not be as tailored to an institution's needs as compared to home-grown rules.
- Keep the information current. Rules must reflect recent clinical practice information.

Order sets

- Update the medication masterfile, then update order sets.
- Ask vendor for system utilities that make similar changes simultaneously to order sets containing the information to be changed.

Future trends

- RxNorm has the potential to eliminate the data translation issues related to interfaces between disparate systems.

tion vocabulary standards. Commitment of significant resources to such projects may not occur until more powerful incentives appear in the health care market. Government health payers such as the Centers for Medicare & Medicaid Services (CMS) may prove to be a significant spur to widespread RxNorm adoption. In 2003, the Medicare Prescription Drug Improvement and Modernization Act (MMA) provided that CMS work toward achieving and incorporating a system of standards that would work toward an ultimate goal of EHR interoperability.[9] However, CMS has yet to mandate use of such standards in transactions made with the agency, although the MMA of 2003 suggests that the agency will require interoperability to improve the efficiency of the system.

References

1. Lai LL. Assessing data quality for decision support-emphasis on secondary analysis. *Pharm Pract Manag Q.* 1998 Apr;18(1):46–51.

2. Mackowiak LR, Hayward SL. Issues of decision support in institutional pharmacy systems. *Pharm Pract Manag Q.* 1998 Apr;18(1):35–45.

3. Mack TA. Decision support considerations in the development and implementation of an electronic medical record. *Pharm Pract Manag Q.* 1998 Apr;18(1):21–34.

4. Broverman C, Kapusnik-Uner J, Shalaby J, Sperzel D. A concept-based medication vocabulary: an essential requirement for pharmacy decision support. *Pharm Pract Manag Q.* 1998 Apr;18(1):1–20.

5. Berlin A, Sorani M, Sim I. A taxonomic description of computer-based clinical decision support systems. *J Biomed Informat.* 2006;39(6):656–667.

6. Payne TH, Hoey PJ, Nichol P, Lovis C. Preparation and use of preconstructed order, order sets, and order menus in a computerized provider order entry system. *J Am Med Inform Assoc.* 2003;10:322–329.

7. Dinning C, Branowicki P, O'Neill JB, Marino BL, Billett A. Chemotherapy error reduction: a multidisciplinary approach to creating templated order sets. *J Pediatr Oncol Nurs.* 2005 Jan-Feb;22(1):20–30.

8. National Library of Medicine. RxNorm Overview. Available at: http://www.nlm.nih.gov/research/umls/rxnorm/overview.html. Accessed February 6, 2007.

9. Centers for Medicare and Medicaid Services. CMS Legislative Summary: MMA of 2003. Available at: http://www.cms.hhs.gov/MMAUpdate/downloads/PL108-173summary.pdf. Accessed February 6, 2007.

CHAPTER 9

A New Frontier
Impact of the Electronic Medical Record and Computerized
Provider Order Entry on Pharmacy Services

Michael Sura

KEY DEFINITIONS

Clinical Decision Support (CDS)—providing clinicians or patients with clinical knowledge and patient-related information, intelligently filtered or presented at appropriate times, to enhance patient care. Clinical knowledge of interest could range from simple facts and relationships to best practices for managing patients with specific disease states, new medical knowledge from clinical research, and other types of information.

Clinical Informatics—the scientific study of the effective analysis, use, and dissemination of information in patient care, clinical research, and medical education.

Clinical Pharmacy Technician—a highly skilled pharmacy technician or "pharmacist assistant" with advanced training and/or pharmacy technician certification completed.

Computerized Provider Order Entry (CPOE)—the portion of a clinical information system that enables a patient's care provider to enter an order for a medication, clinical laboratory, radiology test, or procedure directly into the computer. The system then transmits the order to the appropriate department, or individuals, so that it can be carried out.

Electronic Health Record (EHR)—a longitudinal electronic medical record (EMR) of patient health information generated by one or more encounters in any care delivery setting. It contains episodes of care across multiple care delivery organizations (CDOs) within a community, region, or state.

Electronic Medical Record (EMR)—a computerized legal clinical record created in a CDO, such as a hospital or physician's office. It is an application environment composed of the clinical data repository (CDR), clinical decision support (CDS), controlled medical vocabulary (CMV), computerized provider order entry (CPOE), pharmacy, clinical documentation, and other ancillary applications.

Electronic Prescribing, or e-Prescribing—refers to the use of computing devices to enter, modify, review, and output or communicate drug prescriptions and medication regimens for patients. e-Prescribing is one component of CPOE systems.

Informaticist—someone who applies information technology to a specific discipline (e.g., pharmacy informaticist).

Medication Error—any preventable event that may cause or lead to inappropriate medication use or patient harm while the medication is in the control of the health care professional, patient, or consumer.

Medication-Use System—a complex system involving multiple individuals, processes and technology to manage the ordering, verifying, procurement, preparing, distribution, monitoring, and education of medication therapy.

Personal Health Records (PHR)—an Internet-based set of tools that allows people to access and coordinate their lifelong health information and make appropriate parts of it available to those who need it.

Pharmaceutical Care—the responsible provision of drug therapy for the purpose of achieving outcomes that improve a patient's quality of life.

Technology—anything that is used to replace routine or repetitive tasks previously performed by people, or which extends the capability of people.

Introduction

The Institute of Medicine (IOM) has indicated that access to comprehensive health information through the implementation of electronic health records (EHRs) is critical to ensuring the delivery of high-quality, cost-effective, and safe care to patients.[1] Recommendations to implement computerized provider order entry (CPOE) have also been made by both the IOM[2] and the Leapfrog Group[3] to reduce medication errors. Because of these recommendations, health care systems are implementing these solutions, other related technologies, and automation tools at an accelerated pace. These technological advancements are reshaping patient care and medication use processes, thus impacting the roles and responsibilities within various patient care provider groups,

including pharmacy services. It is critical for pharmacy leaders to adapt to these technologically-induced changes by re-evaluating, redefining, and expanding current pharmacy staff roles to ensure optimal system implementation and support, effective medication management, and improved patient outcomes. This chapter will outline the new frontier of EHR and CPOE implementations, the impact they are likely to have on pharmacy services, and present justification and potential opportunities that will exist in the future for the pharmacy profession. The focus of this content will be relevant on inpatient pharmacy practices, however, impact on pharmacy practice within the primary care ambulatory setting will also be addressed.

Summary of EHR and CPOE

The concepts and benefits of an EHR and CPOE have been outlined in numerous publications over the past decade and details regarding these technologies will be outlined in a separate chapter. However, to summarize these concepts and provide clarification, it should be noted that ongoing confusion exists over the difference between EHRs and electronic medical records (EMRs). EMRs are what currently exist in most practices that have adopted them as their legal medical record, but EHRs are the ultimate goal for care delivery organizations (CDOs). EMRs are created, maintained, and owned within CDOs, such as hospitals and physician offices. An application environment composed of the clinical data repository (CDR), clinical decision support (CDS) tools, controlled medical vocabulary (CMV), CPOE, and clinical documentation applications. The patient's electronic record is supported across inpatient and outpatient environments and is used by healthcare practitioners to document, monitor, and manage care delivery within CDOs. The data in the EMR is the legal record of what happened to the patient during encounters at the CDO. EHRs are a longitudinal electronic medical record (EMR) of patient health information generated by one or more encounters in any care delivery setting, containing episodes of care across multiple CDOs within a community, region, or state.

EHRs represent the ability to easily share medical information among stakeholders, across the continuum of care, and through various modalities of care from different CDOs. For example, a patient's medical information can be shared to a referring physician asked to perform a procedure at another CDO. Stakeholders in this context are patients or consumers, healthcare providers, and employers and payers, including the government. An EHR may also include a personal health record (PHR), which documents information such as symptoms or disease management data inputted and controlled by the patient. PHRs offer an integrated and comprehensive view of health information, including information people generate themselves. This includes symptoms and medication use, information from doctors such as diagnoses and test results, and information from their pharmacies and insurance companies. The EHR has the ability to generate a complete record of all clinical patient encounters across the continuum of care. It also supports other care-related activities directly or indirectly via interface, including evidence-based decision support, quality management, and outcomes reporting. For example, a patient's vaccination history can be maintained within the EHR and corresponding decision support tools can alert clinicians that a scheduled vaccination is forthcoming. This functionality can facilitate ordering and communication processes to drive individual care plans as well as lifetime health maintenance plans. This can therefore improve patient throughput within the clinical arena, clinician productivity, and overall quality of care. The broader EHR term will be utilized for the purposes of outlining the concepts within

this chapter to maintain consistency within its content.

CPOE is the portion of the EHR that enables a patient's care provider to electronically enter an order for a medication, clinical laboratory, radiology test, or procedure. The system then transmits the order to the appropriate department or individuals so that it can be carried out. The most advanced implementations of such systems also provide real-time clinical decision support, such as dosage and alternative medication suggestions, duplicate therapy warnings, as well as drug-drug and drug-allergy interaction checking. Broadly defined, implementations of CPOE will vary from very simple systems, such as PDA-based prescription writing software, to fully integrated EHR systems. However, most CPOE implementations are hospital-based and involve several EHR core components: hospital demographic and registration systems, departmental information systems, billing systems, and/or other integrated clinical information systems such as pharmacy or respiratory care systems.

It should be emphasized that EHRs along with CPOE are clinically based tools that significantly impact clinical workflows and, thus, patient care practices. They should be designed and implemented emphasizing operational process re-design, standardization of workflows, and evidence-based medicine. Incorporating inefficient and ineffective processes into an electronic environment will likely lead to equally problematic and potentially error-prone processes.

These systems are most effective when implemented as part of a global integrated medical record across the continuum of care that may include an electric medication administration record (MAR), medication profile, CDS tools, bar code medication administration (BCMA), and other ancillary clinical information system tools or data. Integrated EHRs operating independently or via HL-7 interfaces allow for the exchange of critical patient information into various automation technologies and across patient care environments. For example, medications ordered and verified can be sent across an interface to automated dispensing cabinets (ADCs) utilized on patient care units to facilitate drug distribution. This helps ensure that only medications intended for a particular patient are visible on a patient's medication profile within an ADC. Bi-directional interfaces can then allow dispensing information from the cabinet to flow back to the EHR for appropriate documentation and auditing. This concept is important in the discussions of how these technologies have and will impact pharmacy services and other departments within CDOs. Global adoption and use of EHRs and CPOE is currently limited in this country primarily due to limited system standards, implementation and support costs, and minimal data supporting the return on investment. However, implementations of these systems appear poised to more broadly and rapidly occur within CDOs over the next decade, bringing significant change to health care environments.

Impact of EHR and CPOE on Pharmacy Roles/Responsibilities

As technological advancements have occurred over recent years, pharmacists and pharmacy technicians have become increasingly concerned that the new frontier of EHRs and CPOE systems will decrease the number of positions required to provide pharmacy-related services. Within CDOs, it is likely that administrators will look to cost-justify new technologies through the reduction of various clinical and ancillary staff positions, including pharmacists and pharmacy technicians. This is especially true when evaluating the costs and anticipated benefits expected with EHR and CPOE implementations. However, organizations that have implemented or are in the process

of implementing EHRs and/or CPOE are finding that these systems can often initiate little or no reductions in staff, particularly in patient-centered pharmaceutical care services. In fact, EHRs and CPOE can force an increase in clinical staff resources as the implementation and support of clinical tools requires unique knowledge about clinical and operational workflows across the continuum of care, medical terminology, and clinical application functionality. This increase in clinical staff resources can be a result of the advancement or development of clinical informatics roles required to implement, maintain, and optimize an EHR within a CDO. Increased clinical resource requirements may also be required to respond to the productivity challenges and workflow changes some clinicians or departments experience with the implementation of an EHR. This can be particularly true for pharmacy services, as organizations have recognized the financial and patient care impact of the clinical pharmacist role across the continuum of care, the advancing age of the U.S. population treated with multiple medications, the increased number and complexity of medications utilized within the patient population, and the knowledge required to manage medication use systems integrated within EHRs and CPOE. However, as EHRs and CPOE technologies advance within organizations, a reduction in the number of pharmacist positions working in the traditional preparing and dispensing roles should be anticipated. At the same time, advancements within a patient-centered pharmaceutical care or non-traditional pharmacy roles, such as pharmacy informatics, have already started, and this trend is expected to continue.

Current Roles in Pharmacy

Significant advances within pharmacy roles and responsibilities have occurred over the past few decades. However, many organizations have not transitioned pharmacy staff resources out of traditional roles and responsibilities due to a number of potential factors including: lack of consensus regarding the profession's scope and goals, resistance to broadening the pharmacist's or pharmacy technician responsibilities beyond dispensing functions, lack of professional competence and/or self-confidence, the false impression that managed care invariably will decrease pharmacist demand, dissension surrounding adoption of the doctor of pharmacy as the sole professional degree, work environments/operational processes or workflows that provide little or no opportunity for patient-centered practice, lack of reimbursement for pharmacists' clinical services, and underdevelopment of practitioners' interpersonal skills.[4] Administrative support and knowledge regarding the benefits pharmacy resources can provide to overall patient care services through advanced pharmaceutical care and leadership of medication use systems is also a significant factor in determining the level of advancement of pharmacy services within an organization.

Despite these barriers, the roles of pharmacists and pharmacy technicians have continued to change immensely over the past number of decades. The practice of pharmacy is evolving away from a focus on traditional dispensing activities to one that focuses on clinical or pharmaceutical care. Pharmaceutical care has been defined as the responsible provision of drug therapy for the purpose of achieving outcomes that improve a patient's quality of life.[5] Thus, pharmaceutical care represents a fundamental paradigm shift highlighting that pharmacy services can help improve patient care and provide more than just a product or ancillary service. This concept also emphasizes the need for pharmacists to accept broader responsibility for the results of patient care that they deliver. Pharmacy training and education programs are attempting to keep pace with the expanding role of pharma-

cists, and pharmacy leaders are working to advance pharmacy technician training as well. Evidence has shown that integrating pharmacists within patient-centered teams with a focus on pharmaceutical care in a variety of patient care settings reduces medication related errors, decreases overall healthcare costs, and improves patient care.[6-13] This information demonstrates how pharmacy services are expanding into new patient care horizons. However, there are arguments that much more work must be done to ensure that pharmacists and pharmacy as a whole are recognized globally as an integral part of the health care team.[14] This will be critical to the ongoing roles and responsibilities of pharmacy services as advancing technologies are implemented.

Pharmacists currently perform many different activities within various CDO settings. These include the traditional order review and entry, product purchasing, preparation and dispensing/distribution activities, clinical monitoring activities, drug utilization review, drug information, and educational services. These responsibilities are well documented, and the American Society of Health-System Pharmacists (ASHP), as well as other pharmacy organizations, has developed best practice policies and standards around these activities to ensure that these are practiced at a high level of quality. A report, "The Pharmacist Workforce: A Study of the Supply and Demand for Pharmacists," by the Department of Health and Human Services, submitted to Congress in 2000, also summarizes many key findings regarding pharmacists' roles in ambulatory care settings, disease management programs, cost containment, managed care, hospitals, and various other health care settings.[15]

Organizations have been successful in re-engineering medication use systems and committing pharmacists' time from distributive to pharmaceutical care roles. However, pharmacists still struggle to break away from the dispensing roles even when positioned within a patient care environment that allows for the advancement of pharmaceutical care. Also, pharmacy technicians are not always positioned in the most efficient or effective roles to maximize their skills and allow for pharmacists to transition away from dispensing or other non-clinically focused roles. These issues are often a result of the issues outlined earlier and must be addressed by pharmacy leaders to ensure success in managing medication use systems and optimizing patient care, especially as technologies such as EHRs and CPOE impact organizations.

Table 9-1 outlines key future roles and responsibilities changes for pharmacy technicians with EHR and/or CPOE.

TABLE 9-1

Key Future Roles/Responsibilities Changes for Pharmacy Technicians with EHR and/or CPOE

Clinical Pharmacy Technician/Pharmacist Assistant
Clinical services

- Perform medication admission histories with appropriate pharmacists oversight and verification.

- Initiate and promote a culture of safety within a CDO.

Distributive services

- Assists pharmacists in verifying patient allergy information, heights and weights, or other specific patient-related information when necessary.

- Decentralized drug distributive roles to coordinate and maximize medication distribution processes, streamline workflows and reduce workload on nursing staff.

EHR/CPOE system implementation

- Participate in EHR/CPOE workflow analysis and re-design activities as they relate to the pharmacy technician role.

- Serve as a CPOE "super user" supportive role to provide real-time order entry support to physicians, physician extenders, and nursing staff during system implementation.

- Initiate and promote a culture of safety within a CDO.

EHR/CPOE system support/optimization

- Decentralized CPOE education and supportive role or "unit-based trainer" to provide real-time order entry support to physicians, physician extenders, and nursing staff.

QA monitoring

- Independently perform PCA checks and document appropriate parameters accordingly.

- Monitor and respond to ADS, BCMA, and other medication use reports to ensure optimal drug distribution.

Pharmacy Informatics Technician
EHR/CPOE system implementation

- Assist in system testing and validation processes.

- Assist with training pharmacy users on workflows and system functionality as they related to EHR, CPOE, and other clinical information systems.

TABLE 9-1 (CONT'D)

Key Future Roles/Responsibilities Changes
for Pharmacy Technicians with EHR and/or CPOE

- Build and maintain medication record, preference list, standardized order set, and clinical decision support tools under the supervision and guidance of a pharmacist informaticist.

- Develop/update training materials, supplemental training information, and competencies related to system functionality and workflows.

- Initiate and promote a culture of safety within a CDO.

EHR/CPOE system support/optimization

- Decentralized CPOE education and supportive role or "unit-based trainer" to provide real-time order entry support to physicians, physician extenders, and nursing staff.

- Maintain and adjust formulary and other miscellaneous databases.

- Management ADS interfaces and integrated workflows within EHR/CPOE or other clinical information systems.

Miscellaneous technology development/support

- Develop and manage pharmacy department website.

- Implement and maintain medication-related web-based resources and other educational/information tools.

QA monitoring

- Report development and management activities to monitor ADS, BCMA, and other medication use processes for quality assurance.

Future Opportunities and Challenges for Pharmacy

There are approximately 250,000 pharmacists practicing in the U.S.,[16] and demand for their services is growing as the population ages, drug utilization increases, and the need for improved medication use processes continues, leading to increasingly diverse and challenging career opportunities for pharmacists. The Pharmacy Manpower project published in 2002 projected that over 400,000 pharmacists will be needed to adequately meet forecasts of market demand for pharmacists in the year 2020.[17] The project assumes that high-quality pharmaceutical care advancements will occur over the next decade through the re-engineering of medication use systems along with pharmacists' roles from distributive functions to more pharmaceutical care and informatics roles. The advancement of pharmacy technician roles and technologies, including automation technology, EHRs, and CPOE, are expected to contribute to this change.

Minimal data and detailed evidence exists to outline the specific impact EHRs and/or CPOE will have on pharmacy services. A case study outlined by Manzo et al.[18] presents an excellent overview outlining the impact that EHRs and CPOE implementations can have on pharmacy staff and medication use processes. This study demonstrated a reduction in overall pharmacy workload in one site while another site noted the workload impact to be neutral. It also cited that each hospital in the study saw an increase in pharmacy personnel expenses required to assist in the implementation and support of the EHR, CPOE, and pharmacy automation. A series of additional articles outlining the design, implementation, and support of EHRs, CPOE, and supporting clinical decision support (CDS) tools also provide useful information regarding pharmacy's perspective on this technology.[19-25] This information is consistent with most other anecdotal information available within the literature and discussed in various organizations' meetings, listservs, commentaries,[26] and other pharmacy information venues. Despite limited data, it is still evident that medication use processes are a part of most patient care environments found within CDOs, justifying the need for pharmacy resources to provide leadership within EHR and CPOE projects, to ensure that these processes are designed, implemented, and maintained in a safe and effective fashion. A summary of the impact with challenges and opportunities that an EHR and CPOE can have on varying pharmacy services follows.

Distributive Roles

It was noted previously that the existence of the pharmacist's traditional distributive roles of preparing and distributing medications will most certainly be reduced as technicians, pharmacy automation technologies, and EHR/CPOE become increasingly responsible for dispensing, communication, and ordering activities. The anticipated time reduction on distributive pharmacist responsibilities is likely to be organizational specific and dependent on technician resources and skill set, the level of advanced automated technology implemented, EHR/CPOE design and level of integration, clinician usability, knowledge base, and acceptance as well as administrative support for advanced pharmaceutical care.

Technician Distributive Role

Also indicated previously, an EHR and CPOE are most effective when implemented as part of an integrated system that may include an electronic MAR. Integration allows for improved communication and information/data exchanges making critical patient care information readily available within multiple applications to all clinicians. Pharmacy-related workflows can be improved significantly, thus creating increased opportunities for pharmaceutical care responsibilities. An integrated EHR has also been shown to streamline medication billing processes within pharmacies when implemented with charge on administration versus the traditional charge on dispense billing method. While posing charge capture risks, if medication documentation practices are poor and without proper monitoring and accountability, this can virtually eliminate pharmacy technician time spent on manual medication billing, crediting, and reconciliation. Manzo et al. indicated an estimated elimination of 12–15 minutes from every patient care unit cart-fill each day.[18] Similar outcomes have been noted by other organizations with a potential to reduce these pharmacy technician billing activities by 4–12 hours each day depending on dispensing volumes. These hours may be re-directed to other distributive or non-traditional activities, thus maximizing technician resources and potentially freeing up pharmacist time to focus on pharmaceutical care activities.

As technology continues to advance, technicians are likely to be expected to oversee primary dispensing and preparation activities, automated dispensing system processes, IV pump management, and pharmacy responsibilities within BCMA systems. Technicians may also take on other medication use system support roles across the continuum of care that will minimize pharmacist involvement with traditional responsibilities. These could include decentralized drug distributive roles that can maximize medication distribution processes, streamline workflows, and reduce workload on nursing staff. Organizations are beginning to utilize pharmacy technicians in nursing assistant–type roles to ensure that medications are readily available in an organized and streamlined fashion on the patient care units. These technicians obtain medications from decentralized automated dispensing cabinets, pharmacy satellites, or central pharmacy services as scheduled and transfer them to nurse medication carts or servers. This can reduce nursing time utilized to search for and gather scheduled medications, thus freeing up their time to provide patient-centered care activities. Others are involving technicians within the medication reconciliation process to perform medication admission histories. For example, Michels et al.[27] developed a pharmacy technician managed medication admission history program that incorporated a pharmacy technician role into the admissions department. The technician telephoned patients scheduled for surgery 1–2 days before admission to obtain a baseline medication history, including nonprescription medications, herbals, vitamins, and other critical patient information. This information was collected and documented on a medication history order form and entered into the pharmacy computer system. Once verified by a pharmacist, the medication history form was made available for the surgeon to review and order necessary prior to admission medications before or after surgery. An analysis of this program reported a statistically significant reduction in medication history–related errors and clinicians perceived the program to be safer, more accurate, and more efficient than the previous nurse-driven program.

Both of these opportunities open up new horizons for technician roles and offer career advancement opportunities outside the routine technician responsibilities. Additional pharmacy technician opportunities within clinical informatics will be outlined later in this chapter.

Pharmacist Distributive and Order Entry Role

The advent of an EHR and CPOE are likely to impact distributive pharmacist responsibilities as well. Assuming effective system design, adherence to mandatory CPOE policies, and adequate physician-focused order entry training, this functionality can eliminate all or a portion of pharmacist-entered orders, thus inducing electronic pharmacist order verification processes. An ASHP shared members group surveyed hospitals across the country to gain knowledge of CPOE verification processes being utilized and their impact on pharmacy roles.[28] This did not provide extensive discrete detail about the impact CPOE has had on various sites. However, most hospitals reported gained efficiencies within pharmacy department medication order processes thus allowing pharmacists to focus on other activities. It should be noted that electronic pharmacist order verification can vary depending on the level of EHR integration. Fully integrated EHRs allow pharmacists to receive medications electronically into a verification queue, thus streamlining the verification process and eliminating transcription. Other systems may require pharmacists to verify physician-placed orders in one system and transcribe those orders into a self-contained pharmacy system.

CPOE has been shown to reduce medication prescribing errors by as much as 50%,[18] and to cut medication turn-around times by approximately 43%–60%.[18,22] These improvements not only improve patient safety but are likely to minimize pharmacist time needed for order clarifications or missing medication follow-up. Turn-around time expectations do change with the insertion of CPOE and the electronic MAR because this puts the rate-limiting step emphasis on pharmacy order verification and dispensing time. This is seen with CPOE and EHRs because the medication order becomes immediately or more readily visible to nursing staff and other clinicians on the electronic MAR or within other medication order review tools. This visibility inherently makes everyone more aware of the medication availability, thus putting emphasis on distributive pharmacy services. This will require an evaluation of medication turn-around time policies and expectations. Decisions regarding these expectations may justify the need to maintain current pharmacy dispensing resources or advance internal distributive and communication technologies, thus neutralizing potential cost savings or the possibility of shifting distributive responsibilities away from pharmacists.

CPOE with CDS can also improve non-formulary and therapeutic substitution decisions within physician ordering processes.[18] These systems can be designed to alert or even prevent physicians from ordering medication therapies defined by hospital formulary policies. This not only improves formulary management and drug costs but reduces pharmacists' time by eliminating follow-up interactions needed to address inappropriate orders. It should be noted that this will vary by organization based on system functionality and design as well as physician training, compliance, and acceptance. For example, some organizations may not be able to design systems to manage medication policies because affiliated hospitals or clinics may share the same system or database but not the same policies or medication formulary.

Pharmacists may still spend significant time involved with the order entry process through frequent corrections of incorrectly entered physician orders encountered during the order verification process. This may be most significant during the initial post-CPOE go-live phase, as physician learning curves increase, but can continue on indefinitely with complex orders, poor system design, or lack of physician adherence to order entry policies. While physi-

cians should positively report fewer clarification interactions from pharmacists, they will desire continued pharmacist presence within the medication ordering processes. Complex or non-standard orders are most likely to continue to require some pharmacist or clinical pharmacy technician intervention. These might include TPN therapy orders, non-standard IV admixtures, or new therapies. Internal policies and procedures around pharmacist order entry corrections must exist to ensure that the integrity of the original order was not misinterpreted or changed. For example, a physician may enter an IV admixture order for a medication using a non-standard base solution. Initial pharmacist interpretation of the order may be that this was entered in error and to modify the order to the standard solution. This assumption may be incorrect and induce a less than desirable clinical outcome if not identified and clarified by a nurse during order verification. Timeliness and communication of order changes must also be addressed to ensure that medication therapy delays are not initiated. This will require system functionality, external communication processes, or standard protocols to ensure that physicians have verified and approved these changes.

CDS tools built within CPOE systems including drug allergy, dose, duplicate therapy and drug interaction alerts all have the potential to improve patient care but can impact clinician workflow and responsibilities. Frequent alerts that may be obvious or even inaccurate can become frustrating for clinicians leading to "alert fatigue." When this occurs, physicians may ignore or override these alerts all together, thus placing the burden on pharmacists to evaluate the significance of these alerts. This can create patient safety concerns if pharmacists do not contact the physician, since they ignored the alert. However, physician backlash may occur if pharmacists frequently call to clarify orders due to these alerts. CDOs need to make sure that system alert settings are appropriately reviewed and approved by a multidisciplinary group of clinicians prior to implementation of CDS tools. Policies and procedures, along with effective training and system design, can also help mitigate the impact alerts may have on pharmacists. For example, systems that allow physicians to document why the alert was overridden may permit pharmacists to easily view these reasons during order verification thus reducing the need for a follow-up phone call. Additionally, responsibilities regarding automatic stop orders and expiring medication orders will need to be defined clearly for pharmacy, nursing, and physician staff. This example points out the importance of pre-implementation system design and planning of CDS tools with proper clinician input and approval to ensure that they effective and efficiently support internal clinical and administrative requirements.

Another area within CPOE that appears to be problematic for pharmacists involves the entry of duplicate medication orders and dispensable product selection errors. Pharmacists should use caution within their verification processes to ensure that duplicate therapy and product selection errors do not occur and must monitor physician order entry carefully. Confirmation of correct product selection is critical to verify that appropriate order components are utilized during product preparation and are important to automated dispensing cabinet drug availability. An example of this occurs with ordering of fentanyl drips which could be ordered using a variety of different concentrations. Physicians will enter the correct rate at which they want to run the drip at but they don't necessary know or care which fentanyl strength, IV solution, or volume to choose. This requires the pharmacist to interpret and modify the order to the appropriate strength and volume and if uncertain a call back to the physician would be required causing delays in patient therapy. Therefore, these

issues have the potential to increase order clarification follow-up time for pharmacists, thus minimizing other positive time-saving opportunities offered by EHRs and CPOE. Pharmacist involvement with system design or optimization may allow for optimal development of system alerts, functional triggers, or robust medication preference lists and order sets to prevent these issues.

Other workflow-related changes that can impact pharmacist dispensing roles include patient transitions across various patient care settings, the transition to an electronic order format and workflow challenges in non-mandatory CPOE environments. Patient care transitions can create difficult medication use processes if the system is not functioning in an integrated fashion well. If medication orders do not transition with the patient in a timely matter, medication dispensing, administration, and billing processes become difficult. Integrated EHRs also open up new ambulatory to inpatient integrated workflow opportunities for pharmacists in dispensing and order verification roles. Ambulatory care areas and other hospital service departments not typically linked to inpatient pharmacy services may be able to send electronic orders directly to the pharmacy for verification, dispensing, and billing. This can potentially streamline processes for these other departments and assist in adherence with pharmacy verification of medication order standards.

However, depending on the level of pharmacy services provided to these care areas prior to implementation of an EHR, an increase in pharmacists' time may be seen since this can increase the overall number of orders being verified and processed. For example, prior to EHR implementation, an ambulatory hospital-based clinic may have stocked and maintained Epogen within the clinic. They may order this in bulk from the pharmacy or an outside pharmaceutical supplier and charge the patient as part of his or her clinic visit. This structure may be non-compliant with medication order verification, preparation, and storage standards as many ambulatory care areas are often challenged to meet the necessary requirements. Also, incorrect or non-compliant billing of these medications may induce significant revenue loss. Therefore, a CDO may decide to utilize an EHR to change this process and allow for pharmacy verification, preparation, and charging of the medication, thus improving adherence to standards related to these processes.

The change from the written to electronic medication order format also presents issues for pharmacy order entry workflows. In the paper order world, pharmacists often identified relevant non-medication orders such as lab values, procedures performed, or clinical consults pending during medication order processing. These orders often help pharmacists assess patient response to medication therapy or plan anticipated pharmaceutical care requirements. However, with CPOE and order verification these non-medication orders may not be readily visible, depending on system design and functionality. Whenever possible, systems need to account for this, and real-time alerts, clinical tools, or reports should be made available for pharmacists to easily review. Pharmacists may also have a difficult time adjusting to electronic order verification, since they will not have a paper order to compare with the electronic order.

Pharmacists have to learn to accept this change and trust the system's design and usability while maintaining appropriate critical thinking. Many clinicians, including pharmacists, working in the EHR and CPOE world become complacent with the data entered into the system because it is computerized information and legible. Just because an order or document is computerized and legible does not mean that it is appropriate. Clinicians can easily select the incorrect medication record or patient, order the wrong dose or frequency, and ignore

a significant system generated alert. It is therefore important to educate clinicians to closely evaluate and scrutinize electronically generated documentation and orders just as they would in the paper world. Change management strategies may be required to gain a delicate balance between clinicians trusting the system and its efficiencies, while continuing to critically evaluate data entered into the system. Significant clinician involvement with system and workflow design, prior to implementation, and post-implementation optimization strategies, should be part of this change management strategy.

Initial CPOE entry errors likely to occur after implementation (especially those related to dispensable product selection) will make this transition difficult for pharmacists. Additional training and change management modalities may need to be utilized to minimize the overall impact of these issues. Organizations functioning in a non-mandatory CPOE environment should expect additional workflow challenges. This initiates dual manual and electronic order processing models for pharmacy and other ancillary service department staff. Medication order verification policies may need to have different requirements if an order is verified through CPOE processes versus non-CPOE ordering processes. Non-standardized processes and workflows can lead to errors since clinicians could follow the same workflow for all ordering processes. Also, these disjointed workflows could collide leading to a medication error. For example, a resident physician utilizing the CPOE system may enter an order for a one-time "stat" IV morphine dose but at the same time the attending physician may verbally order or place a paper order for the same medication on the same patient. Depending on process timing and availability of this medication to the nurse, the patient could inadvertently receive two doses of morphine, if given prior to pharmacist processing, verification, and clarification of each order. Therefore, it is likely that this dual world will increase order processing time and potentially increase the risk of order entry errors. These issues ultimately result in minimizing the anticipated benefits of this technology.

It is difficult to quantify actual time impact on distributive and order entry roles within pharmacy. The extent of impact is likely to vary between different CDOs since system design, current level of pharmacy resources allocated to distributive roles, the level of already implemented automation technology, and CPOE requirements for physicians are inconsistent. With that said, current information suggests that the overall impact on pharmacy distributive and order entry roles is likely to be neutral or reduced, thus initiating the probable transition to more pharmaceutical care activities.

Pharmaceutical Care Roles

As suggested previously, the transition of the pharmacist distributive role to a cognitive provider of pharmaceutical care can be significantly enhanced by EHRs. This technology can efficiently and effectively provide pharmacists real-time and historical patient-specific information about patient diagnosis or disease state, laboratory and culture results, treatment progress and plan, as well as the patient's entire medication history profile. EHRs also provide clinicians with real-time and retrospective data through advanced reporting capabilities. This information is often available across the continuum of care and further improves the wealth of information available to clinically focused pharmacists and other clinicians, allowing for better educated clinical decisions to be made and medication use process improvements.

Pharmacist interactions with other clinicians, and in particular physicians, is likely to change post EHR or CPOE implementation, particularly once physicians become proficient in entering medication orders and document patient care progress notes efficiently. Once an organization is functioning effectively within an EHR environment, direct communications between clinicians may diminish as more real-time documentation and order information becomes readily available within the system and clarification interactions are eliminated. While these systems improve patient communications through improved access to patient information, it should not completely replace the need to effectively interact with other clinicians to ensure optimal patient care. Complacency or reliance on the system as being 100% accurate should be avoided to prevent unpredictable system-induced errors. This further justifies the need for the advancement of pharmaceutical care services as traditional distributive-related communications are likely to be minimized with these technologies. Integrated EHRs and automation technologies can provide pharmacists increased opportunities to work more closely with physicians, other healthcare providers, and patients to assure that optimal pharmaceutical care and patient outcomes if approached correctly. The routine attendance on multidisciplinary patient care rounds, physician or nursing educational sessions, and medication management related committees provide additional opportunities to maintain effective communications and build working relationships with other disciplines.

EHRs and CPOE systems can be built to provide clinicians with extensive and efficient access to drug information, medication formularies, as well as medication-related protocols and guidelines. CDS tools built within these systems will also provide additional prescribing guidance regarding appropriate dosing, product selection, and formulary adherence. This access is likely to diminish pharmacists' time spent communicating or educating other clinicians in these areas. While electronic drug information resources and CDS tools cannot replace pharmacists as a true pharmaceutical care resource, they provide clinicians with easily accessed or automated tools to handle less complex medication-related information efficiently. This should offer more time for clinical pharmacists to focus on medication error reduction initiatives through pharmaceutical care responsibilities such as patient education programs, medication reconciliation, and development of and executing a pharmaceutical care plan or other medication therapy management opportunities. Pharmacists' dedication to patient education programs and medication reconciliation will be particularly valuable as CDOs look to meet the IOM recommendations[29] and Joint Commission standards.[30] These inpatient and ambulatory programs should focus on patient involvement with medication management. This can include medication histories, self-medication programs, reviews of medication administration records, and medication counseling.[31] EHRs can provide tools to facilitate these processes more efficiently and effectively. PHR can also be utilized to involve patients more extensively with medication management by allowing them to monitor medication therapies through lab and vitals monitoring from home. Pharmacists can interact with patient's via PHR technology to engage patient's in self-monitoring of this information, reducing clinic visits and potentially hospital admissions. Table 9-2 provides a listing of additional key post EHR/CPOE clinical inpatient and ambulatory care pharmacist responsibilities as a reference.

It should also be noted that due to the available information and probable communications changes to occur with EHR and CPOE implementations, pharmacist-documented interventions are likely to change in quantity and type. Fewer clarification-type interventions and a shift to more medication management, reconciliation, and patient education interventions are likely to be noted following the implementation of

these technologies. New types of interventions may also need to be developed and incorporated into intervention documentation tools. Order verification type interventions will need to be included to address CPOE-related order issues such as order timing, duration of therapy, and dispensable product selections. Pharmacy leaders that currently monitor and utilize intervention data to justify pharmacy resources will need to evaluate this closely in order to interpret and communicate changes in this data as necessary. The data available through the advent of an EHR and CPOE will also allow pharmacists to take on medication safety monitoring roles by evaluating the frequency of errors and near-misses, so that timely corrections to workflows, policy and procedures, clinical information systems, automated technology and the overall medication use process can be made. This information is therefore valuable in continuously identifying areas for improvement within EHR and CPOE system design and clinician education efforts.

This information demonstrates that clinical pharmacist roles will primarily gain efficiencies following the implementation of EHRs and CPOE. This is not only anticipated in inpatient or hospital-based pharmacist roles, but clinical pharmacists providing pharmaceutical care within ambulatory care settings, disease management programs, and emergency departments can anticipate a similar effect. These changes will continue to challenge pharmacy leaders and pharmacists to advance true pharmaceutical care responsibilities in current settings or look to develop clinical pharmacy services into other non-traditional settings such as clinical informatics.

Clinical Informatics Role

Medical or clinical informatics is the scientific study of the effective analysis, use, and dissemination of information in patient care, clinical research, and medical education. The ultimate goals of clinical informat-

TABLE 9-2

Key Future Roles/Responsibilities Changes
for Pharmacists with EHR and/or CPOE Implementation

Inpatient and Ambulatory Care/Disease Management Clinical Pharmacists

Clinical pharmaceutical care services

- Document all pharmaceutical care provided within the patient's EHR.

- Identify and initiate effective preventative medication management therapies as part of the multi-disciplinary patient care team.

- Initiate or modify medication therapies based on patient responses or clinical interpretations.

- Initiate pharmacokinetic dosing adjustments as necessary.

- Order laboratory tests necessary for monitoring outcomes of medication therapy.

- Perform medication reconciliation activities across the continuum of care (ambulatory visit medication histories, inpatient medication admission histories, inpatient discharge medication order reconciliation, personal medication record reviews, and provide patient teaching).

- Provide collaborative drug therapy management for medications and diseases which require specialized monitoring, patient assessment, and education.

- Coordinate and oversee medication use processes across the continuum of care.

- Facilitate efficient information exchange and continuity of care for patient's medication regimens.

- Routinely monitor medication therapy literature for adverse drug reaction and drug error information and initiate preventative actions.

- Take on medication safety monitoring roles by evaluating the frequency of errors and near-misses, so that timely corrections to workflows, policy and procedures, clinical information systems, automated technology and the overall medication use process can be made.

- Initiate patient education programs that allow pharmacists to focus on patient education and get patients involved with their own medication therapy.

- Interact with patients via PHR technology to engage patients in self-monitoring of key lab values and vitals signs as well as with their overall medication management.

- Initiate and promote a culture of safety within a CDO.

Cost containment/formulary management

- Communicate with health management payers to resolve issues that interfere with access to medications.

- Develop, implement, and oversee programs that ensure cost-effective use of medication therapy.

EHR/CPOE system implementation

- Participate in EHR/CPOE/e-prescribing system design including CDS tools (e.g., rules, alerts, order sets, preference lists, treatment guidelines/plans, etc.).

- Participate in medication use policy activities related to CPOE and other system driven medication use processes.

- Participate in EHR/CPOE workflow analysis and re-design activities.

TABLE 9-2 (CONT'D)

Key Future Roles/Responsibilities Changes
for Pharmacists with EHR and/or CPOE Implementation

- Serve as a CPOE "super user" supportive role to provide real-time order entry support to physicians, physician extenders, and nursing staff during system implementation.

EHR/CPOE system support/optimization

- Participate in clinical informatics activities that support medication use processes.

- Participate on key multidisciplinary committees and provide recommendations for strategies around the development and integration of pharmaceutical care activities using information technology.

- Serve as a CPOE "super user" supportive role to provide real-time order entry support to physicians, physician extenders, and nursing staff post-implementation.

QA monitoring

- Assist in the organizational monitoring of CDS tools to analyze and determine effectiveness and benefits of tools used in production environment. Make recommendations for changes to CDS tools as required.

- Develop, implement, and oversee medication error and adverse drug reaction prevention and reporting programs.

Inpatient Clinical Pharmacists Only
Clinical pharmaceutical care services

- Coordinate services to maximize patient medication therapy compliance, including medication administration teaching and medication counseling.

- Participate in multidisciplinary patient care team rounds to review patient progress and assure the appropriate use of medications.

Cost containment/formulary management

- Maximize timely transitions from intravenous to oral therapy.

Distributive services

- Monitor ADC override activity and verify appropriateness of medications dispensed and administered prior to pharmacist verification.

- Review and verify all physician entered medication orders to verify they are appropriate for a given patient.

Ambulatory Care/Disease Management Clinical Pharmacists Only
Clinical services

- Coordinate services to maximize patient medication therapy compliance including medication administration teaching, counseling, and automated prescription refill reminder and incentive programs.

- Perform limited physical assessments and oversee medication treatments with collaborative drug therapy management authority.

TABLE 9-2 (CONT'D)

Key Future Roles/Responsibilities Changes for Pharmacists with EHR and/or CPOE Implementation

- Provide individualized health promotion and disease prevention, including administration of immunizations in locations that legally and organizationally authorize this.

- Review and clinically respond to electronic medication orders and/or disease management service orders for a given patient.

Informatics Pharmacist

EHR/CPOE system implementation

- Assist in global system functional testing to ensure that the system is working as designed and is efficiently usable for clinicians during the medication order entry process.

- Assist in interface design and planning, especially those key to communications with pharmacy applications and/or automation.

- Assess medication-use systems for vulnerabilities to medication errors and proactively implement strategies to prevent these errors.

- Design, test, and implement CDS tools (e.g., rules, alerts, order sets, preference lists, treatment guidelines/plans, etc.) incorporated into EHR and CPOE systems.

- Develop and implement standards for medication-related vocabularies and terminologies within medication use process and technologies.

- Coordinate training plan and training materials for pharmacy users on workflows and system functionality as they related to EHR, CPOE, and other clinical information systems. Contribute to training processes for other users where medication management processes are utilized within the system.

- Participate in the development and review of CPOE and other medication use process training materials.

- Provide leadership and coordinate EHR/CPOE workflow analysis and re-design activities.

- Provide leadership and coordinate medication use policy development activities related to CPOE and other system driven medication use processes.

- Serve as primary EHR/CPOE support staff for pharmacists, physicians, physician extenders, and nursing staff during system implementation.

- Work closely with information technology, pharmacy staff, and other clinical staff to develop system programming requirements needed to facilitate integrated clinical and distributive workflows.

- Initiate and promote a culture of safety within a CDO.

EHR/CPOE system support/optimization

- Coordinate medication use policy activities related to CPOE and other system driven medication use processes.

- Manage databases related to medication management processes built within EHR and CPOE systems.

- Monitor all existing decision support tools in place throughout the CPOE system to ensure continued scientific and clinical relevance and appropriateness, making modifications to tools as necessary.

TABLE 9-2 (CONT'D)

Key Future Roles/Responsibilities Changes
for Pharmacists with EHR and/or CPOE Implementation

ate and provide leadership in all clinical informatics activities that support medication use
es.

ate in the identification and resolution of system issues utilizing system knowledge,
troubleshooting techniques to provide suggested solutions to identified system problems.

- Participate on key multidisciplinary committees and provide leadership for strategies around the development and integration of pharmaceutical care activities using information technology.

- Provide system support and optimization processes to ensure safe, efficient, and effective use of EHR and CPOE systems.

- Serve as primary EHR/CPOE support staff for pharmacists, physicians, physician extenders, and nursing staff post-implementation.

- Serve as primary communication conduit to medical, pharmacy, nursing, and IT staff with regard to the implementation of new or modified CPOE clinical decision support tools.

- Support safe drug administrative, documentation, ordering, and reconciliation practices through leadership and development of EHR and CPOE system workflow design, build, validation, and staff education.

- Initiate and promote a culture of safety within a CDO.

Miscellaneous technology development/support

- Manage medication-related, web-based resources and other educational or information tools.

- Oversee pharmacy department website design, implementation, and support.

- Provide a unique understanding of patient care workflows and medication use processes as well as project and time management, data analysis, and pharmaceutical care skills.

- Provide oversight of all pharmacy technician informaticist activities.

- Provide recommendations for various device solutions that can effectively accommodate clinician workflows and medication use processes in a variety of different patient care environments.

- Serve as liaison between IT, pharmacy, and other hospital departments, as well as vendor representatives during CPOE application research, design, implementation, and maintenance processes.

QA monitoring

- Assist in the mining, collating, analyzing, and interpreting of data from these systems to improve patient outcomes.

- Oversee report monitoring activities to monitor clinical decision support activity and medication use processes for effectiveness and quality assurance.

- Take on medication safety monitoring roles by evaluating the frequency of errors and near-misses, so that timely corrections to workflows, policy and procedures, clinical information systems, automated technology, and the overall medication use process can be made.

ics are to streamline the processes of patient care, to provide clinicians with accurate data in a timely manner, improve the quality of care, and to reduce costs. The broad definition of clinical informatics and the number of varying disciplines involved present ongoing opportunities for the advancement of pharmacy as a member of the clinical informatics field. Pharmacy informatics can be defined as the use and integration of data, information, knowledge, technology, and automation in the medication use process for the purpose of improving health outcomes.[29] While clinical informatics growth has tended to create subspecialties of informaticians, it is critical to integrate the knowledge base of these individuals, especially with today's more advanced technologies. A clinical informatician must possess a unique combination of knowledge about clinical workflows, clinical information systems, and related technologies and the issues of medical terminology, codification, and data measurements. This knowledge allows informaticians to play an important role in translating the clinical knowledge and workflow needs of clinicians into the functional system requirements and specifications for the design of the database, clinical operation and business processes, and user interface that are essential for technologies, such as EHRs, to successfully improve patient care services. While pharmacy probably has more experience in using technology than other clinicians including physicians and nurses, these other groups have made more significant advancements in integrating and expanding their knowledge base and involvement within a global clinical informatics community. Therefore, it is important for pharmacy and other clinician communities to embrace a more global role within clinical informatics and avoid a subspecialty silo. This is particularly important as EHRs and CPOE systems become more integrated.

Informatician roles may or may not fall under the information technology (IT) umbrella, but either way must maintain knowledge of their sub-specialty practice standards and workflows, gain global understanding of other sub-specialty workflows, and become proficient with system functionality and requirements in order to play a key role in the decision-making processes involved with the implementation and support of EHRs. All departments need to accept that an integrated EHR is not "their" system but "everyone's" system, including the patient. A key benefit of newer EHR and CPOE systems is that pharmacy and other clinicians involved in the medication use process will no longer be separate from each other. These systems will have applications, modules, and tools that are interwoven, with boundaries that are absent or fluid.[30] This concept is much different from the department specific clinical information system managed internally. Medication use processes within EHRs and CPOE become part of and impact all department workflows across the continuum of care. This justifies the need for the advancement of pharmacists and pharmacy technicians into the global clinical informatics team.

Pharmacy resources from all patient care settings must be involved with the implementation of an EHR and CPOE. These roles could be less time intensive such as "super user" roles, part-time implementation and optimization team roles, or more dedicated full-time informatics pharmacist and technician roles. There also needs to be appropriate pharmacy leadership involvement or a "pharmacy champion" for these projects. This can be the director of pharmacy, pharmacy informatics manager, or another pharmacy leader that can effectively represent pharmacy, make key pharmacy-related decisions, and provide recommendations and other contributions to global EHR and CPOE processes.

The number of pharmacy resources needed for an EHR and/or CPOE implementation can vary depending on size of

CDO, scope of system implementation, organization commitment/priority, vendor variances, and timeline of project and support requirements. Experience is showing that these implementations can require very large numbers of IT and clinical resources and more successful implementations typically dedicate more clinical resources to these efforts. CDOs should consult with vendors for implementation and support resource recommendations as different vendors follow different implementation models. It is also recommended to utilize internal staff versus consultants whenever possible to implement and support EHR and CPOE implementations. While dedicating full-time employees to these efforts can be costly, consultant resources are equally expensive. Consultants hold little accountability to produce high-quality results and often leave without proper knowledge transfer to internal resources. This can leave an organization open to future functionality risks if system issues develop, and it minimizes potential optimization opportunities.

This all leads to the idea that clinical operations and financial groups, rather than IT, should manage today's more complex EHRs, CPOE, and other integrated clinical information systems. Implementation, support, and optimization responsibilities will require non-IT evaluations to ensure that system design or changes meet clinical, policy, and billing requirements within a CDO. IT still plays a critical role in the implementation and support of these systems but should focus on hardware, security, and network infrastructure requirements to ensure that the EHR clinical tools in today's healthcare can be used efficiently and effectively without performance concerns.

Pharmacist Informaticists

Pharmacists have historically worked with clinical information systems more extensively than most other clinician groups. This experience serves pharmacists well with the advancement of EHRs, CPOE, CDS, and other integrated technologies. This is particularly true with CPOE implementations as up to 40% of all orders within a CDO can be medication orders.[30] Pharmacists can provide a unique understanding of patient care workflows and medication use processes as well as project and time management, data analysis, and pharmaceutical care skills.[30] This blend of expertise allows pharmacists to play a pivotal role in the success of CPOE and other technology-related implementations.

Currently, there are many paths to becoming a pharmacy informaticist, with a growing number of training and residency programs focusing on this area. Although some pharmacy informaticists have formal academic or experiential training, the typical pharmacy informaticist is a pharmacist who has knowledge of computer systems, medication-use processes and safety issues, clinical management of medications, drug distribution, and administration, and has developed extensive expertise in using technology to support these activities by participating and supporting previous pharmacy system and automated technology implementations.[29]

Medication order entry appears to be more difficult to implement, maintain, and support than other ordering processes for procedures or lab orders. Carpenter et al. completed a multi-site observational study of CPOE evaluating the differences with medication order entry versus other CPOE components.[32] Four primary challenges with medication orders were identified:

1. The complexity of medication orders and consequences of any errors.

2. Changes in professional relationships and roles.

3. Difficulties imposed by prescribing in different settings.

4. Impact of medication administration technologies.[32]

Medication order entry requires choosing an appropriate drug, dose, route, frequency, duration, and other possible dispensable components into an order. This process has been managed by pharmacists for many decades, however, this is a very new concept for physicians and other patient care providers that typically have had less experience utilizing computers and are not concerned with most medication order details. In order to ensure safe entry of orders, CPOE systems should be designed with discrete data fields to eliminate potential typing errors a free-text order entry model can induce. These discrete data fields are also the foundation for CDS tools and automated dispensing systems to work effectively and allow for robust reporting capabilities. The development of standardized order sets can also facilitate and simplify medication order entry practices for physicians and other health care providers. While these concepts are good to ensure safe order entry practices, ordering processes appear rigid and challenging for physicians. Pharmacists and pharmacy informaticists need to provide guidance and leadership for medication order entry processes to ensure that physicians and other clinicians effectively adapt to the challenges posed by CPOE, and the safety measures offered by this technology are realized.

ASHP published a statement on the pharmacist's role in informatics in 2007 that outlines the purpose, responsibilities, leadership requirements, and educational recommendations for pharmacists within clinical informatics roles.[33] In summary, this document outlines the pharmacist informatics roles and responsibilities including active participation and leadership in all clinical informatics activities related to the implementation, support, optimization, and education of medication use processes built within the system. It points out that pharmacists must be involved in:

- The development and implementation of standards for medication-related vocabularies and terminologies.

- Overseeing databases related to medication management systems (including CPOE and e-prescribing).

- Performing risk assessments for medication use systems.

- The development and prioritization of CDS systems.

- Assisting in data mining, collating, and analyzing.

- Providing leadership and direction within organizations as they relate to EHRs, CPOE, and related technologies.

Pharmacy informatics resources should also be part of global device solution selection and interface design and planning, especially those key to communications with pharmacy applications and/or automation. It is also critical for pharmacy informatics to assist in system testing to ensure that the system is functioning as designed and is efficiently usable for clinicians during the medication order entry process in both ambulatory and inpatient care environments. Pharmacist informaticists should also participate in the development and review of CPOE and e-prescribing training materials. These activities are essential to ensure provider knowledge of the medication related tools and workflows and enhance user acceptance and satisfaction of this technology. Ultimately, pharmacy informatics resources can optimize system utilization which in turn, may reduce medication related errors and improve patient outcomes. Documented research to evaluate the overall value of pharmacist informaticists should be performed to support this claim.

Active participation of pharmacists in all aspects of clinical informatics regarding system design, testing, support and optimization, workflow re-design, and proper global education regarding EHR medication-use processes is imperative for safe and effective medication use. This participation must be collaborative and comprehensive with other clinical services departments, physicians, and IT. Key responsibilities for pharmacists practicing in a clinical informatics role are provided in Table 9-2 as a reference.

Pharmacy Technician Informaticists

As previously outlined, technicians are likely to be expected to oversee a variety of different distributive-related activities with the advent of EHRs and CPOE. This expanded level of experience, along with knowledge and expertise of pharmacy-related workflows, computer software programs, and other related pharmacy technologies, can provide pharmacy technicians with opportunities within clinical informatics. This may be particularly true for more advanced pharmacy technicians that have had medication order entry responsibilities and/or experience with computer programming. No formal training for pharmacy technician informaticists currently exists, however, pharmacy technician certification, computer-training courses, clinical application training, and certification and vendor provided advanced automation training can all assist in advancing the basic informatics competence level of a pharmacy technician. These should be required of technicians placed into informatics roles, not only to verify their level of competence with basic informatics concepts and application knowledge, but to also ensure extensive knowledge of core pharmacy technician responsibilities and workflows.

Pharmacy technicians working in an informatics role can prove to be excellent system design, implementation, and support resources for pharmacy departments and CDOs. Their role can be structured to include automation technology within pharmacy, thus inserting a resource with an understanding of integration requirements needed to successfully bridge these technologies and streamline medication use systems. During EHR and CPOE implementation, pharmacy technician informaticists can manage a number of system build and maintenance responsibilities. These can include but are not limited to:

- Medication record build and maintenance.

- Formulary database management.

- Standard order set and medication preference list build.

- System testing and validation.

- Management of ADS interfaces and integrated workflows with EHR/CPOE or other clinical information systems.

- Pharmacy department website management, implementation, and maintenance of medication-related web-based resources and other educational or information tools.

- System report management as well as development of pharmacy staff training materials.

All of the responsibilities should be performed under the guidance and verification of a pharmacy informatics manager or pharmacist informaticist to ensure quality assurance.

Pharmacy technician informaticians can also contribute significantly in assisting with training pharmacy users on workflows and system functionality as they relate to the EHR and CPOE. Additional opportunities for technicians with advanced skills and experience with medication order entry also exist. Decentralized CPOE education and supportive roles are being developed within CDOs during and after system implementations. This "unit-based trainer" or "superuser" role can offer real-time order entry support to physicians, physician extenders, and nursing staff. While most beneficial immediately after EHR or CPOE implementation, this can serve as a full-time supportive role, especially in teaching organizations, where constant turnover of physician residents and medical students creates a need for on-going order entry support. This serves as a career advancement or transition opportunity for technicians that has not been part of traditional pharmacy technician roles and allows them to expand their roles outside of pharmacy support.

Required Resources

The key question in this discussion is how many clinical providers, including pharmacy staff, are needed to provide appropriate clinical informatics support within an organization. There is likely to be no single, correct answer, since this can vary considerably depending on CDO size, clinical services provided, EHR and/or CPOE project scope, designated implementation timeline, the selected vendor, and the system build or design imposed by an organization—a standardized vs. a highly customized system. The organizational commitment made to an EHR and/or CPOE implementation can also impact the volume of clinical informatics resources needed because organizations that commit global resources to these projects can potentially minimize dedicated informatics resources, particularly go-live support resources, by utilizing online clinical and support staff effectively within system implementation, education, and support processes. The extent to which clinical informatics has developed within an organization will also impact this, as IT may receive the bulk of resource allocations to manage these implementations. A. Miller outlined resources required during a CPOE implementation at a large university medical center to serve as a reference point[21]; however, it is difficult to transpose this information to other organizations for all of the reasons mentioned above. CDOs should consult with other EHR- and CPOE-experienced CDOs utilizing similar vendor-specific EHR and/or CPOE solutions to gain insight into their implementation and support resource requirements as well as the overall clinical resource staffing impact that

may be observed.

It should also be noted that EHR and/or CPOE technology are still in their infancy and will continue to advance over time. This will force governmental, legal and other healthcare agencies to adapt and modify existing documentation and order management requirements for the patient healthcare record, patient safety standards, and scope of practice requirements. These changes, along with the continual advancement of technology, are likely to drive additional workflow and EHR/CPOE system development changes that will require healthcare providers, including pharmacy, to continually re-evaluate, identify, justify, and advance their roles, responsibilities and resources. Ultimately, each organization and pharmacy department should anticipate and evaluate the potential impact and required informatics-related responsibilities as a result of EHR and/or CPOE implementations to justify the required resources needed to ensure optimal patient care and outcomes.

Conclusion

The modern pharmacist is experiencing a new frontier of evolving and changing roles and responsibilities in both old and new practice environments. To be successful in the future, the profession of pharmacy will need to provide leadership within organizations to assure that technologies such as EHRs and CPOE are implemented, supported, and optimized effectively and safely. Risks associated with implementing these systems must be considered and monitored as unanticipated adverse events are always a concern with new technologies.

Pharmacy departments will be challenged to take on a more global role in order to meet the Institute of Medicine (IOM) recommendations for preventing medication errors.[29] Pharmacists and pharmacy technicians will face opportunities for expanded practice scopes that will require and demand interdisciplinary training in

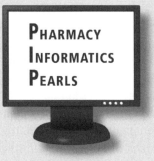

IMPACT OF THE EHR AND CPOE ON PHARMACY SERVICES

Summary of EHR and CPOE

- EHRs along with CPOE (including e-prescribing) are clinically based tools that significantly impact clinical workflows and, thus, patient care practices.
- These technologies should be designed and implemented emphasizing operational process re-design, standardization of workflows, and evidence-based medicine.
- Incorporating inefficient and ineffective processes into an electronic environment will likely lead to equally problematic and potentially error-prone processes.
- Implementations of these systems appear poised to more broadly and rapidly occur within organizations over the next decade, bringing significant change to healthcare environments.

Impact of EHR and CPOE on pharmacy roles/responsibilities

- Technicians are likely to be expected to oversee primary dispensing and preparation activities, automated dispensing system processes, IV pump management, and pharmacy responsibilities within BCMA systems.
- EHRs and CPOE advancements are likely to reduce the number of pharmacist positions working in the traditional preparing and dispensing roles in the future.
- The anticipated time reduction on distributive pharmacist responsibilities is likely to be organizational specific and will include multiple other internal factors.
- Pharmacists in distributive roles are likely to see reductions in time spent on order processing, order clarifications, and formulary management issues.
- Distributive or order entry-focused pharmacists may see increases in time spent correcting incorrect or duplicate physician entered medication orders, alert evaluation interpretation time and follow-up, and/or medication order management with patient transitions.
- Clinical pharmacist roles will primarily gain efficiencies following the implementation of EHRs and CPOE, allowing them to focus on pharmaceutical care responsibilities.

Future opportunities and challenges for pharmacy

- EHRs and CPOE will challenge pharmacy leaders and pharmacists to advance true pharmaceutical care responsibilities across the continuum of care.
- Expanding medication use processes within EHRs and CPOE (including e-prescribing) justify the need for the advancement of pharmacists and pharmacy technicians into global clinical informatics teams.
- The number of pharmacy resources needed for an EHR and/or CPOE implementation is variable.
- CDOs should consult with vendors for implementation and support resource recommendations.
- Utilize internal staff vs. consultants to implement and support EHR and CPOE implementations.
- Pharmacy informaticists must provide guidance in electronic medication use processes to ensure clinicians effectively adapt to CPOE and e-prescribing challenges and safety measures are realized.
- Departments must accept that an integrated EHR is not "their" system but "everyone's" system.
- Reliance on systems as being 100% accurate must be avoided to prevent system-induced errors.
- Pharmacist interactions and communication processes will change post EHR/CPOE implementation.
- Pharmacists may struggle with workflow changes and the adjustment to electronic order verification.

- The number of clinical providers needed to provide appropriate clinical informatics support within an organization is variable.
- Pharmacy departments will be challenged to take on a more global role in order to meet the IOM recommendations for preventing medication errors.[29]

Overall impact of EHR and CPOE implementations

- Organizations that work with EHRs and/or CPOE are finding that these systems can often initiate little or no reductions in staff, particularly in patient-centered pharmaceutical care services.
- EHRs and CPOE often force an increase of clinical staff resources as the implementation and support of clinical tools requires unique knowledge about clinical and operational workflows, medical terminology, and clinical application functionality.
- Organizations functioning in a non-mandatory CPOE environment should expect workflow challenges.
- The advancements and implementations of EHRs and CPOE will not replace pharmacists and pharmacy technicians in optimizing overall pharmaceutical care and patient outcomes.

areas beyond current standards. Future roles and responsibilities for pharmacists and pharmacy technicians will also be very organizational specific. Each CDO will have its own perception and requirements of pharmaceutical services based on organizational culture and vision, financial status, resource commitment, and workflows or medication use processes built within their EHR and CPOE systems. Pharmacy leaders will need to respond to these perceptions to ensure that the future health care environment continually holds many opportunities for pharmacists and pharmacy technicians, thus allowing pharmacy services to focus the profession's efforts on improving patients' drug therapy outcomes through effective pharmaceutical care and medication use system management. Learning to effectively initiate and promote a culture of safety within a CDO while utilizing and integrating an EHR and CPOE tools into everyday responsibilities will streamline and optimize distributive functions, improve medication use processes, advance communication and information sharing, and enhance pharmacists pharmaceutical care opportunities, leading to improved patient care and outcomes.

Clinical informaticians, by being both healthcare providers and clinical information technology professionals, are uniquely situated to identify, advise, and solve clinician requirements across the continuum of care with a high degree of credibility. Pharmacists and pharmacy technicians, just as nursing and physicians, need to actively be part of these roles in order to set current and future directions of EHR and CPOE strategies. Pharmacy informatics responsibilities can incorporate global medication use processes within these systems that align with pharmacy-specific technology oversight. This will bring greater efficiency and effectiveness into the implementations and support of these technologies, thus lowering healthcare IT costs and improving patient care results.

Different pharmacy department structures and pharmacy practice philosophies exist within various CDOs and will often integrate distributive, clinical, and even informatics roles within their pharmacy staff. This is important to note when evaluating, interpreting, and referencing the above summaries on pharmacy roles in determining the full impact of EHRs and CPOE. The above information also demonstrates that with effective pharmacy initiative and leadership, it is anticipated that future opportunities can and will exist within key pharmacy staffing roles and new roles will be developed as a result of the impact EHRs and CPOE will have on pharmacy services.

Technological advancements with the EMR and CPOE will be an ongoing endeavor that will challenge traditional pharmacy roles and responsibilities. However, through effective pharmacy leadership, new challenges and opportunities will exist and pharmacy services can continue to play a pivotal role in providing efficient and effective pharmaceutical care. It is vital to keep in mind that the advancements and implementations of EHRs and CPOE, while having the ability to prevent medication-related errors and improve patient care, will not replace pharmacists and pharmacy technicians in optimizing overall pharmaceutical care and patient outcomes.

References

1. Chassin MR, Galvin RW. The urgent need to improve health care quality: Institute of Medicine National Roundtable on Health Care Quality. *JAMA*. 1998;280:1000–1005.

2. Kohn LT, Corrigan JM, Donaldson MS, ed. To err is human: building a safer health system. Washington, DC: National Academy Press; 1999.

3. Milstein A, Galvin RS, Delbanco SF, et al. Improving the safety of health care : the Leapfrog initiative. *Eff Clin Pract*. 2000;3:313–316.

4. American College of Clinical Pharmacy White Paper: A vision of pharmacy's future roles, responsibilities, and manpower needs in the United States. *Pharmacotherapy*. 2000;20(8):991–1022.

5. Hepler CD, Strand LM. Opportunities and responsibilities in pharmaceutical care. *Am J Hosp Pharm*. 1990;47:533–543.

6. Johnson JA, Bootman JL. Drug-related morbidity and mortality: a cost-of-illness model. *Arch Intern Med*. 1995;155:1949–1956.

7. Chiquette E, Amato MG, Bussey HI. Comparison of an anticoagulation clinic with usual medical care. *Arch Intern Med*. 1998;158:1641–1647.

8. Bond CA, Raehl CL, Franke T. Clinical pharmacy services and hospital mortality rates. *Pharmacotherapy*. 1999;19:556–564.

9. Leape LL, Cullen DJ, Clapp MD, et al. Pharmacist participation on physician rounds and adverse drug events in the intensive care unit. *JAMA*. 1999;282:267–270.

10. Kucukarslan SN, Peters M, Mlynarek M, et al. Pharmacists on rounding teams reduce preventable adverse drug events in hospital general medicine units. *Arch Intern Med*. 2003;163:2014–2018.

11. Locke C, Ravnan SL, Patel R, et al. Reduction in warfarin adverse events requiring hospitalization after implementation of a pharmacist-managed anticoagulation service. *Pharmacotherapy*. 2005;25:685–689.

12. Schnipper JL, Kirwin JL, Cotugno MC, et al. Role of pharmacist counseling in preventing adverse drug events after hospitalization. *Arch Intern Med*. 2006;166:565–571.

13. Helling DK. Implementing yesterday's promises. *Am J Hosp Pharm*. 2000;57:576–581.

14. Schumock GT, Butler MG, Meek PD, et al. Evidence of the economic benefit of clinical pharmacy services: 1996-2000. *Pharmacotherapy*. 2003;23:113–132.

15. Report to Congress: The Pharmacist Workforce: A Study of the Supply and Demand for Pharmacists. Department of Health and Human Services Health Resources and Services Administration, Bureau of Health Professions. December 2000. Available at http://bhpr.hrsa.gov/healthworkforce/reports/pharmacist.htm Accessed 5/27/07.

16. U.S. Department of Labor Bureau of Labor Statistics. Occupational Outlook Handbook 2006–2007 Edition. http://www.bls.gov/home.htm Accessed 5/27/2007.

17. Knapp, DA. Professionally determined need for pharmacy services in 2020. *Am J Pharm Educ*. 2002;66:421–429.

18. Manzo J, Sinnett MJ, Sosnowski F, et al. Case study : Challenges, successes and lessons learned from implementing computerized physician order entry (CPOE) at two distinct health systems : Implications of CPOE on the pharmacy and medication-use process. *Hosp Pharm*. 2005;40:420–429.

19. Grisso AG, Wright L, Hargrove FR. computerized prescriber order entry: A pharmacist's role in CPOE: A pediatric perspective. *Hosp Pharm*. 2003;38:1086–1090.

20. Grisso AG, Wright L, Rosenbloom ST. Computerized prescriber order entry: Expansion of pharmacokinetic services through the electronic health record using CPOE and computerized note capture tools. *Hosp Pharm*. 2004;39:184–187.

21. Miller AS. Computerized prescriber order entry: Pharmacy work plan. *Hosp Pharm*. 2003;38:981–985.

22. Miller AS. Computerized Prescriber Order Entry: Quality and operations improvement: Medication turnaround time. *Hosp Pharm.* 2002;37:644–646, 695.

23. Miller AS. Prescriber computer order entry: Team structure and physician impact. *Hosp Pharm.* 2000;35:822–824.

24. Miller AS. Prescriber computer order entry: System design. *Hosp Pharm.* 2000;35:1008–1010.

25. Miller AS. Prescriber computer order entry: Hardware configuration and pharmacy issues. *Hosp Pharm.* 2000;35:1114–1117.

26. Shane R. Computerized physician order entry: Challenges and opportunities. *Am J Health-Syst Pharm.* 2002;59:286–288.

27. Michels RD, Meisel S. Program using pharmacy technicians to obtain medication histories. *Am J Health-Syst Pharm.* 2003;60:1982–1986.

28. ASHP Shared Member Resources. Computerized Prescriber Order Entry: Order Verification Process survey. Available at: http://www.ashp.org/emplibrary/R-CPOE-OrdVerifProc.pdf Accessed 5/30/2007.

29. Bates DW. Preventing medication errors: A summary. *Am J Health-Syst Pharm.* 2007;64(Suppl 9):S3–9.

30. The Joint Commission. 2008 National Patient Safety Goals. Available at: http://www.jointcommission.org/PatientSafety/NationalPatientSafetyGoals/

31. Schneider PJ. Opportunities for pharmacy. *Am J Health-Syst Pharm.* 2007; 64(Suppl 9):S10–16.

32. Carpenter JD, Gorman PN. What's so special about medications: A pharmacist's observation from the POE study. *Proc AMIA Symp.* 2001;95–99.

33. ASHP Section of Pharmacy Practice Managers. ASHP Statement on the pharmacist's role in informatics. 2007;64:200–203.

Medication Safety

Stan Kent and Lynn Boecler

CHAPTER OUTLINE

KEY DEFINITIONS

Adverse Drug Event—an injury resulting from a medication or lack of intended medication.

Electronic Health Record (EHR)—a longitudinal electronic record of patient health information generated by one or more encounters in any care delivery setting. Included in this information are patient demographics, progress notes, problems, medications, vital signs, past medical history, immunizations, laboratory data, and radiology reports.

Improper Dose Error—administration to the patient of a dose that is greater than or less than the amount ordered by the prescriber or administration of duplicate doses to the patient, i.e., one or more dosage units in addition to those that were ordered.

Medication Error—any preventable event that may cause or lead to inappropriate medication use or patient harm while the medication is in the control of the health care professional, patient, or consumer.

Medication Reconciliation—the process of identifying the most accurate list of all medications a patient is taking, including name, dosage, frequency, and route, and using this list to provide correct medications for patients anywhere within the health care system. Reconciliation involves comparing the patient's current list of medications against admission, transfer, and/or discharge orders.

Monitoring Error—failure to review a prescribed regimen for appropriateness and detection of problems, or failure to use appropriate clinical or laboratory data for adequate assessment of patient response to prescribed therapy.

Omission Error—failure to administer an ordered dose to a patient before the next scheduled dose, if any.

Order Set—compilation of medication and procedure orders that can be accessed and ordered from a single source in the EHR. These are analogous to paper pre-printed order forms.

Prescribing Error—incorrect drug selection (based on indications, contraindications, known allergies, existing drug therapy, and other factors), dose, dosage form, quantity, route, concentration, rate of administration, or instructions for use of a drug product ordered or authorized by physician (or other legitimate prescriber); illegible prescriptions or medication orders that lead to errors that reach the patient.

Unauthorized Drug Error—administration to the patient of medication not authorized by a legitimate prescriber for the patient.

Wrong Dosage-Form Error—administration to the patient of a drug product in a different dosage form than ordered by the prescriber.

Wrong Drug-Preparation Error—drug product incorrectly formulated or manipulated before administration.

Wrong Time Error—administration of medication outside a predefined time interval from its scheduled administration time (this interval should be established by each individual health care facility).

Introduction

A case could be made that the safe use of medications should be the highest priority for everyone who touches the medication use process. Those who prescribe, prepare, dispense, administer, and monitor drug therapy are all in key positions to make or break the good intended by the use of medications. Assuring that medications are used safely is certainly every pharmacist's responsibility and priority. For decades, pharmacists and pharmacy technicians have witnessed the problems that result from medication errors and adverse reactions. Michael Cohen and Neil Davis were shepherds for our profession in this field of study.[1-2] Through articles and editorials published over the past 40 years, they raised the level of awareness by frequently pointing out where things went wrong and made suggestions for improvement. Many health-system pharmacies incorporated those suggestions toward the goal of improving the quality of patient care.

Attention to the problem of medication errors, and medication safety in general, began to increase in 1989 when Manasse

published two articles that framed the subject.[3-4] These landmark articles on "drug misadventures" placed the issue in a different, and higher, perspective for pharmacists. These articles pointed out how the problem was really much larger than previously imagined, and it certainly extended beyond the walls of the nations' hospitals. Attention again increased in 1995 when Bates and Leape published data that quantified the impact of adverse events.[5-6] Then in 1997, Classen and Bates published cost information that really garnered the attention of decision-makers in health care.[7-8] These two studies, conducted simultaneously at two separate prestigious institutions, yielded remarkably similar results that could be extrapolated to hospitals across the nation. They began to solidify the economic case for investing in medication safety in health systems. When these costs are adjusted for today's dollars, these numbers are approximately double. The financial impact is compelling and cannot be ignored.

The Institute of Medicine then published the landmark "To Err is Human" report in 1999. This report brought the problem of safe medication use to the highest level of national attention ever seen.[9] The report pointed out that annually, up to 100,000 lives are lost and millions of others affected by medical errors, with medication errors leading the way. Thus began the most recent national focus and endeavor to improve medication safety. Since this publication, virtually every provider and accrediting organization has embarked upon a journey to make improvements in the safe use of medications.

The vast majority of efforts to improve medication safety have focused on changing systems and processes, encouraged increased reporting of actual and near miss events, examined the root causes of errors, teamwork and communication, and human factors. These efforts are increasingly turning to technology to help us "error-proof" our practices. Over the past 10 years, an explosion of technological advances has occurred that can help with prescribing, dispensing, administering, and monitoring medication use. From CPOE with decision support, to bar-coding systems that assist with patient identification at the point of care, these systems are rapidly being adopted and improved.

The extent of issues surrounding medication safety are very broad and beyond the scope of this book. Readers are encouraged to explore more comprehensive texts and other resources for assistance.[10-11] Similarly, in another chapter in this book, Rough and Melroy discuss the use of automation and technology to improve patient safety.[12] The purpose of this chapter is to point out how medication safety can be maximized using an electronic medical record (EMR). It is important to remember that communication surrounding adverse drug events can be confusing, especially as you work with nonclinicians. Several tools exist which can help you to communicate these issues with others in your organization.[13-14] As pharmacists, we are uniquely positioned to provide leadership to our organizations regarding enhancements in patient safety that can be achieved through the process of implementing an EMR.

Why Focus on the EMR and CPOE?

While there are several areas of the medication use process where improvements in safety can be made, the EMR offers perhaps the best opportunity to demonstrate the most impact on several stages in the medication use process. Bates demonstrated that 49% of all ADEs, and 56% of preventable ADEs, have their genesis in the prescribing stage; that 42% of serious ADEs are preventable; and that errors are much more likely to be intercepted earlier rather than later in the medication use process (see Table 10-1).[8] Whether the cause is that a drug is prescribed to which a patient is allergic, or a known drug interaction exists that could lead to patient harm, the error could be

stopped at this stage. Early studies evaluating the impact of institution-developed CPOE systems which employed basic decision support features demonstrated reductions in medication errors.[15] Thus, of all the efforts to make medication use safer, the most logical place to start is at the beginning with the prescribing process. Unfortunately, implementing a comprehensive, integrated EMR is an expensive and daunting task. To date, less than 0.5% of health systems fully employ this type of technology.[16] But given the hope of improved safety, improved quality, and lower costs, increased efforts are being made in health-systems across the country to develop and implement the EMR.

While EMRs are best known for their functionality that allows for CPOE and the errors that can be prevented, there are many types of errors that can be avoided using these systems more comprehensively. The types of errors include:

Prescribing Errors

- Incorrect drug selection—specific drugs can be associated with specific indications for use and tying that to the patient's problem list. Most contemporary CPOE systems allow for customization of naming to support tall man lettering and other actions to differentiate medication names in the look-up lists. Many systems also allow for displaying different naming conventions throughout the system to provide user-appropriate drug descriptions, e.g., pharmacy technicians need to understand product level details and physicians are primarily focused on the drug name and not the details of the product to be dispensed.

- Contraindications—reminders can be built to alert prescribers about absolute contraindications for use, and automatically appear when the drug is ordered. The prescriber can then check to see if the patient has any of those contraindications.

TABLE 10-1

ADEs That Can Be Prevented with an EMR

Prescribing errors	■ Incorrect drug selection
	■ Contraindications
	■ Drug-allergy ordering conflicts
	■ Drug-drug interactions
	■ Wrong dose prescribed
	■ Wrong administration techniques or instructions
	■ Illegible prescriptions
	■ Wrong dosage-form error
Dispensing errors	■ Wrong dose-preparation error
Administration errors	■ Omissions
	■ Wrong time error
	■ Improper dose administered error
Monitoring errors	■ Monitoring error

■ Allergies—drugs to which a patient is allergic can be avoided by matching the allergy database with the drug database. Assuring that the system has current patient-specific information is key to the success of these tools. By requiring a clinician to update allergies in the EMR periodically, it can be assured that these safety tools are used effectively and as intended. The system should be designed to block entry of medication orders if there is no allergy information documented. When designing the system, it is important to think through which point in the process the drug order-allergy conflict will be presented to the clinician: at the time of medication selection or at the time of final order signing. Consideration should also be given to whether the alert will be presented separately in order for it to stand out, or at the same time as other ordering alerts.

■ Drug-drug interactions—many contemporary CPOE systems allow prescribers to set the sensitivity of their drug-drug interaction settings to only trigger and display the most likely and severe interactions. This reduces alert fatigue and increases the chances that an important alert will not be over-ridden. Flexibility in the alerting system is an important consideration to ensure that all clinicians are alerted to drug-interaction conflicts as appropriate for their role.

■ Wrong dose prescribed—the system can be built so that common default doses and frequencies automatically appear. Even more helpful is the functionality that can calculate weight-based or body-surface-area doses, thereby avoiding calculation errors. A comprehensive EMR and CPOE system can use patient specific information like weight or BMI, age, concurrent disease states or lab values to direct prescribers to appropriate doses or notify clinicians when adjustments to therapy are required.

- Wrong administration techniques or instructions—information about specific administration techniques or special instructions can be pre-built into an administration instructions field associated with the drug.

- Illegible prescriptions—since the information in an EMR is in a typed format, legibility is no longer a concern. However, this does not mean that the intent of orders will always be clear. It is also possible to have look-alike, sound-alike errors in a CPOE system, and these should be addressed through the implementation and maintenance processes.

- Wrong dosage-form error—restrictions can be built into CPOE systems to ensure that route of administration is appropriate for the drug product associated with the order. For example, oral solution products should not allow for the intravenous route to be selected.

Dispensing Errors

- Wrong drug-preparation error—interfaces between the CPOE system, the pharmacy dispensing system, and the total parenteral nutrition compounder eliminate the transcription step reducing the potential for introducing error at this stage in the dispensing process. Another example is to ensure that the appropriate concentration of a drip is prepared and administered at the correct dose. This can be achieved through the use of the system by eliminating transcription steps from order entry to pharmacy dispensing to documentation of administration. All affected clinicians interacting with this medication are looking at the same drug order thereby eliminating the confusion about what is needed.

Administration Errors

- Omissions—a reminder time window can be established so that if a medication is past the scheduled administration time the nurse is notified to give the medication.

- Wrong time errors—EMRs can employ functionality that tell a nurse if she is about to administer a medication at the wrong time. However, this may require a change in nursing workflow related to medication administration since most nursing policies call for charting immediately after a dose is given. Bar coded medication administration (BCMA) incorporated with the EMR is an effective way to prevent these errors.

- Improper dose administered error—in order to prevent these types of error, a BCMA system must be incorporated with the electronic MAR in the EMR system. Additional safeguards can be put in place by linking an automated dispensing system (ADS) with the pharmacy computer system that is integrated or interfaced with the EMR system.

Monitoring Errors

- Monitoring error—EMRs are excellent tools for prompting clinicians to gather essential patient laboratory or physical assessment data and for notifying clinicians of situations that require further evaluation.

New Sources of Error

Typically, new technology or systems are introduced to improve quality or performance. However, whenever a new system is implemented, there exists a potential for new sources of error. Some of these errors are related to the change process itself (i.e., because something is being done differently from the way it has been done in the past). Other new errors are related to the new technology itself. As technology continues to mature and systems become more integrated, the downstream effects of any change must be thoroughly evaluated. In order to identify and prevent potential new sources of error, it is important to flowchart processes related to the new system. The process of flowcharting your work is important because it forces consideration of how processes will work and where they might go wrong in the new system. An EMR is no exception. While it improves many aspects of medication use, there are some areas where new sources of error can occur. The following are examples of some new errors that can be introduced with this technology.

Prescribing

Prescribing with electronic systems typically provides lists of drugs from which physicians can choose. This increases the possibility that they will select the wrong medication from a long list of drugs with similar names or the same name but a different dosage form. This may result in the wrong strength or dosage form of a drug being prescribed, often unbeknownst to the prescriber. Another potential error that can occur in the prescribing phase relates to dependence on other pieces of information in the record. Some medication orders can automatically integrate a patient's weight, height, age, prior allergies or adverse reactions, medication lists, laboratory values, diagnosis, etc. If these pieces of information are missing or, worse yet, outdated, then the resultant medication order may not be as intended. Therefore it is important to ensure that patient demographic data is accurately entered by all healthcare providers.

Transcribing

It should be the goal of the organization to minimize the need for transcription by maximizing the use of the EMR and CPOE and integrating the pharmacy dispensing system. Currently, many organizations are choosing to roll-out various components of the EMR over several years and using double entry workflows in the interim. All temporary workflows should be evaluated and risks considered as the organization plans for the roll-out of the technology. While manual transcription in the traditional

sense from paper orders into the pharmacy computer system does not occur in an EMR, pharmacists still review and verify medication orders. In the paper-to-computer-system transcription process the pharmacist entered the order into the pharmacy computer system as he wanted it to appear to ensure accurate dispensing and charging. The electronic verification of CPOE orders process involves the pharmacist modifying pieces of the order to ensure that the order is appropriate for dispensing and charging. In many systems these minor changes to the order by the pharmacist are allowed as they were in the paper world as long as the intent of the order written by the physician is not changed. This review process often results in modification by the pharmacist, during which error can be introduced.

Dispensing

One of the most challenging aspects of an EMR is seamlessly interfacing prescribing software with pharmacy dispensing systems and processes. In systems that maintain separate medication databases for these two functions, this process is almost impossible to keep synchronized. This often results in electronically entered orders being printed and then re-entered into the pharmacy system. Not only is this process more labor intensive, but it introduces the potential for more errors. These authors believe that maintaining an integrated, single-medication database, owned by pharmacy and used by both systems, is the best approach. It is also important that the drug master file be built and maintained properly. If the system is not continuously updated with new information, it can lead to problems with interfaces to dispensing systems or drug preparation devices.

Administering

The dynamic nature of the electronic MAR requires nursing staff to take a different approach to medication administration. Prior to the electronic MAR, even with daily computer-generated paper MARs, the nurse controlled changes to the MAR. The electronic MAR is updated as changes to orders are made, and it requires a shift in how nurses determine which medications are due and when. It is imperative to have active participation by nursing staff when deciding how the electronic MAR will function. The order in which the information is presented, as well as the descriptions used for the medications, are important considerations to ensure a safe transition to an electronic MAR. When frequently prescribed medication orders can be pre-built, it is often tempting to include significant amounts of information in the administration instructions (e.g., scales for insulin administration, heparin dosing, instructions for administering pain medication, etc.). Prescribers will sometimes also add even more information to the order (while anecdotal, this seems to happen more with electronic orders than it did in paper systems). Also, depending upon the time frame chosen for medications to remain on the MAR after their stop date, the number of medications listed can be quite large. Therefore, the amount of data that displays on an electronic MAR can be significant. This often results in confusion for nurses and leads to potential administration of wrong medications or doses. Aspects of what will appear on the MAR and for how long needs to be carefully considered.

Monitoring

One of the benefits of the EMR is that information from prior patient encounters is often readily available. However, one of the challenges is to ensure that clinicians can easily determine the source of this information. For example, patient allergies may be stored in the system with the patient and appear each time that patient is seen. It therefore becomes important to know when the patient was last asked if the list was accurate. This is a concern with lab values and patient weights as well. In traditional paper systems,

a challenge of monitoring drug therapy was lack of information. Conversely, in the EMR there is often information overload due to the efficiency with which one can see a patient's entire medical history which may or may not be relevant to the issue at hand. Clinicians must develop systems to efficiently focus on the most important pieces of data needed to monitor a drug's effectiveness. One function in a computer system that can confound monitoring, as well as create information overload due to repeated notes, is indiscriminate use of "cut/copy and paste." In an effort to save time, some clinicians will copy a progress note from a prior encounter or date and paste it into the current day's note. If this is not carefully updated then old information might be used to make a decision about therapy. The medication administration record (MAR) is another piece of the EMR that has great potential for information overload if not carefully implemented. There are often requests to push much information to the user, however, the MAR can get crowded very quickly with product information, drug information for nurses, hyperlinks to more information, and patient education information.

Using EMR and CPOE Systems to Meet Medication-related National Patient Safety Goals of The Joint Commission[17]

The 2007 Medication-related National Patient Safety Goals of the Joint Commission are to:

- Accurately and completely reconcile medications across the continuum of care
- Improve the accuracy of patient identification
- Communication amongst caregivers
- Improve the safety of medications
  EMR can be used to address these goals by accurately and completely reconciling medications across the continuum of care.

Following the introduction of a national patient safety goal by The Joint Commission, considerable attention has been directed to the reconciliation of medications across the continuum of care.[18] Several articles have shown the lack of accuracy and completeness of medication lists as patients move through the health-care system.[19-23] Currently available technology can address many of the steps involved in a comprehensive medication reconciliation program, however, it is how the clinicians interact with this technology that will determine its success. Although the integrated EMR offers the promise of access to information and improved communication across the continuum, a complex process like medication reconciliation requires each clinician and the patient to all do their part to ensure the accuracy of the information. Until major changes occur in the way patient-specific health care data is stored and shared in this country, success in this area depends on working within the restraints of our current systems.

Even in integrated systems where the prescription information may be electronically available from the primary care physician, there remains the need to clarify the medication history list. Health care professionals must clarify any discrepancies between what the patient states and what is listed in the EMR. Additionally, the existing lists of prescriptions entered by another provider make some clinicians wary about removing a medication from the list simply because the patient states he is not taking it. Procedures must be developed to determine how to handle medications the patient should be taking but is not and medications for which the patient is not following the physician prescribed regimen. Although having a longitudinal, dynamic medication list within an integrated computer system seems ideal for accomplishing medication reconciliation, it is often more complex. First, not starting from scratch with each

admission as occurs in most paper and partial paper systems means that there is more information to sort through. Not only is reconciliation of the history with the inpatient orders required, but also reconciliation of prescription history documented in the EMR with the patient-stated history must also occur. The dilemma that faces clinicians is which source to believe; the computer system maintained by various clinicians over time or the list the patient is providing at this moment. Computerized systems that store medication history lists should be able to support storing the vitamins, OTCs, and nutraceuticals that the patient states they are taking. Many CPOE systems allow this medication history list to be converted into inpatient orders as the medications are reconciled at admission.

Historically, a challenging and error-prone process was dealing with medication orders as patients were transferred to different levels of care within an organization. For many years, the standard operating procedure for inpatient care was to expect that all orders be re-written upon transfer to ensure that the patient was receiving exactly what was intended. The EMR and CPOE provide an opportunity to make this process safer and less complex. All orders can be clearly listed. Providers can then select which orders to continue, modify, or discontinue upon transfer, and the computer system can hold these changes until the transfer actually occurs. For example, consider a post-surgical patient in the recovery room who will be transferring to the general floor. That patient may continue to receive the more intensive pain medications for the duration he is in the recovery room despite the fact that the clinician has completed his transfer note. In the paper world this process was often accomplished by the pharmacist waiting to enter the new orders until the patient appeared as transferred to their new room on the floor which sometimes resulted in medication delays on the floor.

The EMR and CPOE also allow for effective communication to the patient and subsequent care givers at the point of discharge. By generating the list of medications from the computer system, the transcription step in which errors can be introduced is eliminated. The computer-generated list can also clearly state which pre-admission medications should continue, which pre-admission medications have been modified during the stay, which pre-admission meds should be discontinued, and which new medications have been added. It is essential that the computer generated list provided to the patient be written in patient-friendly language. For example, the directions must state "take twice daily" as opposed to "BID."

To date, many organizations have some level of computerization of the patient record have demonstrated improvements using electronic systems to achieve medication reconciliation.[24] More research is needed to determine if the EMR improves the reconciliation of medications compared with manual systems, stand-alone electronic medication reconciliation systems, and a combination electronic and paper systems.

Improve the Accuracy of Patient Identification

Employing bar-coded medication administration (BCMA) in conjunction with an electronic MAR allows positive patient identification reducing the potential for wrong patient errors related to medication administration. Additionally, many EMR systems allow configuration of patient look-up lists and configuration of presentation of patient identifiers to reduce the risk of wrong-patient errors.

Communication Amongst Caregivers

An integrated CPOE and EMR system can address many issues to enhance communication between various care providers. Unsafe abbreviations can be eliminated from medication orders through careful decisions on system build. Additionally, some systems can now identify unsafe abbreviations in free-text parts of the system and recommend replacement words to the users. Systems allow multiple means of communication to more quickly and accurately communicate critical test results to the appropriate clinicians so that action may be taken in a timely manner. Tools can be built to concisely pull relevant information to enhance handoff communications. Brief summary reports of current patient status or priority issues can be reviewed by clinicians supplementing, or in some cases replacing, the verbal handoffs between clinicians.

Improve the Safety of Using Medications

CPOE systems can use information about the patient or the prescriber to direct the prescriber to order the appropriate medication for the patient, minimizing the potential for an incorrect concentration of a drug to be selected in order entry. Both passive (e.g., drug name displays) and active (e.g., pop-up alerts or requiring an action by user) steps can be taken to address look-alike, sound-alike medication pairs.

Conclusion

EMRs with CPOE are increasingly employed by health-systems and physician practices as a means to improve patient safety and the overall quality of care. These systems are continuously improving in performance, reliability, and functionality. It is important to keep in mind that medications are used in many places in the EMR for prescribing, medication administration (eMAR), allergy files, vaccination documentation, decision support, and monitoring tools used by various clinicians. Thus pharmacists must become knowledgeable about and involved with more than just the traditional pharmacy components of these systems in order to maximize the potential related to medication safety. It is critical for pharmacists to be involved in the design, build, and implementation of an EMR in your health systems.

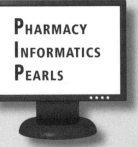

PHARMACY
INFORMATICS
PEARLS

MEDICATION SAFETY ISSUES

- Be aware of too many alerts or warnings otherwise alert fatigue will set in and prescribers will not read any alerts. (Prescribing or Administering)
- Establish a comprehensive checklist of both usual and unusual order types to test after every software upgrade. (Prescribing)
- Make sure that synonyms/abbreviations used for allergies are all appropriate (e.g., PCN is the brand name of a grape-seed extract product, not just penicillin). (Prescribing and Monitoring)
- Set up the system so that allergies are identified when a prescriber first selects a drug rather than after completion of the ordering process. (Prescribing)
- Integrating the pharmacy dispensing application with the rest of the EMR is preferable because pharmacy can control the entire medication master file. (Dispensing)
- Involve physicians early and often in decisions related to how the CPOE function will work in your system. (Prescribing and Monitoring)
- Involve nurses early and often in decisions related to how the eMAR function will work in your system. (Dispensing, Administering, and Monitoring)
- Establish a procedure for identifying look-alike, sound-alike medications on drug look-up screens and implement a system to avoid potential errors. (Prescribing, Dispensing, and Administering)
- Be aware of how much information is being presented in a single screen so users can focus on the key information they need at that time. (Prescribing, Dispensing, Administering, and Monitoring)
- Responsibility for drug master file maintenance should reside in the pharmacy operations department. (Prescribing and Ordering)

References

1. Cohen M, ed. *Medication Errors.* Washington, DC: American Pharmacists Association; 2007.

2. Davis N. *Medical Abbreviations: 28,000 Conveniences at the Expense of Communication and Safety.* Warminster, PA: Neil N. Davis Associates; 2006.

3. Manasse HR. Medication use in an imperfect world: drug misadventuring as an issue of public policy, part 1. *Am J Hosp Pharm.* 1989;46:929–944.

4. Manasse HR. Medication use in an imperfect world: drug misadventuring as an issue of public policy, part 2. *Am J Hosp Pharm.* 1989;46:1141–1152.

5. Bates DW, Cullen DJ, Laird NM, et al. Incidence of adverse events and potential adverse events: implications for prevention. *JAMA.* 1995;274:29–34.

6. Leape LL, Bates DW, Cullen DJ, et al. Systems analysis of adverse drug events. *JAMA.* 1995;274:35–43.

7. Bates DW, Spell N, Cullen DJ, et al. The costs of adverse drug events in hospitalized patients. *JAMA.* 1997;277:307–311.

8. Classen DC, Pestotnik SL, Evans RS, et al. Adverse drug events in hospitalized patients. *JAMA.* 1997;277:301–306.

9. Kohn L, Corrigan J, Donaldson M, eds. Committee on Quality of Health Care in America. Institute of Medicine. "To Err is Human: Building a Safer Health System." Washington, DC: National Academy Press; 1999.

10. Manasse HR, Thompson KK. *Medication Safety: A Guide for Health Care Facilities.* Bethesda, MD: American Society of Health-System Pharmacists; 2005.

11. Institute for Safe Medication Practices. Available at: www.ISMP.org. Accessed May 31, 2007.

12. Rough SR, Melroy J. Pharmacy automation systems. In: Dumitru D, ed. *A Pharmacy Informatics Primer.* Bethesda, MD: American Society of Health-System Pharmacists; 2008.

13. ASHP Reports. Suggested definitions and relationships among misadventures, medication errors, adverse drug events, and adverse drug reactions. *Am J Health-Syst Pharm.* 1998;55:165–166.

14. American Society of Hospital Pharmacists. ASHP guidelines on preventing medication errors in hospitals. *Am J Hosp Pharm.* 1993;50:305–314.

15. Bates DW, Teich JM, Lee J, et al. The impact of computerized physician order entry on medication error prevention. *J Am Med Inform Assoc.* 1999;6:313–321.

16. HIMSS website. http://www.himssanalytics.org/docs/EMRAM.pdf. Accessed May 30, 2007

17. The Joint Commission. National Patient Safety Goals. Available at: http://www.jointcommission.org/PatientSafety/NationalPatientSafetyGoals/07_hap_cah_npsgs.htm Accessed May 31, 2007.

18. Piscoran S, ed. *Medication Reconciliation Handbook.* Oakbrook Terrace, IL: Joint Commission Resources; 2006.

19. Gleason KM, Groszek JM, Sullivan C, et al. Reconciliation of discrepancies in medication histories and admission orders of newly hospitalized patients. *Am J Health-Syst Pharm.* 2004;61:1689–1695.

20. Lau HS, Florax C, Porsius AJ, et al. The completeness of medication histories in hospital medical records of patients admitted to general internal medicine wards. *Br J Clin Pharmacol.* 2000;49:597–603.

21. Cornish PL, Knowles SR, Marchesano R, et al. Unintended medication discrepancies at the time of hospital admission. *Arch Intern Med.* 2005;165:424–429.

22. Pronovost P, Weast B, Schwarz M, et al. Medication reconciliation: A practical tool to reduce the risk of medication errors. *J Crit Care.* 2003:18(4): 201–205.

23. Kaboli PJ, McClimon BJ, Hoth AB, etal. Assessing the accuracy of computerized medication histories. *Am J Med Care.* 2004;10(part 2):872–877.

24. Kramer JS, Hopkins PJ, Rosendale JC, et al. Implementation of an electronic system for medication reconciliation. *Am J Health-Syst Pharm.* 2007;64:404–422.

Reporting and Data Mining

Michael E. McGregory and Scott R. McCreadie

CHAPTER OUTLINE

KEY DEFINITIONS

Business Intelligence—an umbrella term that describes the strategic integration of technology and processes that allow organizations to leverage their data to make better decisions.

Dashboard—common report format used to quickly evaluate the performance of a business process. Dashboards commonly use visuals such as dials, gauges, or stoplights to represent results.

Data Integrity—the accuracy, completeness, consistency, and validity of data.

Data Mining—broad term that encompasses numerous methods used to identify patterns and relationships in data. Examples of data mining techniques include neural networks, rule induction, and genetic algorithms.

Data Warehouse—centralized repository of data from an organization's individual information systems that is organized into integrated subject domains for reporting or data mining. Data warehouses may be implemented with relational or dimensional data models.

Database Query—general term to describe a "search" of a database that returns data for use in reporting or other analyses.

Dimensional Database Model—an approach to designing databases for the purpose of maximizing end-user friendliness and query performance as well as to preserve data history. These features stand in contrast to the strengths of the relational database model (see below).

ePHI—electronically protected health information. Individually identifiable health information stored electronically by healthcare providers.

Fitness for Purpose—a property of data that is appropriate for a given use. In reporting or other data analysis, fitness for purpose is evaluated along dimensions of timeliness and relevancy for the task at hand.

On Line Analytical Processing (OLAP)—a class of applications to support complex queries and analysis across multiple dimensions. OLAP systems often implement a dimensional data model and are closely related to data warehouses.

On Line Transaction Processing (OLTP)—a class of applications designed to support transaction based operational processes such as order entry or packaging. OLTP systems often rely on databases that implement a relational data model.

Open Database Connectivity (ODBC)—standard interface for accessing modern database systems.

Relational Database Model—an approach to designing databases based on mathematical set theory. Proper application of the model helps ensure data integrity is maintained during transactions that update, add, or remove data.

Reporting—the concise presentation of relevant operational or clinical data for decision making or performance review purposes.

Structured Query Language (SQL)—standard language used to query and manage databases. Pronounced "sequel."

Introduction

Data generated during the provision of patient care continue to migrate away from paper-based formats to electronic methods of storage, usage, and retrieval. While this continued conversion presents its own sets of challenges, the ability to assemble, aggregate, and analyze this data is greatly enhanced. Data and information once locked into paper formats that are difficult to share can quickly be made available to multiple users in different locations and transformed for use in new ways. Electronic data and information can be analyzed, compared, contrasted, trended, and shared faster than ever before. Unlocking our data and information in this manner helps us better understand how healthcare is being provided and our impact on both patient outcomes and institutional operations.

By examining the data through techniques such as reporting and data mining, the pharmacy manager can discover new opportunities to improve services and meet patient needs. These analyses help reduce the use of intuition or guessing in evaluating a pharmacy's performance. Instead, the data can be used to compute accurate and consistent metrics of performance and efficiency. Appropriately applied, the pharmacy manager can use these tools to make objective comparisons and target improvements where they can have the greatest impact.

While the continued conversion of paper-based records to electronic records has many positive benefits, there is also a need for increased control and monitoring of how that data is used. Safeguards must be in place to limit access to the data and information to those with a valid reason to use it and ensure that the use is appropriate. Patients put their trust in healthcare providers to protect their health information and use it effectively. As such, pharmacy managers not only use the data and information but, in many cases serve as stewards of that information to protect patients' trust.

The new flood of electronic data sources available to pharmacy managers present new opportunities but also new challenges that must be addressed. It's critical that the pharmacy manager understand the quality, attributes, and limitations of the data prior to relying on it to make business decisions. In this chapter, we'll explore reporting and data mining and offer practical advice on using them effectively to evaluate departmental performance and improve the care of patients.

Data, Information, and Knowledge

Healthcare systems are very good at producing data. In fact, managers are often drowning in data and have a hard time analyzing it. Data by itself is useless until it is transformed into useful information. The main purpose of reporting and data mining is to turn data into information. Information is data that actually makes a difference. The root of the word is to "inform" or give shape to the data so that it is meaningful when delivered to a receiver. Data is converted to information when it is contextualized, categorized, calculated, corrected, and condensed.[1] Reporting and data mining can help managers do exactly that. They allow managers to use those vast collections of laboratory and drug data to create meaningful information that help pharmacists make better decisions and take appropriate actions.

Knowledge is a step beyond information and is largely a human element. Knowledge is information that is connected and compared to other information or historical context. Knowledge is what people develop with experience and cannot be completely reduced into a set of codified rules.[2] Healthcare, like many other professions, relies heavily on the knowledge of workers such as pharmacists who cannot be replaced by technology and automation. When pharmacists interact with reports or the output of a data mining algorithm, new knowledge is created. As you read this chapter, keep this hierarchy in mind (see Figure 11-1). While those that manage data and reporting processes are primarily concerned with the conversion from data to information, it is the use of that information which is important.

Reporting vs. Data Mining

Reporting and data mining are often considered components of business intelligence (BI). In fact, many commercially available software tools used to support reporting and data mining are marketed as BI applications. BI is an umbrella term to describe the strategic integration of technology and processes that allow organizations to leverage their data to make better decisions.[3] A form of business intelligence that is more familiar to pharmacists and other healthcare professionals is decision support. However, since the concepts of reporting and data mining describe several different types of analysis, it's easy to see how the boundaries between these similar concepts are blurred. For managers new to the field of informat-

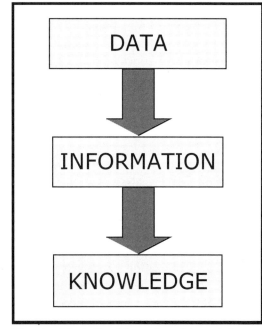

Figure 11-1. The hierarchy of data, information, and knowledge.

ics and experienced professionals looking to cut through the buzzwords, we recommend leaving the taxonomy behind. Focusing on the outcome of using data to make better decisions will help lead managers to the right analytical method for the right job regardless of its classification.

Understanding and Evaluating Data Quality

Understanding the data available in your institution is a prerequisite for establishing effective reporting or data mining solutions. Data of clinical, operational, and financial interest may be located in a single repository or scattered across multiple information systems. Regardless of the number of sources or the complexity of your institution's data, they must be assessed for both data integrity and fitness for purpose. Otherwise, the synthesized information will be inaccurate and misleading.

Data integrity refers to the accuracy, completeness, consistency, and validity of data while its fitness for purpose is evaluated along dimensions of timeliness and relevancy for the task at hand. In practice, these concepts should be considered along a scale as opposed to dichotomous classifications, as few actual healthcare information systems would perfectly meet all definitions. Table 11-1 provides examples for each component of data integrity and fitness for purpose. [4,5]

A manager's assessment of data quality will depend on the analysis at hand. Consider an inpatient pharmacy information system that records the number of doses sent and the scheduled administration time. This data is likely to be of sufficient quality to assess drug utilization trends at a product level and could even be used to evaluate the number of technicians per shift needed to deliver the medications to the nursing units.

However, the scheduled administration times are not accurate enough to monitor processes that require actual administration time data. For example, it may be tempting to combine the pharmacy dispensing information with laboratory data to perform a quality assurance check on the pharmacokinetic calculations performed by a dosing service. However, if a drug concentration was drawn by the phlebotomy team 5 minutes before the scheduled administration time (as ordered), but the dose was actually given 30 minutes early (which many medication administration policies allow), a reported trough level would be subject to gross miscalculation on the QA report. In this new context, the scheduled administration time data is no longer fit for use.

TABLE 11-1

Elements of Data Quality

Data Quality Element	Definition	Example of Data Quality Issue
Accuracy	Data that correctly represents its real-world value.	An automated dispensing machine's calculated quantity on hand of 50 tablets that corresponds to an actual count of 45 tablets.
Completeness	Data that contains all expected values.	The user name of the pharmacist who verified an order is missing.
Consistency	Data that is represented the same way in all systems.	Male gender is coded as 1 in the billing system and 0 in the pharmacy information system.
Validity	Data that is recorded within an acceptable range or format.	Dates that are expected as MM/DD/YYYY being entered as DD/MM/YYYY.
Timeliness	Data that is an appropriate age for its intended use.	Using reports of yesterday's IV compounding workload to drive staffing assignments today.
Relevancy	Data that is useful for a given task.	Using the number of orders entered per day to measure the workload of pharmacists assigned to a pharmacokinetic dosing service.

Identifying Data Quality Issues

Once the importance of data quality is understood, managers must learn to identify and address potential data quality issues. The majority of data quality issues encountered in healthcare information systems can be uncovered by considering both the processes that generate the data, and the methods used to store and retrieve them.

Familiarity with the day-to-day processes that generate data is critical to evaluating its overall quality. Unfortunately, an institution's intended use for an information system does not always correlate to the actual use.[6] Workarounds that jeopardize data accuracy and relevancy have been documented for many healthcare technologies in use.[7-10] For example, barcode medication administration systems (BCMA) require the nurse to scan a barcode on the patient's wristband prior to administering a medication to ensure that the right patient is getting the right drug. However, when a barcode is difficult to scan due to curvature around a wrist or other impediment, one observed workaround is to print extra wristbands and scan the copies. Reports generated from this data would probably indicate a high compliance rate for the bedside scanning process when, in fact, it is being circumvented.

In addition to local knowledge of the processes that generate the data in a repository, a general understanding of the common data storage and modeling strategies used in healthcare information systems will also help identify and address many data quality issues. One of the most common issues encountered with healthcare data is the loss of "point in time" history from transaction based (OLTP) systems. OLTP systems are designed to efficiently support a high volume of short operations or transactions like order entry and packaging.[11,12] Even though many of these systems provide valuable reporting capabilities, they generally do not maintain a "snapshot history" of relevant configuration settings that may change over time. For example, status flags indicating if a medication is on the formulary or stocked in an ADM generally refer to the current state of the product. A report of all non-formulary medications dispensed over the past year would have to use the current formulary to determine the status of previous orders. Medications that changed status over that time frame would be incorrectly classified.

Valuable data might even be stored or processed by users in spreadsheets or desktop database applications. Outcomes research or medication use evaluation (MUE) data is often maintained in this manner. These custom or home-grown grown tools should be evaluated carefully for data quality issues. One meta-review reported that an average of 24% of spreadsheets used for activities such as capital budgeting contained material errors.[13]

Data quality is essential to producing relevant and actionable information and should be in the forefront of a manager's mind when developing or evaluating a reporting or data mining solution.

Reporting

The underlying goal of reporting and data mining is to use data to make better decisions. Reporting techniques accomplish this task by consolidating large amounts of data into a format that is easier for managers or clinicians to interpret. This section discusses the types of reports commonly seen in healthcare management, the visual elements used to present the data, and the methods used to deliver the final product to end-users.

Report Types

Most reports used in healthcare management can be grouped into three categories: ad-hoc, pre-defined, and drill-down.[14] Ad-hoc reports are often exploratory in nature. Someone will ask "Can we get a report that tells us how many…" which begins the process. The actual reports are usually simple, perhaps only containing a table of summary data or a basic graph. Ad-hoc reports tend to be very specific to the question at hand and may provide the basis for new pre-defined reports. As their name implies, pre-defined reports were designed at some point in the past and can quickly be regenerated with updated information. For these reports to be of repeated value, they typically present information of a more general nature to support multiple types of analysis or are needed to manage a routine operational process. The reports that vendors provide with information systems usually fall into this category. Drill-down reports allow a user to start with a high level overview of the data and then drill down into specific areas of interest with increasing detail. Management dashboards often provide this type of drill-down feature. See Figure 11-2 for an example of a dashboard report.

Visual Elements

Common visual elements used in reports include data tables, cross tab matrices, and charts. These are the specific data presentation tools used to build the report. The selection of the visual elements used depends on the needs and preferences of report's audience, the type of analysis to be performed, and the information a manager wishes to convey.

Tables are common elements found in reports. They are useful for presenting higher level, aggregated data as well as transaction level details. Most reporting tools make it easy to group rows of data according to a common attribute and to calculate summary values such as sums, averages, and counts. In this manner, a report of acquisition costs could be grouped by drug class and then sub-grouped by fiscal year to get an overall

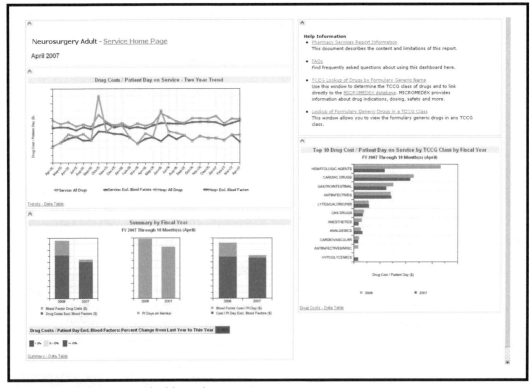

Figure 11-2. Drug cost dashboard.

picture of drug expenses (see Figure 11-3). A more advanced table structure is the cross tab or pivot table. Here, data variables are arranged both across the top of the columns (similar to a standard table) and along the side in rows. The intersection of each pair of variables contains a summary measure. Continuing with the previous example, the fiscal years could be used as column headings and drug classes used as row headings (see Figure 11-4). As with standard or "flat"

data tables, many reporting tools make generating cross tabs relatively easy and can calculate totals across the columns and rows with a mouse click. Cross tabs are an excellent way to summarize large amounts of data.

Charts and graphs are also common elements of reporting used to visualize data. Basic charts include bar, line, and pie charts. They allow for data to be compared across groups, trended over time, and related to

DRUG CLASS	ANTICOAGULANT/THROMBIN INHIBITORS		
FISCAL YEAR		**2006**	
SUB CLASS	ANTICOAGULANTS,COUMARIN TYPE		
	DRUG	**FISCAL QTR**	**DRUG COST**
	WARFARIN	1	$2,582.79
	WARFARIN	2	$2,674.04
	WARFARIN	3	$2,523.24
	WARFARIN	4	$2,240.05
Sum			10020.1175
SUB CLASS	HEPARIN AND RELATED PREPARATIONS		
	DRUG	**FISCAL QTR**	**DRUG COST**
	ENOXAPARIN	1	$97,706.43
	ENOXAPARIN	2	$93,797.43
	ENOXAPARIN	3	$104,303.71
	ENOXAPARIN	4	$104,889.52
	FONDAPARINUX	1	$649.30
	FONDAPARINUX	2	$588.90
	FONDAPARINUX	3	$226.50
	FONDAPARINUX	4	$513.40
	HEPARIN	1	$15,333.09
	HEPARIN	2	$17,426.79
	HEPARIN	3	$16,644.50
	HEPARIN	4	$17,459.78
Sum			469539.3476

Figure 11-3. Report grouped by drug class, fiscal year, and sub-class.

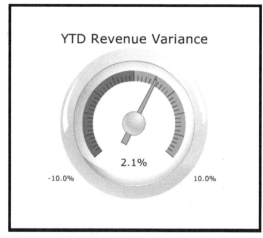

Figure 11-4. Cross-tab table.

The spreadsheet image shows:

Drug Cost Cross-Tab Table

Drug Class	Fiscal Year	
	2006	2007
GP 2b3a Inhibitors	$ 60,417.92	$ 66,592.74
Anticoagulant/Thrombin Inhibitors	$ 722,996.27	$ 889,723.37
Antiemetics	$ 1,107,976.60	$ 1,204,597.83
Antimicrobials	$ 3,388,399.46	$ 3,491,576.02
Colony Stimulating Factors	$ 448,547.22	$ 520,909.38
CRRT Solutions	$ 372,905.85	$ 400,325.91
Erythropoietic Agents	$ 473,813.56	$ 593,538.26
Factor VII	$ 1,544,355.67	$ 1,289,043.54
Injectible Anesthetics	$ 299,865.72	$ 160,040.29
IVIG Products	$ 497,832.40	$ 505,914.64
Neuromuscular Blockers	$ 55,248.29	$ 74,284.63
PPIs/H2 Receptor Antagonists	$ 166,252.15	$ 172,881.87
Thrombolytic Agents	$ 35,720.64	$ 98,451.74
Total Parenteral Nutrition	$ 291,699.53	$ 294,551.52
Transplant Immunosuppressants	$ 1,620,182.07	$ 2,024,503.84

the whole, respectively. Graphical indicators such as stoplights, dials, or gauges can be used to indicate the overall status of a process or key performance metric (see Figure 11-5). These elements are often incorporated into dashboard reports. Visuals like charts and graphs are an effective means of summarizing data and conveying results quickly. It's a good idea to keep the visuals clean and to the point to reduce the chances that an end-user will misinterpret the report and draw inappropriate conclusions. Excessive decoration or 3-D charts that don't actually use the extra dimension can be distracting to an audience.[15,16] Managers should also guard against chart designs that can inadvertently mislead a reader. For example, using a non-zero baseline or otherwise altering the scale of an axis might cause your audience to draw an incorrect conclusion due to the visual presentation even though the data points are labeled accurately. This tactic is often seen in marketing materials

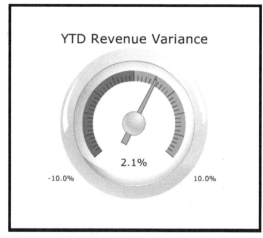

Figure 11-5. Gauge used to display data.

for products and services to sway the viewer's conclusion.

Controls are visual elements only found on electronic reports and allow a user to specify various parameters for the report to further refine its output. The most common controls used in electronic reports include drop-down lists, check boxes, radio buttons, and date selectors. Limiting a report to data collected within a specific, user-selected time frame is a common use for a control. Others include filters that limit a formulary listing report to only those medications beginning with 'sulfa' or to sort a flat data table by brand or generic name. These advanced elements allow an electronic report to offer a greater level of interactivity.

Report Layout and Design

A finished report is more than a random collection of tables and graphs. The layout and design of a report can also influence how the information is received. Keeping a report simple and to the point will help ensure that the intended message is communicated clearly and effectively. Start by clarifying the specific decisions or analyses a report will support. Is the purpose strategic, analytical, or operational in nature? Who are the intended users? Will the results of the report cause additional questions to be asked? Answers to these questions will help determine the types of information, elements and controls needed for your report or dashboard. Next, consider the organization of the report content. If two graphs are intended to be contrasted, group them together visually. This might include a common border or color scheme. Likewise, separate out the distinct domains of information to avoid misleading or inappropriate comparisons of the information. Also, seek regular feedback from users. Do *they* see the logic in the layout?[17]

Delivery Methods

Reports, like other aspects of healthcare, are moving towards an electronic platform. This isn't to suggest a goal of eliminating paper reports (in fact many reports should be designed for easy printing), but rather that new mechanisms for requesting, retrieving, and customizing reports are now available. Delivery mechanisms can be divided into push and pull techniques. Push techniques deliver information to the user without an explicit user interaction. Automated delivery of a weekly workload report via e-mail is a push method. Pull methods require the user to seek the information. In a pull scenario, a user must access the reporting website or request an updated report from an application's menu.

A number of factors can play into a decision to use a push vs. pull delivery method. A push mechanism can serve as a regular reminder and makes it easier for the user to take responsibility by reading and responding to the report. However, care should be taken to avoid "report fatigue." A limitless barrage of automated reports being sent to a manager's in-box can also have negative impact on follow-up.

Reporting Tools

Custom reporting capabilities are now available from a variety of applications to supplement the pre-defined reports provided by a source system (e.g., a pharmacy information system). Reporting tools can range from common office software to desktop report authoring programs, web-based portals, and enterprise-wide business intelligence suites. In most cases, your choice of reporting tools will be limited to what your institution provides and what your information system vendor supports. This section will focus on common functions found in general reporting applications.

Data Access

A mechanism must be provided for a reporting to tool to retrieve data from a source system. Open database connectivity (ODBC) connections and "flat file" imports are the most common methods used in healthcare reporting. A flat file is a data extract from a source system (usually a delimited text file) that is subsequently imported into the reporting tool. Flat files avoid a host of database security issues for the source system. However, reports built around this type of data access are harder to keep current. New extracts have to be requested, generated, transmitted to the user, and then re-imported into the reporting tool. While some of these steps can be automated to reduce the time lag, reports that depend on current data need real-time access to the source database. ODBC connections provide a conduit for this direct data access and are supported by the majority of databases and reporting tools on the market today. With a connection established, the reporting tool uses input from a user-friendly graphical interface or menu to generate a database SQL command that retrieves the requested data. Of course, report authors and users must have sufficient security credentials to access the source database.

Export Formats/Office Suite Integration

Most reporting tools will offer several export options. A popular export format is the portable document format (.pdf) which is easily read by free software and maintains your original formatting for consistent printing. In other cases, easy exporting of the underlying data for further analysis is desired. In that situation, a comma delimited data file that can be used in a desktop spreadsheet program would be appropriate. In the case of desktop applications where a copy of the original application is needed to open the report, the report author will need to perform the export and distribute the resulting files. Conversely, web-based reporting tools will typically allow users to select a desired export format on demand.

Seamless integration with other business applications is another common feature found in modern reporting tools. This type of integration might allow a user to access a report, manipulate the underlying data in a spreadsheet, and immediately see the modifications in the original report. Software vendors that offer of suites of complimentary business applications frequently tout the productivity enhancements of tight integration.

User Friendliness

The user-friendliness of any software application is in the eye of the beholder. That said, many powerful reporting tools have been developed to the point where non-technically oriented personnel can produce quite sophisticated reports and dashboards. Tools targeted at these end users offer familiar interfaces and toolbars that mimic popular word processors or e-mail programs. However, with more advanced tools there is likely to be a steeper learning curve. The reporting needs of managers, clinicians and other staff will likely drive tool selection for your department. Certain advanced reporting scenarios may require investment in training and tools to achieve success.

Data Warehouses/Data Marts

Overview

So far, this chapter has discussed reports based on individual source systems such as order entry systems, automated dispensing machines, or cartfill robots. However, some health-systems also have data warehouses available. These warehouses aggregate data from a hospital's individual information systems to facilitate reporting and data analysis. The ability to access data from several source systems from a single warehouse allows managers to develop more extensive reports. For example, a report showing an increased use of a restricted antibiotic (using data from the pharmacy) can be enhanced by overlaying diagnosis data (from the billing department or microbiology data (from the lab). A report showing the increased drug use trend alone may leave a manger wondering if there is an increased need for the drug or if an antibiotic stewardship policy is not being enforced. However, these additional overlays may help guide managers to the actual reasons for the increased antibiotic use.

A data warehouse can be broadly defined as an organized collection of data specifically modeled and designed for large-volumes of data to support management decision making within an organization. A data warehouse is modeled differently than transaction-based systems (which run most operational systems in healthcare) in that a data warehouse can present historical views of the data at any point in time. Data warehouses serve to increase the accessibility of the organization's data and also increase the consistency of that data for longitudinal reporting. Data warehouses are often designed to be the primary source of data and information for decision-making within an organization and many healthcare organizations have implemented data warehouses to support clinical and operational analyses.

Data warehouses are set up around business subjects such as sales, costs, and marketing as opposed to which operational computer system the data originated. In healthcare, the warehouse is usually set up for the areas of financial management and clinical outcomes which may be further broken down by pharmacy, laboratory, and other areas.

Data marts are very similar to data warehouses. They are designed the same way but have a narrower scope. A data warehouse tends to reflect enterprise-wide data whereas a data mart is limited to a particular subject area with the company. An example is a data mart that includes only the purchasing data from the pharmacy.

Structure of a Data Warehouse

A data warehouse is built differently than transaction database systems by using what's called a dimensional model. This model consists of two types of information: facts and dimensions. Facts are numerical measurements about the business and are often continuously valued and additive. It is critical for the facts to have these properties as many queries of the data will attempt to add or average large volumes of the data. Some examples of fact data include dollars sold, units sold, cost, and other business measures.[18]

Dimensions are ways to slice the facts through textual descriptions. They are often used to group or limit fact data for a report.

Some examples include time, products, and stores.[18] In healthcare, dimensions are subjects such as drugs, medical services, patients, diagnoses, procedures, or other attributes. It is a common data warehouse structure to have a single fact table linked to many dimension tables. This allows the end user to slice the data by many dimensions of the business.

The mechanics of developing a data warehouse are beyond the scope of this chapter, as it generally requires a large and sustained organizational commitment with data specialists that guide the process.

Using a Data Warehouse

A data warehouse can be accessed through the types reporting tools discussed previously in this chapter. In many organizations, the team that manages the data warehouse will also have tools available for users. With an understanding of the contents of the data warehouse and knowledge of the tools to access that content, a manager can use the data to help make more informed decisions.

Data Mining

Data mining is a broad term that encompasses automated methods of "knowledge discovery." Generally, these are data-driven, machine learning techniques used to extract previously unknown patterns and relationships from large databases.[19] Data mining is complementary to other forms of business intelligence such as reporting but is usually considered to be a distinct discipline.[20]

Data mining methods commonly address tasks of classifying, clustering, associating, and predicting data. The algorithms developed to perform each of these tasks are rooted in advanced statistical methodologies and have been applied to both clinical and operational aspects of healthcare. Silver and colleagues describe the use of data mining to explore the financial losses associated with a specific diagnosis related group (DRG). They were able to identify a specific subset of cases that accounted for the majority of the losses and recommend administrative actions.[21] A more pharmacy-centric example is the work of Rudman and colleagues who applied data mining techniques to adverse drug event (ADE) reports. Their analysis revealed which predictor variables (type of drug, person involved, location of the event, etc.) were more closely associated with the severity of an ADE.[22] Other healthcare applications include infection control and biosurveillance.[19]

Of particular interest in healthcare are predictive models that apply data mining techniques. The outputs of these models indicate the probability of an outcome (e.g., "this patient will generate a financial loss for the institution"). Common predictive modeling techniques include decision trees, rule induction, and neural networks. All of these require large data samples that can be separated into training and validation sets. This provides one set of cases for the algorithm to "learn from" and build the model and an independent set to test the model's performance.[23] One of the key differences between the algorithms is their ability to explain a conclusion. The decision trees and if/then rules developed by decision tree and rule induction algorithms can be readily understood. In those cases a manager or analyst could examine the process used by the algorithm to help understand the outcome. In contract, neural networks act as a "black box" that provides an answer with little justification. Here, no such examination is possible.[19]

Data mining techniques are powerful analytical tools that often require the assistance of model building experts. This is due to both the complexity of software used to perform these analyses and the potential for spurious models. The latter is particularly true when data mining is used in an exploratory manner since the performance of the model is limited by the quality (particularly the completeness) of the training data. Also, users should be aware of how conclusions

are reached. As with other statistically based methodologies, *statistical* significance does not necessarily imply *clinical* significance.

Practical Challenges

There are many challenges that must be understood and addressed to ensure meaningful reports and accurate data mining models. As we mentioned in our earlier discussion of data quality, a thorough understanding of your data is critical to ensure that any assumptions are correct and that the output accurately reflects the purpose of the report. Additionally, there are a number of practical issues faced by pharmacy managers looking to leverage reporting and data mining tools that must be considered.

Common Denominators

The expression "comparing apples to apples" is used as a figure of speech when someone is making a comparison among groups. This same thought is important to consider when working with data in a reporting scenario. In many industries, common denominators often boil down to monetary terms or inventory units but healthcare is a bit more complicated. While the monetary and inventory units exist, there are a number of other denominators, such as quality of life, which are much harder to define.

In the pharmacy environment, reporting might look at utilization patterns of a drug or particular group of drugs. In such cases, managers need to make sure they are using common units of measure. For example, if a drug is recorded both as milligrams and grams for a dosage unit, the data must be converted so that the units are the same in order to produce accurate aggregate results (e.g., sums or averages). A similar challenge may be seen when reporting on patients' age if the data is stored based on years, months, or days, depending on the age of the patient. In this case, it makes more sense to use the date of birth to calculate age in a common unit so the data will be consistent.

Multiple Sources of Truth

This challenge arises in environments such as healthcare where data is widely distributed among various information systems. This can result in data that isn't consistent between the sources due to modifications in one system and not the other. This often surfaces when reports generated from two separate sources that measure a common element disagree. For example, purchasing systems and dispensing systems both record quantities of drugs. Even if they both measured a given drug in the same units of measure, a report of yearly utilization from each system will likely yield different answers. One source of variation is that waste may not be accounted for in the dispensing system when partial vials are used to prepare a dose. In most cases these variations will be small. However, reconciling these differences can be a major source of frustration for managers trying to use the information to make decisions or explain organizational performance.

If a health system has a dedicated reporting environment or a consolidated data warehouse, some of these challenges may have been addressed. If an institution does not have a reporting environment or data warehouse, it is a significant initial effort to establish one. A big challenge to setting up these systems is determining the most accurate sources of truth and to clean the data of issues before it is loaded in the final form for reporting. While this is a significant undertaking it greatly improves the accuracy and consistency of reports.

Attribution Bias

One of the key challenges with decision making is attribution bias. This occurs when an event is attributed to another event even though the first event did not cause the second. Attribution bias is a common folly in decision making across all industries. It is very much a factor in healthcare because so many things are related. An example might be attributing a reduced length of stay to a new drug. While it could be true, there are many other factors that impact length of stay. Perhaps the health system implemented a new scheduling system that helped move patients through their care more efficiently. It is usually very difficult to measure the true impact of a single change in healthcare.

Changing Environment

Another challenge is that the environment changes over reporting periods. An example is drug costs. A common report is to trend drug costs or usage over time in an attempt to see how well medication use policies are working. However, there are many variables that impact the overall cost or consumption of a medication. Patient volume changes, drug cost inflation, new alternative therapies, and patent expirations can all affect the total costs of drugs over time. In this example, a technique such as variance analysis can help sort out the individual effects of these changes and improve the interpretation of the report.

Privacy and Confidentiality Rules

The awareness of the need for privacy and confidentiality of healthcare data has grown as healthcare data has becoming increasingly electronic. In the early 1990s, a group of healthcare industry leaders gathered to discuss strategies to reduce administrative healthcare costs. Much of that early work focused on data transmission standards and code sets in healthcare as well as the creation of such things as the national provider ID. That work turned into the HIPAA regulations we know today and is administered by the U.S. Department of Health and Human Services (DHHS).[24]

Key parts of the HIPAA legislation and rules that affect reporting and data mining are the security and privacy rules. The security rule established in 2003 requires a consistent level of protection of all individually-identifiable health information (ePHI) that is stored or transmitted electronically. The security rule requires that safeguards be in place in the forms of appropriate policies and procedures to protect data, restricted physical access to ePHI, and ensuring that technical security measures are in place to protect networks, computers, and other electronic devices.[24]

The Privacy Rule was created to protect the privacy of ePHI in the hands of covered entities. The Privacy Rule is broad and contains a number of provisions protecting patients' healthcare data. It:

- Provides patients the right to access their medical records.

- Allows patients to restrict who can see their medical records.

- Allows patients to know who has accessed their medical records.

- Limits disclosures of medical records to those who need to know for treatment and operations use.

- Limits use of ePHI for research without proper notification and permission.

- Requires the activities of healthcare entities (including training and education programs for employees and formal business associate agreements with partners) understand and follow the Privacy Rule.

- Sets up penalties for violations of the Privacy Rule.

Pharmacy managers must understand that they are data stewards of the ePHI and must protect it accordingly. The privacy and confidentiality rules do allow broad access to ePHI for treatment and operational or billing uses which allows the pharmacy manager to use it for reporting.

Case Study: Putting it all together— supplementing vendor reports

In response to a staffing shortage, a large pharmacy department implemented technician order entry. In this model, during high volume shifts, technicians would triage incoming orders (via fax machine) and perform the initial entry into the dispensing system. Hard copies of technician entered orders were placed in a queue for pharmacist verification which would trigger the label printing and dose preparation processes. This was intended as an interim solution until workload in a CPOE environment was evaluated following its implementation in 6 months. One week after technician order entry began the number of missing doses reported by nursing staff increased sharply. Many of these missing doses were traced to orders that were entered by technicians but were lost in the paper shuffle and never verified.

In addition to improving the flow and handoffs of the hardcopy orders, the pharmacy managers wanted a mechanism to help the satellite pharmacists identify orders awaiting verification and for them to monitor the number of unverified orders at the end of each shift. While the pharmacy system did not provide such a report of unverified orders, it did allow ODBC access to the underlying database. The pharmacy information systems manager used a reporting tool licensed by the hospital for enterprise reporting to retrieve and share the desired information. The body of the report was a simple table of unverified orders grouped by the location of the original technician entry location and ordered by time of entry and priority (STAT, now, regular). The report was accessible on-demand via a web browser for satellite pharmacists and emailed as a spreadsheet at the end of each shift to the appropriate supervisors. Pharmacists were expected to check the report at regular intervals during their shifts. It was decided not to e-mail the report to the satellite personnel because there was no electronic mechanism to consistently identify the individuals working in a given location and the managers wanted to avoid spamming all pharmacists with the report. Managers reviewed the reports as part of their regular duties to check for compliance with the process and aid in troubleshooting missing medication reports filed by nurses.

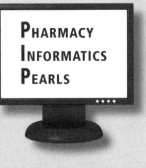

PHARMACY INFORMATICS PEARLS

REPORTING AND DATA MINING

- Data quality is critical to any analysis. Quality refers to both data integrity (accuracy, completeness, consistency, and validity of data) and its fitness for purpose (timeliness and relevancy).
- Keep your reports simple and actionable.
- Data warehouses and data marts usually provide a ready source of high quality data that is optimized for reporting and data mining. Use them whenever possible.
- Data mining techniques are powerful, but remember to assess the models for "clinical significance" not just "statistical significance."
- Watch out for multiple sources of truth. If two different information systems capture similar types of data be sure to identify one as the source of truth for reporting and analysis purposes.
- HIPAA privacy and security rules apply to the electronic data sources used for reporting and data mining, and pharmacy managers must act as responsible stewards.

The reports provided the satellite pharmacists with the information they needed to proactively identify and respond to the unverified technician–entered orders before the nursing staff needed to administer the dose. After a few weeks of using the reports, pharmacy managers noted that missing medication reports were back to pre-technician entry levels. Further, the end-of-shift reports indicated that pharmacists were reviewing technician orders within an appropriate time frame which led mangers to conclude that the verification process was now working as planned.

References

1. Davenport TH, Laurence P. *Working Knowledge: How Organizations Manage What They Know.* Boston: Harvard Business School Press; 1998:2–5.

2. Hostmann B, Rayner N, Friedman T. Gartner's Business Intelligence and Performance Management Framework. Gartner, October 9, 2006, p. 3.

3. Tiwana A. *The Knowledge Management Tookit: Orchestrating IT, Strategy, and Knowledge Platforms.* 2nd ed. Upper Saddle River, NJ: Prentice Hall; 2002:36–38.

4. Fisher C, Lauria E, Chengalur-Smith S, Wang R. *Introduction to Information Quality.* Cambridge, MA: MIT Information Quality Program; 2006:44–48.

5. Lee YW, Pipino LL, Funk JD, Wang R. *Journey to Data Quality.* Cambridge, MA: MIT Press; 2006:9–10.

6. Lee YW, Pipino LL, Funk JD, Wang R. *Journey to Data Quality.* Cambridge, MA: MIT Press; 2006:80–81.

7. Mills PD, Neily J, Mims E. et al. Improving the bar-coded medication administration system at the Department of Veterans Affairs. *Am J Health-Syst Pharm.* 2006;63:1442–1447.

8. Cummings J, Bush P, Smith D. Bar-coding medication administration overview and consensus recommendations. *Am J Health Syst. Pharm.* 2005;62:2626–2629.

9. Ash JS, Berg M., Coiera E. Some unintended consequences of information technology in health care: the nature of patient care information system-related errors. *J Am Med Inform. Assoc.* 2004;11(2):104–112.

10. Pederson CA, Schneider PJ, Scheckelhoff DJ. ASHP national survey of pharmacy practice in hospital settings: Dispensing and administration—2005. *Am J Health-Syst Pharm.* 2006;63:327–345.

11. Riordan RM. *Designing Effective Database Systems.* Upper Saddle River, NJ: Addison Wesley Professional; 2005. Section 6.1 accessed via Safari Books Online.

12. Kimball R, Ross M, Thornthwaite W. *The Data Warehouse Lifecycle Toolkit: Expert Methods for Designing, Developing, and Deploying Data Warehouses.* New York: Wiley; 1998:139–144.

13. Panko R. What We Know About Spreadsheet Errors. http://panko.cba.hawaii.edu/ssr/Mypapers/whatknow.htm, accessed May 2007.

14. Bergeron BP. *Performance Management in Healthcare: From Key Performance Indicators to Balanced Scorecard.* Chicago: Healthcare Information and Management Systems Society; 2006:103.

15. Few S. Common Mistakes in Data Presentation. http://www.intelligententerprise.com/showArticle.jhtml?articleID=26100530, accessed May 2007.

16. Knight G. *Analyzing Business Data with Excel.* Sebastopol, CA: O'Reilly; 2006. Section 12.3 accessed via Safari Books Online.

17. Few S. *Information Dashboard Design.* Sebastopol, CA: O'Reilly; 2006. Section 7.1 accessed via Safari Books Online.

18. Kimball R. *The Data Warehouse Toolkit: Practical Techniques for Building Dimensional Data Warehouses.* New York: Wiley; 1996: 12–13.

19. Coiera E. *Guide to Health Informatics.* 2nd ed. London: Arnold; 2003:337–338, 350–354.

20. Mena J. Data Mining FAQ's. *DM Review.* January 1998.

21. Silver M, Sakata T, Su H, et al. Case Study: How to apply data mining techniques in a healthcare data warehouse. *J Healthcare Info Manage.* 2001;15(2):155–164.

22. Rudman WJ, Brown CA, Hewitt CR, et al. The use of data mining tools in identifying medication error near misses and adverse drug events. *Top Health Inform Manage.* 2002;23(2):94–103.

23. Hobbs G. Data mining and healthcare informatics. *Am J Health Behav.* 2001;25(3):285–289.

24. Phoenix Health Systems. *HIPAA Primer.* http://www.hipaadvisory.com/REGS/HIPAAprimer.htm, accessed May 2007.

Planning for Downtime

Alicia S. Miller[*]

KEY DEFINITIONS

Affected Systems—identification of pharmacy information/automation systems as well as hospital information systems that support pharmacy operations and the medication use process. These systems usually consist of the pharmacy information system (PIS), automated dispensing cabinets (ADM), pharmacy robot, TPN compounding machine, pharmacy's intranet and/or hospital's internet sites, admitting/ registration system (ADT/registration) for patient access, financial systems, carousel inventory cabinets, bar code medication administration systems (BCMA), clinical decision support (CDS), computerized provider order entry (CPOE), electronic medication administration record (eMAR), clinical results/electronic healthcare record, laboratory information systems, etc.

Cost of Downtime—associated costs including: (1) direct costs—staff salary, downtime equipment, lost revenue, downtime supplies, and (2) indirect costs—delays in medication delivery, increase in medication errors, staff stress levels, etc.

Evaluation/Outcomes Measure—post downtime review to determine if existing policies and procedures, planning, and staffing worked, and what needs to be changed.

Levels of Downtime—duration of downtime that will require different activation of the downtime plan to maintain pharmacy operations, for example: (1) short duration—up to 2 hours, (2) medium duration—2 to 7 hours, and (3) long duration—greater than 8 hours.

Recovery Period—time period post downtime for entry of data generated during downtime to update pharmacy information/automations systems that were affected during downtime.

Scheduled Downtime—system outage that is scheduled for pharmacy information/automation systems allowing for

*The author wishes to recognize the assistance of Jill Lemke Zimmerman, Pharm.D., M.S., for her preparation of the downtime policy and procedure.

prospective downtime planning; most common reasons include planned hardware or software upgrades.

Unscheduled Downtime—system outage that is not scheduled for pharmacy information/automation systems, resulting in no prospective downtime planning. Most common reasons include unplanned hardware or software failures, power outages, and extreme weather conditions.

Background

In the ideal technical environment, downtime of pharmacy information systems, automation, or associated information systems involving the medication use process would not be an issue. There would be sufficient redundancy for hardware and software, as well as the necessary information system infrastructure (power, network, routers, and hubs) to eliminate a single source of failure which would lead to downtime. As reliance on clinical information systems increases and becomes entrenched in normal workflow, the more difficult it becomes to work without 100% available computer systems.[1] Senior staff will forget how to work in a paper environment while younger staff may have never worked without technology, leading to chaos if proper paper backup systems are not available.[2] This dependency on technology should never outweigh the fundamental role of the pharmacist in providing safe, cost-effective pharmaceutical care to the patient. Around-the-clock system access is now considered a necessity, which increases the staff's concern about downtime.[3]

Currently, scheduled downtime occurs because of the need for software and hardware upgrades, routine maintenance activities, infrastructure maintenance and upgrades, and any other planned occurrence that would cause the systems to be unavailable.[4] Unscheduled downtime occurs randomly and without warning, and different responses are required based on the time of day, duration of downtime, and what systems are affected. The main advantage of scheduled downtime is the ability to pre-plan, review, and staff for the downtime. However, even scheduled downtimes can turn into mini-unscheduled downtimes when unexpected problems are encountered that can extend the downtime or create unintended consequences.

Unfortunately, downtime (scheduled and unscheduled) will occur and planning for such events is crucial. Downtime plans can also be requested during surveys by the Joint Commission on Accreditation of Healthcare Organizations especially as the survey relates to automated dispensing cabinets access during system inaccessibility.[5]

The content and examples in this chapter are to be used as a reference or starting point for development of downtime plans, policies and procedures, and workflows specific to each individual's organizational and departmental information systems and operational environments.

Downtime Policy

The fundamental role of a downtime policy is to ensure continuity of the medication use process by a structured, methodical plan that will enable the staff to revert to a manual process with minimal disruption to patient care. Most pharmacies are operating with minimum staffing levels, so transitioning to a manual process while trying to maintain normal operations is a stretch without prospective planning. A downtime policy template with its major categories can be seen in Figure 12-1. The major categories include notification of system outages, scheduled versus unscheduled downtime and duration, patient profiles, handling of existing and new medication orders, label options, shift procedures, contents of a downtime box, testing methodology, recovery processes, post downtime assessment and identification of affected systems. This template can be used as a starting point for customization and addition of specific issues by individual hospital pharmacies. The purpose of each category will be discussed briefly.

Pharmacy Information System Downtime Policy

POLICY: The Department of Pharmacy is responsible for providing safe and effective patient care in a timely matter, despite the presence or absence of automated systems. In consideration of the possibility of a pharmacy system outage, the following policy will help ensure that patient needs are met with both accuracy and timeliness. Pharmacy system outages should be handled only in accordance with the following procedures.

TABLE OF CONTENTS

PROCESS:

1.0   NOTIFICATION OF SYSTEM OUTAGE

1.1 Pharmacy administrator on-call will be contacted immediately upon realization of a pharmacy system outage.

1.2 Pharmacy administrator will determine which downtime process plan will be implemented.

2.0   SCHEDULED VERSUS UNSCHEDULED DOWNTIME; DURATION

2.1 Scheduled downtime is defined as system outages that are planned.

2.2 Non-scheduled downtime is defined as a system outage that is not planned.

2.3 Duration of downtime.

3.0   PATIENT PROFILES

3.1 Patient medication profiles can be obtained from the following sources:

Figure 12-1. Pharmacy downtime policy—downtime.

Pharmacy Information System Downtime Policy (cont'd)

4.0   EXISTING MEDICATION ORDERS

     4.1 IV admixtures

     4.2 Medications

5.0   NEW ORDERS

     5.1 IV Admixtures

     5.2 Medications

6.0   LABELS

     6.1 IV admixtures

     6.2 Medications

     6.3 Syringe medications

7.0   SHIFT PROCEDURES

     7.1 Procedures and Resource Checklist

8.0   DOWNTIME BOX

     8.1 Contents of box

9.0   TESTING

     9.1 Frequency

     9.2 Duration

     9.3 Shifts/days of week

10.0   RECOVERY

     10.1 Form recovery team

     10.2 Identify recovery areas

     10.3 Prepare recovery procedures

11.0   POST DOWNTIME ASSESSMENT

12.0   AFFECTED SYSTEMS

     12.1 ADT

     12.2 Automated dispensing cabinets

     12.3 CPOE

     12.4 Network

     12.5 Patient financial

     12.6 Bedside point of care

Figure 12-1 (cont'd). Pharmacy downtime policy—downtime.

1. Notification of system outage: Used to establish a hierarchy of reporting structure within the department. One person should be identified as the activator of the downtime policy after determining cause, duration, and extent of the downtime. Communication of pharmacy's downtime to external parties should also be considered. This could include information systems, nursing, medical staff, and even administration, depending on the length and impact of downtime. The communication should include the cause of the downtime, if known, the anticipated recovery time, and if changes have to be made in the medication ordering process (for example, faxing orders or reverting to manually written medication orders). Throughout an extended downtime, periodic updates should be provided to all affected departments. Methods of communication can include email, phone calls, and establishment of a dedicated phone number where updates can be recorded for users to access. After the recovery phase has been completed, a communication announcing the end of the downtime and resumption of normal workflow should be sent to all affected parties.

2. Scheduled versus unscheduled; duration: Provide hospital specific definition of these terms as there is no standard agreement as to what constitutes a short, medium, or long duration or what system unavailability is included in an unscheduled downtime. Medication order processing during downtime can also be defined here. For example, during a short duration, only first doses or STAT and emergency medications should be dispensed. For long duration downtime, doses should be dispensed to cover the next unit dose chart exchange or IV batch fill. Orders with start times beyond the anticipated downtime duration should be filed and be processed post downtime. Managing dispensing activities parallel to the length of the downtime duration provides a structured framework to assist the pharmacy staff in determining what orders are to be processed and what doses are to be sent, which reduces confusion and potential lost charges.

3. Patient profile generation options (Figure 12-2): Defines backup access method for current medication profiles for a patient based on system availability and hospital's CPOE and ADM functionality. This can include nightly printing of all current medication profiles for current patients, nightly electronic transfer of current medication profiles to alternative software applications, patient profile access via CPOE or eMAR if stand-alone from PIS, ADM profiles if all medications orders are sent to the ADM, and clinical data repository/electronic healthcare record if real time. The method can vary depending on scheduled versus unscheduled downtime, and the hospital's information systems capability.

4. Existing medication orders: Defines how existing unit dose and IV orders will be identified for the next batch processing if downtime continues beyond the last generated batch fill. Options include using the last printed unit dose cartfill list, IV fill reports and/or IV profiles, or using the patient profile to differentiate between IV and unit dose medications.

5. New orders: Defines the process for handling new orders usually separated out between unit dose medications and IVs. Further delineation can occur between drugs needing to be dispensed from pharmacy and what is available in ADM. Considerations include documentation of start time, number of doses sent, and sorting and filing of orders.

6. Label printing options (Figure 12-3): Identification of alternative methods of

Potential Patient Profile Solutions

	Option 1—CPOE, ADM Functional	Option 2—CPOE, ADM Functional	Option 3—CPOE Not Functional, ADM Functional	Option 4—CPOE and ADM Not Functional
Plan	■ Print Unit ADM Inventory for RPhs once. ■ View patient profiles on CPOE. ■ Create labels for IV dose due in the 8 hours following the last IV batch time or since the last RPh did hand labels for. ■ Create labels for all UD due in the 8 hours following the last cart fill or since the last RPh did hand labels for. ■ Other RPh(s) creates labels for all new doses and notifies other RPhs of DCs.	■ Print Unit ADM Inventory for RPhs once. ■ Print CPOE "MAR print for specified window" for 24 hours each 8 hours. ■ Highlight IV dose due in the 8 hours following the last IV batch time or since the last RPh did hand labels for. ■ Highlight all UD due in the 8 hours following the last cart fill or since the last RPh did hand labels for. ■ Hand write or type labels for medications identified. ■ Other RPh(s) creates labels for all new doses and notifies other RPhs of DCs.	■ Print Unit ADM Inventory for RPhs once. ■ Print patient med profile from ADM once. ■ Highlight IV dose due in the 8 hours following the last IV batch time or since the last RPh did hand labels for. ■ Highlight all UD due in the 8 hours following the last cart fill or since the last RPh did hand labels for. ■ Hand write or type labels for medications identified. ■ Other RPh(s) creates labels for all new doses and notifies other RPhs of DCs from paper orders.	■ Obtain copies of nursing worklists from the nursing units. ■ Highlight IV dose due in the 8 hours following the last IV batch time or since the last RPh did hand labels for. ■ Highlight all UD due in the 8 hours following the last cart fill or since the last RPh did hand labels for. ■ Hand write or type labels for medications identified. ■ Other RPh(s) creates labels for all new doses and notifies other RPhs of DCs from paper orders.

Figure 12-2. Potential patient profile solutions—downtime.

Potential Patient Profile Solutions (cont'd)

	Option 1—CPOE, ADM Functional	Option 2—CPOE, ADM Functional	Option 3—CPOE Not Functional, ADM Functional	Option 4—CPOE and ADM Not Functional
Monetary Cost Now	■ None	■ None	■ None	■ None
Time Cost Now	■ None	■ None	■ None	■ None
Monetary Cost Later	■ Cost of paper used to print ADM inventory.	■ Cost of paper used to print patient profiles and ADM inventory.	■ Cost of paper used to print patient profiles and ADM inventory.	■ Cost of copies.
Time Cost Later	■ Handwriting/ Typing	■ Handwriting/ Typing	■ Handwriting/ Typing	
Potential Problems	■ ADM and CPOE may not be available during a network outage. ■ How will billing be tracked?	■ Profile RPhs are using is not the most up-to-date. ■ ADM and CPOE may not be available during a network outage.	■ Profile RPhs are using is not the most up-to-date. ■ ADM may not be available during a network outage.	■ 24-hour nursing worklists may not be available.

Figure 12-2 (cont'd). Potential patient profile solutions—downtime.

label generation for new and existing medication orders. These can include using pre-printed IV labels for the most frequently ordered drugs, creation of word processing templates, use of typewriters, printing an extra set of IV labels if time permits, and, the most rudimentary method of generating labels, manually writing the information on a label.

7. Shift procedures: Identify any downtime variation between shifts, different resource requirements by shift, and hand-off criteria when downtime extends beyond a single shift.

8. Downtime box contents (Figure 12-4): Defines what should be contained in the box and the number and location of the required boxes. The benefit of a downtime box is to provide the staff a consolidated method of obtaining all the necessary information, forms, and processes for managing a downtime. Other contents of the downtime box can include flashlights, batteries, walkie-talkies, or other supplies deemed necessary to support operations during the downtime.

9. Testing: Defines when downtime testing of the plan will occur. Periodic testing of

Potential Label Solutions

Requirements	Option 1	Option 2	Option 3
Plan	■ Print blank labels from PIS now and store until needed for handwriting or typing.	■ Create blank labels in MS Word and print them on regular labels when needed for handwriting or typing.	■ Hand write or type labels on labels purchased from office product supplier when needed.
Monetary Cost	■ Cost of labels	■ None	■ None
Time Cost Now	■ Time to print labels. ■ Time to develop blank label on PIS.	■ Time to create label blanks in MS Word. ■ Time to install drivers and network connections to be able to print from Word to current label printers.	■ None
Monetary Cost Later	■ None	■ None	■ Cost of labels from office supplier.
Time Cost Later	■ Handwriting/ typing	■ Handwriting/ typing	■ Handwriting/ typing ■ Time to get labels from supplier. ■ Time to develop blank label if possible during outage.
Potential Problems	■ Staff may not be able to locate pre-printed labels when needed.	■ Staff may not have MS Word available if the entire network has an outage.	■ Relying on supplier to have sufficient quantity of labels. ■ May not be able to develop a blank label if entire network is out.

Figure 12-3. Potential label solutions—downtime.

Downtime Box Contents

Check	Content
	Downtime Box(es)—(identify number and location of boxes)
	1. IV labels
	2. Bin labels
	3. Syringe labels
	4. Downtime accordion order file
	5. Telephone order documentation forms
	6. Instructions on printing patient profiles from either PIS or CPOE
	7. Instructions on accessing ADM inventory
	8. Policy and procedure for downtime
	9. Downtime flow sheet
	10. Specialized reports; for example, Epidural and DUE lists
	11. Current record of ordered IV/reports
	12. Standardized administration times

Figure 12-4. Downtime box contents—downtime.

the downtime plan should be conducted even though there might be an impact on patient care and staff resources. Downtime testing should be viewed in the same light as conducting periodic disaster preparedness drills within the hospital. Select pharmacy staff should be identified as key resources who maintain their downtime competency and assist pharmacy staff during the initial phase of an unscheduled downtime. Downtime instruction should also occur during orientation of new employees and annual mandatory modules. It is also important to get administrative recognition and approval for downtime drills to help justify the potential disruption on patient care activities for pharmacy and nursing.

10. Recovery: Identify components, processes, and resources needed for the recovery phase, which commences post downtime and concludes when all affected systems have been updated and operations have returned to normal processing.

11. Post downtime assessment: Defines team structure, assessment tool, period of discovery, and re-training process if the downtime plan is revised.

12. Affected systems: List systems that, if unavailable, can impact the technology used in supporting the medication use process. This should also include any hardware, network, power, or environmental failures.

One final consideration in the downtime policy is determining whether any allowable data loss is acceptable. Data loss can include not entering completed orders during a downtime, not capturing all of the charges that occurred during a downtime, documentation of pharmacists' clinical activities and interventions, and accurate inventory utilization. If there is zero tolerance for any of the aforementioned categories, then more resources, testing, and planning will be required.

Affected Systems

The complexity of clinical information systems within the health system has increased exponentially over the last decade with more technology being used to improve patient care and increase pharmacy departmental efficiency. Downtime can no longer be viewed as an isolated incident internal to pharmacy. Even though standalone pharmacy information systems are being replaced with integrated platforms, those that are still interfaced are reliant on interface engines, ADT/registration systems, patient financial systems, and CPOE systems to remain 100% operational. An example of system interoperability to and from a pharmacy information system can be seen in Diagram 12-1. Any one of these systems, if not available, can cause negative impact on the PIS, which will require some portion of the downtime plan to be triggered.

In addition to downtime of pharmacy information systems, automation supporting other facets of the medication use process need to have downtime plans developed, as they are just as critical in supporting patient care as information systems. Automated dispensing cabinets and bedside point of care systems are two examples of such automation that have become embedded into pharmacy and nursing operations. Both have their own importance in the medication use process and their own individual downtime requirements beyond the usual PIS downtime plan. Automated dispensing cabinets should be on emergency power, and the server should be located in a protected area. System backups should be done daily and stored separate from the server room. Operational impact should be identified; for example, the need to go on critical override when the pharmacy

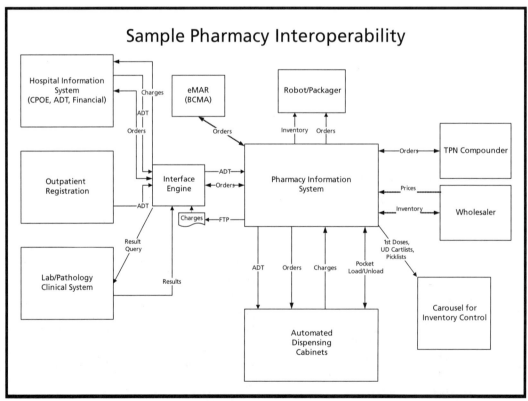

Diagram 12-1. Pharmacy interoperability—downtime.

system information is unavailable. Bar code medication administration systems, which are also dependant on PIS for medication orders, need the ability for overrides during a downtime so nurses can still administer medications to patients. If BCMA is down, then nurses need to revert to manual documentation of medication administration.

Another, often ignored, aspect of downtime is the ability to access the internet, intranet, and/or drug knowledge databases during a power or hardware failure. Intranets are being used for centralized storage of policies and procedures, instructional manuals, drug information databases, and other operational facts. Without the intranet, pharmacy personnel would be stymied in their ability to review, verify, or search the critical information available on the intranet. Redundancy and a secure location for the intranet server should be part of the downtime plan. It is also advisable to have critical policies and procedures or other key operational documents in paper format in case of a total system outage.

The hospital's network and hardware infrastructure, even though they are outside pharmacy's domain and are transparent to most clinicians, provide the foundation for clinical systems' connectivity and access of clinical systems throughout the hospital. The pharmacy information system could be 100% operational but inaccessible if there are network issues. Determining where the network has failed and the scope of the failure could allow pharmacy personnel to keep processing medication orders in areas unaffected by the network outage.

Additional sources of non-related system downtime are the loss of utilities, heating, ventilation and air conditioning (HVAC), elevator, and telecommunications outages. Verification of emergency power connectivity is imperative to provide at least a minimum number of workstations, printers, and other critical hardware such as intranet servers that are available when nor-

mal power is interrupted. Facilities management departments should be contacted for an inventory and assessment of pharmacy's emergency power requirements. HVAC outages become an issue if the room temperature becomes excessive for computer equipment, requiring systems to be powered down before they overheat. Even an elevator outage can create disruptions in the medication use process by impeding delivery of medications from the wholesaler, transport of unit dose carts to nursing units, or ability of disabled staff to navigate within the hospital. The use of land line and wireless phones are a crucial part of communication within the hospital. A telecommunication outage can create major disruptions in maintaining patient care. There should be downtime phones available in all patient care areas and ancillary departments. A list of all downtime phone numbers should be posted in close proximity to the downtime phone and included in the downtime box. Walkie-talkies can also be used as an alternative communication method if the downtime phones are compromised.

It is imperative, therefore, to ask more detailed questions when notification is received of an apparent unscheduled downtime. Is it truly the clinical system experiencing the downtime, or is it network problems? Troubleshooting and tracing the problem to determine the underlying source of the downtime is usually the first step to undertake before starting downtime procedures.

Each affected system and its interdependency on other systems does warrant inclusion in the departmental downtime policy and procedure to provide coverage for the inevitable failure of these systems.

Downtime Procedure

Development of a downtime procedure is necessary to provide a step-by-step process of activities that will be performed during either a scheduled or unscheduled downtime. A work group should be formed consisting of staff that represents various shifts, areas, and tasks within the department, with their primary objective the identification of daily functions that are dependant on automation/technology for support of the medication use process. A pre-planning downtime template as seen in Figure 12-5 is an example of a deliverable for scheduled downtime by the work group. Within the template, computer generated output should be listed along with information on how long it takes to print each job, when the printing should commence prior to downtime, what will be its coverage period and in what priority should the job run. For example, if there is only one report printer and the duration of printing all output (unit dose cart lists, medication administration records, pick lists, food/drug interactions, patient profiles, etc.) is calculated to be 12 hours, then pharmacy needs to identify additional printers or realize the generated reports could be at least 12 hours old. In this same scenario, a priority might be given to printing the MAR (ICU before medical-surgical units) first, followed by unit dose cart fill lists, patient profiles, and any remaining reports if time permits. The template should also recognize any variance in job generation by listing the various areas or pharmacies that require additional processing. Other deliverables include creation of the downtime procedure manual (Figure 12-6), including the order workflow and resource checklist. The pharmacy information systems downtime procedure manual should incorporate and address anticipated concerns for changes to processes that will occur during a downtime.

The downtime procedure manual provides the detailed framework for activities, resources, equipment, and processes required in a downtime, in a logical, easy to follow, concise manner. There should be no ambiguity in responsibilities, roles, and functions necessary to support pharmacy operations during a downtime.

The following auxiliary equipment needs to be readily accessible and functional even though it will be rarely used in normal pharmacy operations: typewriters with good ribbons, stand-alone label maker with labels, and correct size containers for placement of paper orders and requisitions. Periodic inspection and inventory of these items is recommended to ascertain functional status and that the equipment has not disappeared over time.

Extra staff will be needed to supplement normal pharmacy operations staffing levels to support the additional workload required from reverting to a manual process. There is no formula, standard, or benchmark to determine what the additional staffing requirement should be but, at a minimum, one to two extra staff per shift during the downtime and two to three extra staff per shift during the recovery phase, with a slant towards more pharmacists, is not unrealistic. Of course, this is dependant on the duration of the downtime, day of week, census at the hospital, and time of day. Justification of overtime is usually not an issue when used in conjunction with a downtime.

Another decision point is where all the downtime policies and procedures, manuals, and template documents should be stored. A centralized location to access key information and resources required to efficiently and knowledgeably carry out the downtime plan is preferred. This can include creation of a downtime directory on a shared network drive containing the policy and procedure, label templates, forms, templates, etc., printing out the contents of the shared directory and placing the output in the downtime boxes, creating web pages on the departmental intranet server, and/or inclusion in the departmental disaster manual. All four options might be utilized to mitigate the inaccessibility during a downtime but requires more maintenance to ensure that all four locations contain the same version and updates.

Downtime Pre-Planning Template

FUNCTIONS	Main Pharmacy	IV Room	Satellite Pharmacy	2nd Facility Pharmacy	Ambulatory Pharmacy	Purchasing
UD cart list 1. Printing duration 2. Start time 3. Coverage period						
UD cart ex-change 1. Printing duration 2. Start time						
UD pick list 1. Printing duration 2. Start time						
UD bin list 1. Printing duration 2. Start time						
MAR 1. Printing duration 2. Start time						
IV batch labels 1. Printing duration 2. Start time 3. Coverage period						
IV batch pro-duction 1. Printing duration 2. Start time						

Figure 12-5. Downtime pre-planning template—downtime.

Downtime Pre-Planning Template (cont'd)

FUNCTIONS	Main Pharmacy	IV Room	Satellite Pharmacy	2nd Facility Pharmacy	Ambulatory Pharmacy	Purchasing
Syringe production						
Patient profiles 1. Printing duration 2. Start time						
DUE reports (vanco, gent, tob) runs at 5 a.m. 1. Printing duration 2. Start time 3. Hold new orders						
Allergy pending 1. Printing duration 2. Start time						
Epidural list 1. Printing duration 2. Start time						
Food-drug interaction 1. Printing duration 2. Start time						

Figure 12-5 (cont'd). Downtime pre-planning template—downtime.

An occasionally overlooked factor in downtime planning is reviewing backup procedures, storage, and testing methodology. A backup is a routine process whereby the data on the PIS computer is copied to another medium. Complete backups include the operating system, application software and patient data. Incremental backups can also be performed which only include new patient data from the last backup. Backups

Downtime Pre-Planning Template (cont'd)						
FUNCTIONS	**Main Pharmacy**	**IV Room**	**Satellite Pharmacy**	**2nd Facility Pharmacy**	**Ambulatory Pharmacy**	**Purchasing**
ADM inventory 1. Printing duration 2. Start time 3. Turn on critical override						
Vertical purchasing cabinets						
Downtime boxes						
Typewriters						

Figure 12-5 (cont'd). Downtime pre-planning template—downtime.

are an insurance policy that is necessary in case of hardware failure. Backup procedures should include the frequency of backups (daily, weekly, monthly), what types of backup (incremental versus complete), determination if users need to be logged off for backups, length and impact on system performance during backups, automatic or manually scheduled backups, backup medium (tape, externally connected hard drives, centralized disk sharing), what is being backed up (application programs, operating system, data), number of saved backups, and identification of responsible staff. Storage of backup media should never be in the same location as the application being backed up, and it should be stored in a location safe from water, fire, and heat damage.

Backups that are never tested aren't really backups. The worst time to discover your backups are worthless is during a restoration after a hardware failure or system upgrade. The existing downtime anxiety level caused by the hardware failure or system upgrade will increase exponentially. Ideally, testing would occur on redundant hardware so as not to impact the production environment. However, this can be unrealistic due to cost of hardware, additional licensing fees, and vendor support time. Using the production server is an option but will probably result in a scheduled downtime of a medium duration. You also risk corrupting the production database, which could result in re-entry of lost or erroneous data resulting in an extended recovery period. Information systems should be involved in these discussions because they have the expertise to determine what backup options would work better based on the hospital's hardware configuration.

Recovery Procedure

In most downtimes, the recovery period is where the greatest need for additional staff, coordination, and confusion resides. The benefits of recovery planning include being

```
                                                    Effective Date _____

                                                    Revision Date _____

                        PROCEDURE MANUAL
──────────────────────────────────────────────────────────────────────
           Title: Pharmacy Information System Downtime
──────────────────────────────────────────────────────────────────────

SCHEDULED DOWNTIME PROCEDURE

1.0  PHARMACIST IN CHARGE

     1.1   Designate the pharmacist in charge of downtime operations for each shift.

     1.2   The pharmacist-in-charge responsibilities include:

           1.2.1  Coordinate the flow of orders (refer to Appendix A flow sheet)

           1.2.2  Designate a technician responsible for coordinating report printing 12 hours
                  prior to PIS downtime. Use the checklist (refer to Appendix B) included to
                  track the report printing. After the central pharmacy reports are printed, the
                  technician can coordinate other facility report printing. Patient profiles can be
                  printed from CPOE/eMAR to reduce the time necessary to print reports on PIS.

           1.2.3  Designate a pharmacist and technician to type medication and IV labels. Their
                  sole responsibility is the processing of orders; they are not to be pulled for
                  other jobs.

           1.2.4  Designate a technician to review orders and determine which medications are
                  in ADM using an ADM report.

           1.2.5  Pharmacist in charge will have the authority to send extra employees home,
                  when it is necessary.

2.0  DOWNTIME SET-UP

     2.1   Verify that all the necessary staffing, labels, typewriters, and other items are available
           (refer to Box Contents and Checklist).

     2.2   Retrieve typewriters from specified area. The typewriters should be placed prior to
           downtime. The placement and number of the typewriters should also be identified.

     2.3   Common pre-printed IV labels are in the Downtime Box. To print more IV labels,
           syringe labels, or any policy and procedures, the files are located in the shared drive
           under Downtime Folder.

     2.4   To keep track of verbal orders, use the verbal order log included in the Downtime Box
           or on the shared drive.

     2.5   To keep track of epidural orders, use the epidural list included in the Downtime Box
           or on the shared drive.

     2.6   To keep track of drug usage evaluations and/or pharmacokinetic monitoring started
           during downtime, use the DUE list included in the Downtime Box or on the shared
           drive.
```

Figure 12-6. Procedure manual—downtime.

2.7 Collect the prior day's cart list sheets for reference and cart fill.

2.8 Place a copy of the default administration times next to each typewriter for the pharmacist to write on the order (included in the Downtime Box).

3.0 PROCESSING ORDERS

3.1 For the complete processing of orders, refer to the flow chart in the Downtime Box.

3.2 After the pharmacist types the IV labels for the batch and first dose hood, they all should be paper-clipped to the order. The labels and the order will go to the first dose hood to be filled. The pharmacist checks the first dose IV and initials the order and the IV to indicate it has been checked. Once the first dose IV is complete, then the order and the IV batch labels will be transferred to the IV room.

3.3 When the IV batch labels are checked and the pharmacist places their initials on the order, it can be filed alphabetically in the accordion included in the Downtime Box.

3.4 For unit dose medications dispensed from the pharmacy, the label should include the patient name and location (refer to the flow chart).

4.0 PIS RECOVERY

4.1 Enter manual written orders into PIS prior to the entry of the CPOE orders. This will allow for a double check of orders put into CPOE by the house staff. (This is only if both CPOE and PIS are down.)

4.2 Downtime CPOE orders are defined as orders that were manually written during the downtime and are put in CPOE when the systems recover. DT or Downtime written in the Comment Section will denote a downtime order.

4.3 New orders written after the downtime will not have DT or Downtime written in the comment section.

4.4 Enter orders written during a PIS downtime using standard order entry procedure for the following types of orders:

4.4.1 New Medication Order, Scheduled or PRN

4.4.1.2 Cancel label print for doses that were dispensed during the down-time.

4.4.2 New IV Order

4.4.2.1 Enter order with start time per order start time. Discard labels for bags that were dispensed during the downtime.

4.4.2.2 (Alternate) Enter order with post-downtime start time. Manually charge for doses dispensed during the downtime.

4.5 Use ADHOC charging to charge for the following types of orders:

4.5.1 Non-ADM one-time medication/IV orders

4.5.2 Orders started and discontinued during the downtime

4.5.3 Replacement doses dispensed during the downtime

Figure 12-6 (cont'd). Procedure manual—downtime.

4.6 Do not enter one-time ADM orders into PIS as the ADM system will charge for these items.

5.0 UNSCHEDULED DOWNTIME PROCEDURE

5.1 All things remain the same as a planned downtime except report printing. To fill unit dose medications it will be necessary to keep the cart list report from the prior day.

5.2 To fill batch IVs, an IV summary report should be printed daily in case of a PIS downtime.

6.0 DOWNTIME PROCEDURES SUPPLEMENTAL INSTRUCTIONS

Pre-Downtime and During Downtime

I. **Filing** of CPOE orders received during the pharmacy downtime:

   a. Staff in the central pharmacy should use bins to separate orders received during the downtime as follows:

      i. Routine orders—For scheduled medication and IV orders

      ii. PRN orders—For PRN orders that are in ADM or available on demand

      iii. Bill only—For orders that were sent, e.g., ONCE orders, and need to be billed only

   b. If a printed page contains more than one order, the page should be placed in the bin that will receive the highest priority for order entry after PIS becomes available (see I.c.).

   c. When the PIS application becomes available, order entry of downtime orders should be prioritized in the following order:

      i. Routine orders—first

      ii. PRN orders—second

      iii. Bill only—third

II. **ADM inventories**

   a. Pre-downtime, a hard copy of ADM station inventories will be printed and placed in a binder and kept in pharmacy.

III. **Bin labels**

   a. Extra sets of bin labels will be printed pre-downtime to be used for labeling drug doses dispensed during the downtime.

IV. **Documentation** on CPOE orders received during the pharmacy downtime:

   a. <u>Clinical Interventions</u>—Document on the CPOE order if any interventions, e.g., lab review, allergy checks, were performed at the point of order receipt and drug dispensing, so that this does not have to be repeated at the time of order entry when Centricity becomes available.

Figure 12-6 (cont'd). Procedure manual—downtime.

    b.   <u>IV Doses Dispensed</u>—Document on the CPOE order how many doses were dispensed for IV orders to allow for proper billing when PIS becomes available (See VI.b., VII.c.).

V. **Expensive/time-slotted IVs**

    a.   Notify the IV pharmacist (or place notification in a designated folder) when an order is received during the downtime to discontinue an expensive/time-slotted IV, so that the dose will not be made and wasted.

VI. **IV Doses** sent during the downtime

    a.   IV batch labels will be printed pre-downtime for a coverage period of at least 6 hours beyond planned downtime period.

    b.   During the downtime, dispense enough IV doses to cover the interval for which the IV batch has printed.

Recovery Period

VII. **Post downtime order entry** of orders received during the downtime

    a.   <u>Scheduled medication orders</u> (e.g., Q8H, BID)

        i.   Use start time listed on the CPOE order or manually record on order to allow for automated processing and billing of doses dispensed during the downtime.

    b.   <u>PRN medication orders</u>

        i.   Use PIS default start time OR start time listed on the CPOE order.

    c.   <u>Scheduled and PRN IV orders</u>

        i.   Use start time listed on the CPOE order.

        ii.   Verify correct number of doses are billed.

Figure 12-6 (cont'd). Procedure manual—downtime.

able to revert back to normal operations as quickly as possible; ensuring an orderly, systematic, and timely recovery; reducing legal liability; and minimizing potential lost revenue. Recovery should be expedited in a formal manner whereby prerequisites are identified, re-entry of orders is done in a consistent method, and specific tasks are assigned to individual recovery staff.

A recovery team should be formed consisting of a team leader, site team leader, and recovery personnel. The team leader responsibilities include notification to the staff that downtime is over and recovery should be commenced, verification that pre-requisite systems are available and updated (ADT,

CPOE), coordination of the recovery effort regarding staffing and entry of orders, problem resolution, and providing assistance to the recovery personnel. The site team leader reports to the team leader and provides a more direct, hands-on responsibility during the recovery period at each recovery entry location. The recovery personnel are responsible for entry of downtime orders and should be located in a sequestered area of pharmacy to work uninterrupted and be removed from normal operations.

The first step in the recovery process is to have updated ADT information within the PIS if ADT was one of the affected downtime systems. This can take several hours, depending on the length of the downtime. Once ADT is complete, then orders can be entered. The priority of order entry should be (1) entry of scheduled orders, (2) PRN orders, (3) one-time and completed orders, and (4) replacement doses that were sent and require charging. If at all possible, downtime orders should be completed before entry of any new orders is entered on the patient. It is beneficial to have a logical, structured plan so that downtime orders are sorted by unit and then by patient, in chronological order, followed by entry of the downtime orders by each patient in the unit. A checklist by unit can then be used to monitor status of the recovery period as well as when new orders can be entered on a unit.

One detail that can be overlooked during the recovery period is removing the override status from automated dispensing cabinets. Usually, ADM are set to critical override during the PIS downtime to allow nurses to access medications for patients. Once the downtime is over and PIS order entry is complete, the critical override needs to be removed.

In some situations, even though this can add time to the total downtime/recovery period, a complete backup of the system should be performed if the downtime was for an extended period or caused by a hardware failure. To complete the recovery procedure, it is important to inform the affected parties that the downtime is over and normal workflow has resumed. This re-establishes routine operation methodology and serves as a notification to physicians and nurses that all medication orders are deemed current within pharmacy. If a discrepancy is identified, the pharmacy needs to be contacted.

Post Downtime Assessment

An evaluation of the downtime plan should be conducted after each downtime (scheduled and unscheduled) to determine the effectiveness of the plan and to make any necessary changes to enhance the downtime process. Downtime should be considered an integral part of pharmacy's continuous quality improvement program because of (1) its impact on patient care, and (2) its infrequent occurrence. The evaluation methodology should include dialogue with all pharmacy shifts and areas as well as any external departments affected by the downtime including ADT, nursing, dietary, medical staff, laboratory, finance, etc. All comments should be viewed as constructive without any repercussions.

Questions that should be asked include the following:

- Was there adequate staffing?
- Were downtime boxes complete and accessible?
- Was communication effective during downtime?
- Was staff prepared for the downtime?
- Was chaos kept to a minimum?
- Was patient care impacted?
- Was recovery effectively accomplished?
- What worked well?
- What did not work well?

These questions can be asked during group meetings, distributed as a survey document, or available electronically on the hospital's intranet site. The responses to the questions should be reviewed and appropriate changes made to the downtime plan. Feedback should be provided to the participants as to the outcomes of their comments and revisions made to the downtime plan. Scoring cards can also be distributed in addition to the questions to determine a numeric score for each downtime that can serve as a benchmark.

Cost of Downtime

A final consideration in downtime planning is to calculate the financial impact of the various components of downtime: prevention, downtime and recovery resource consumption, medication errors, and lost revenue. As tolerance for downtime decreases, the cost to prevent downtime increases. Assessment of risk should be undertaken of the technology supporting the medication use process to determine what risks can be mitigated, as some risk is acceptable when the cost of eliminating downtime exceeds the inherent benefit. This assessment begins by looking at what business functions will be affected (order entry, dispensing), what process dependencies are involved (inputs—ADT, outputs—order requisition to ADM), what is the impact of interruption (low, medium, high), and what is the downtime tolerance (0 to 5). Values can be assigned to each category to calculate a cost to benefit ratio. This will allow prioritization of downtime dollars for the most critical technology.

Another method to determine risk assessment is the use of the following calculation[6]:

- Single loss expectancy (SLE)—how much do we stand to lose if an identified risk comes to pass?

- Annualized rate of occurrence (ARO)—what is the probability of an identified risk coming to pass annually?

- Annualized loss expectancy (ALE)—how much do we expect to lose each year?

$$ALE = SLE \times ARO$$

ALE example:

Risk identified: pharmacy information system is on a single server

Risk scenario: server crashes and is unavailable for 1 day and results in 5% lost charges

SLE—$100,000 (based on daily revenue generation of $2,000,000)

ARO—0.5%

$$ALE = \$100,000 \times 0.5\% = \$500$$

An annualized loss expectancy of $500 in this scenario means that the risk of downtime is minimal and does not require major downtime investment. However this formula does not take into consideration additional tangible dollars such as overtime or the intangible impact on patient care, staff morale, and departmental credibility.

Calculating the cost of downtime should involve information systems, facilities engineering, finance, and hospital administration, as capital dollars might need to be budgeted, emergency power might need to be expanded, or backup or offsite solutions may need to be made available within IS.

Computerized Provider Order Entry Considerations

The implementation of CPOE in healthcare organizations adds another layer of complexity to a downtime plan due to the interdisciplinary nature of the application. Basic principles of downtime still apply with CPOE, but additional processes must be considered as well as the need for additional resources during the downtime and recovery phases.

First, a hospital notification list needs to be created to include key contacts for all departments that will be affected by downtime. The key contacts will then be responsible for notifying their personnel of either scheduled or unscheduled downtime. These key contacts include representatives from the medical staff, residents, nursing, ancillary departments, and hospital administration. Overhead announcements and screen updates on unit workstations can also be utilized to notify staff of downtime within the hospital and provide status updates. A downtime phone line is another option to provide status updates. Communication is critical as so many personnel are involved, most departments are affected, and patient care must be maintained during downtime.

Medication order processing is the next consideration with CPOE downtime.

During short downtime duration, physicians should limit their prescribing to only orders that are necessary for the patient during the downtime. Pre-printed order forms, including admission order sets, should be maintained on the unit to support the physician in transitioning to paper orders. Pharmacy will need to maintain fax machines for receipt of paper orders and revert to retrieving orders while making medication delivery rounds.

The final consideration for CPOE downtime is the recovery phase. Personnel responsible for re-entry of orders have to be identified. Ideally, it will be an interdisciplin-ary process and the healthcare professional writing the order enters the order into the CPOE system. Realistically, physicians may not be as readily available to participate in the recovery process, which leaves the entry of orders to either the nurse or pharmacist.

A decision needs to be made if all downtime orders are to be entered or only recurrent orders. If one time orders or orders completed during the downtime are not entered, then a complete electronic health record is not maintained for the patient.[7] A paper medical record would need to be created for those non-entered orders and a

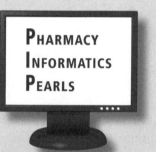

Downtime

Scheduled downtime

- The preferred method of downtime as staff have time to prepare for the downtime. Scheduled downtime should occur when there is the least impact on patient care and occur as infrequently as possible

Unscheduled downtime

- Unexpected downtime leads to a more chaotic implementation of downtime procedures. Causes can consist of power outages, storm damage, floods, hardware failure, software failure, and fires. The impact of unscheduled downtime can be reduced by creating downtime procedures and scheduling periodic downtime drills.

Affected systems

- Pharmacy needs to look beyond the pharmacy information system when preparing for downtime, because other technology and information systems within the hospital and pharmacy can impact patient care if unavailable. These can include:
  - CPOE
  - ADT
  - ADM
  - Pharmacy robot
  - TPN compounding
  - Carousels for inventory control
  - Clinical decision support
  - Intranet/Internet
  - Clinical results
  - Information systems infrastructure—network, routers, hubs, interface engine

Levels of downtime

- The duration of the downtime (known if a scheduled downtime, or estimated if unscheduled) requires different downtime responses from pharmacy. This can include turning on the critical override in the ADM, increase staffing levels, more accurate documentation on downtime forms, increased communication between affected parties, and more structured processes.

Cost of downtime

■ There are expected costs associated with downtime. These include direct costs such as overtime, additional equipment, supplies (back-up labels, printing hardcopy patient profiles), and lost revenue as well as indirect costs, which include delays in medication delivery, increase in medication errors, and staff's stress levels. Costs of preventing downtime can also be calculated using a cost-benefit analysis.

Recovery period

■ The phase of downtime when systems are available and downtime orders are processed in a timely manner to return to normal operations as quickly as possible.

Post downtime assessment

■ The effectiveness of the downtime plan should be reviewed after each downtime by soliciting input from affected parties using methods such as meetings, questionnaires or emails. Revisions to the downtime plan should occur based on valid suggestions.

notation should be made in the electronic health record that a downtime occurred and orders could be incomplete. Also, if CPOE and PIS are not interfaced or integrated, there should be a notation on the entered order stating this was a downtime order as a trigger to pharmacy that the order should already be in the PIS. Another decision to be made is whether downtime orders need to be co-signed by the physician if entered by another licensed healthcare professional. If they do, then downtime orders should be entered and verified before new orders are entered on the patient.

Conclusion

It is inevitable that downtime in some form or another will eventually occur that will impact the PIS and/or medication use technology. Downtime planning must be addressed and considered part of the department's disaster planning process. Involving the staff, reviewing the downtime

plan with changes or additions to pharmacy technology/automation, periodic testing of the plan, and reassessment of the plan post downtime are key success factors in minimizing the impact of downtime on delivery of quality, timely, and safe pharmaceutical care to patients. The spectrum of downtime can range from one malfunctioning workstation to a total system failure and loss of emergency power. Planning for the worst case scenario is vital.

Technology/automation systems are only very important tools used routinely by healthcare professionals to deliver care. Fundamentally, it is people who provide the care—not technology.

References

1. Kilbridge P. Computer crash: Lessons from a system failure. *N Engl J Med.* 2003;348(10):881–882.

2. Campbell E, Sittig D, Ash J, et al. Types of unintended consequences related to computerized provider order entry. *J Am Med Inform Assoc.* 2006;13(5):547–556.

Appendix A. Downtime Order Flow Chart

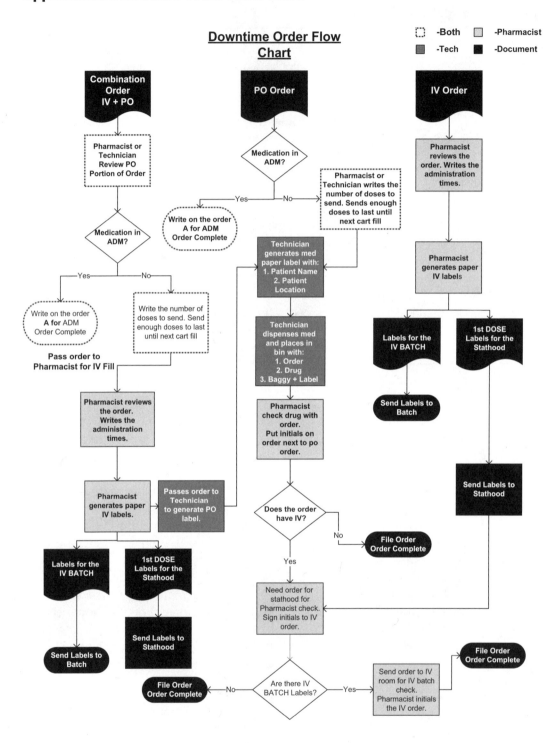

Appendix B. Resource Checklist

Resource Checklist

Check	Resource
	Downtime box(es)
	Typewriters (# and location)
	Reports
	1. Unit dose (UD) cart list
	2. UD bin labels
	3. IV order summary
	4. IV batch production list
	5. Patient profiles
	6. Specialized reports generated—food/drug interactions, pending allergies
	Staffing
	1. Extra pharmacist on each shift during downtime (1)
	2. Extra technician(s) at each shift during downtime (1–2)
	3. Extra pharmacist(s) for recovery period (4)
	Labels on Hand
	1. IV admixture labels (determine quantity)
	2. Med/syringe labels (determine quantity)

3. Weiner M, Gress T, Thiemann D, et al. Contrasting views of physicians and nurses about an inpatient computer-based provider order-entry system. *J Am Med Inform Assoc.* 1999;6:234–244.

4. Miller A. Downtime procedures (part 1). *Hosp Pharm.* 2003;38(6):608–610.

5. Garrelts J, Koehn L, Snyder V, et al. Automated medication distribution systems and compliance with Joint Commission standards. *Am J Health Syst Pharm.* 2001;58:2267–2272.

6. Brown M. Things do go wrong: business continuity planning. Paper presented at HIMSS RHIO/HIE Forum; December 5, 2006; Salt Lake City, NV.

7. Miller, A. Downtime procedures (part 2) *Hosp Pharm.* 2003;38(7):694–697.

CHAPTER 13

Management Issues*

Marc Young

KEY DEFINITIONS

Health Insurance Portability and Accountability Act (HIPAA)—law enacted in 1996 by the U.S. Congress in order to protect patient medical information. Title II of HIPAA, the Administrative Simplification (AS) provisions, requires the establishment of national standards for electronic health care transactions and national identifiers for providers, health insurance plans, and employers to address the security and privacy of health data.

Change Management—a discipline in information systems service that seeks to ensure that standard methods and procedures are used when making changes to information technology infrastructure, attempting to balance the need for change with the potential negative impact changes can produce.

Human Factors—physical, mental, or behavioral properties of people that may have critical influence on how people interact with technological systems, organizations, or their environment.

Implementation—the execution of a plan that, when referring to a technology system, generally encompasses requirements analysis, determination of project scope, integration plan, user training, policy development, and delivery.

Integration—in information technology, the physical or functional linking of two separate systems in order to achieve a desired new functionality or capability, often through the use of interfaces. (Note: For the purposes of this chapter, we will use the preceding definition of "integration." The definition is still a matter of debate in the informatics community.)

Interface—internal communication between two separate entities, i.e., hardware or software, that allows information and resources to be shared without affecting how external entities, i.e., a user, interacts with each system.

---

*The views expressed in this chapter are those of the author and do not necessarily reflect the official policy or position of the Department of the Navy, Department of Defense, nor the U.S. Government.

Patient Care Information System (PCIS)—
technology system used by a health care professional for the provision of care to a patient, either directly through decision support or in a support role such as informational storage or management of information function. PCIS supports the provision of care for patients.

Medication Management System—an automated system that is often connected to other healthcare systems, that supports patient safety, and that improves the quality of care by reducing practice errors and misuse. A medication management system does so by providing access to medications only by authorized personnel and (usually) only if a validated order exists within the system.

This chapter will focus in a stair-step fashion on some of the main points to consider when updating or acquiring a new technology for a pharmacy. The sections will highlight some key determinants and areas that might cause the reader to go in one direction or another or in some cases decide not to act altogether. Rather than focus on day-to-day management techniques, the following sections will emphasize the need to know what the problem is and clearly state desired objectives in order to know when success is achieved or more importantly when not try in the first place. In addition, this chapter also contains review of the basic fundamentals of project planning and relationships with people or representative parties that will be useful in the process for the system determination.

System Determination

Today's health care practitioners find themselves in a world of ever-increasing technological advances that seem to be coming at a more rapid pace. Health information technology (HIT) expenditures are estimated to reach nearly $40 billion by the year 2008.[1] There is a national push to reduce the number of medical errors, including medication errors, through the use of information technology and systems such as electronic

health records (EHR) and computerized provider order entry (CPOE). President Bush has called upon healthcare institutions and organizations to implement electronic health records and systems, designed to improve efficiency and effectiveness of health care delivery, by the year 2014.[2] It is generally recognized that many areas in the health care delivery process could be improved through the increased use of HIT, e.g., automation or CPOE, which increases knowledge or replaces humans in certain situations that have a tendency for errors of commission or omission.[3] In some healthcare settings it is not uncommon to see physicians, nurses, and pharmacists replacing their manual paper methods of the past with various types of HIT, often with handheld or portable versions, to provide real-time data entry and retrieval of information as they care for patients. Regardless of the size, shape or location or whether it is a new system or a change to a legacy system, a successful HIT implementation requires adequate planning in order to ensure that the system becomes a tool not a deterrent or barrier for the healthcare practitioner.

Description of the Problem

Before any system change is undertaken, there should be a clear description of the problem for the technology to solve. The time spent in the determination phase of new system acquisition answering the hard questions of "who, what, when, where and how" is a critical factor in the system's success or failure. This may seem elementary but with all of the benefits of HIT, it is often thought to be a magic solution for the problems (such as staffing shortages) facing many organizations today. Before embarking down the road to new system acquisition, the first question that needs to be asked is "What is the problem we are trying to fix?" Is it actually a problem that is solvable with technology. A technology solution, such as telepharmacy, might address certain events such as staffing shortages by providing a means to extend staff at times and to locations not previously possible. But this extension might come at a substantially higher cost and result in the need to manage additional personnel in a new and more labor intense manner. In contrast, the primary cause(s) could be addressed without necessarily applying a technology but relying on simpler more traditional methods such as flexible staffing or modifications to services offered until staffing challenges are resolved. Proper understanding and description of the root problem is critical to avoid using resources in the various steps and procedures necessary for HIT acquisition that could actually produce a negative impact if the HIT implementation ends in failure.

Elements of the System

Development of Requirements

After a decision is made to implement technology for a particular problem, then the decision of which technology to use is a pre-implementation step or phase that encompasses development and analysis of requirements that start a sequence of events that will lead to system acquisition depicted in Figure 13-1. The requirements and analysis phase focuses on defining the technical, functional, and business requirements that the technology will need to perform. Many hours may be spent in this phase discussing what the HIT needs to do and for whom it should be done. End-users of the HIT will provide the functional requirements, the business requirements will often be provided by management or administrators and information systems (IS) support personnel can assist with the technical requirements. It is critical that all users that will interact with the system or will receive data or other services from this system have a chance to define requirements. Excluding one potential user group due to time constraints or lack of planning might prove problematic later. For example, selection of an inpatient medication management system should not rely solely on the pharmacy for determination but also include nursing staff, IS department, administrators, quality assurance department, etc. to ensure that all vantage points get included. Table 13-1 lists potential users or influencers for selecting a pharmacy system.[4]

Work in a clinical environment is so complex that there needs to be a very solid fit between the users, tasks, and technology.

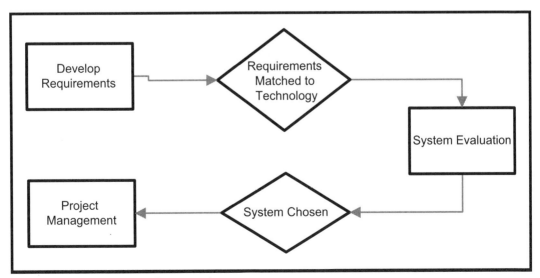

Figure 13-1. Elements of system determination.

TABLE 13-1

Users/Influencers for a Pharmacy System

Group	Reason for Inclusion
Nursing staff	User of the system/influencer of process
IS department	Support system performance
Physicians	User of system or influencer of process
Pharmacists/pharmacy technicians	User of system or influencer of process
State board of pharmacy	Influencer of process
Patient safety/quality assurance	Influencer of process
Administrators	Influencer of process/funding source
Patients/consumer associations	User of system/influencer
Insurance companies/payers	Influencer

In order to obtain the most optimal use of HIT, an organization should balance the needs of the users and their tasks with the available technology. An example of this balance is depicted in the FITT model in Figure 13-2. The FITT model emphasizes the importance of end-user involvement in the early stages of development.[5] Failures in HIT implementations, such as the infamous implementation and subsequent abandoning of CPOE at Cedars Sinai Hospital in Los Angeles, are often the result of inadequate requirements gathering and involvement of the intended health care professionals that will use the technology.[6,7] Once all of the requirements have been gathered, they need prioritization. A simple way to prioritize is to delineate things that the system must do and things that you would like it to do but won't negatively impact your operation if not done. In doing this, you will later be able to narrow to a specific product and also ensure that the system implemented will meet the needs and not hinder any of the users. Ultimately, user involvement helps ensure that all tasks are included in the pre-implementation phase, which will also be a critical component to acceptance after installation or integration.

Matching Requirements to a Technology

Once all of the requirements have been fully vetted among the various stakeholders, then the next phase of implementation begins. This phase is known as the development or evaluation phase. The objectives and planned functions for the HIT detailed in the requirements may or may not exist in a currently available product. With the large number of companies and systems on the market, it is important to quickly find and evaluate all existing technologies. One way to cast a wide net for information gathering is to send out either a request for information (RFI) or request for proposal (RFP). In both cases, it is an invitation for suppliers to submit proposals to describe how they can meet the stated requirements or objectives. Often an RFP includes pricing information but an RFI usually does not. Answers to the RFP or RFI will often let you know if a product exists that meets your needs. If none of the responses will meet the requirements, further searching through the internet, professional associations or contacts, etc., may be required to ensure that no product exists. If one truly does not, then either the requirements will need revising or the system or application would have to be developed specifically for the organization.

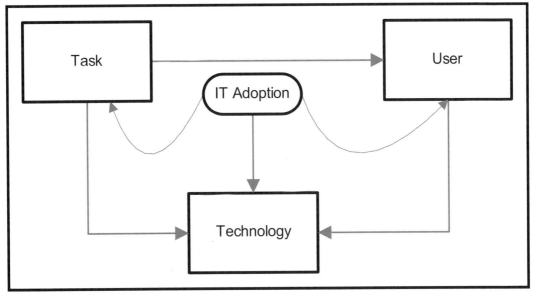

Figure 13-2. FITT framework. *Source:* Adapted from reference 5.

Vendor/System Evaluation

The evaluation of vendors and systems should occur both before and after the implementation of any HIT. In both cases, the previously developed requirements serve as the guidelines for developing evaluation criteria. Both objective and subjective criteria provide value to any assessment for determining success or failure. The objective measures could focus on selected key features of the HIT, financial considerations, support, and infrastructure required by the organization, maintenance and support provided by vendor, availability of the technology, and technical performance (interfaces, security, etc.). Subjective factors measurement might include areas such as the ease of use, impact on safety, and reliability. However, a user group might not understand or appreciate the benefits of change that a technology represents. In some cases the subjective measures might overshadow any level of technical success since the opinions of users and managers often begin arriving before other data and thus serve as the lasting first impression.[4,8]

Evaluation: The Money

Healthcare, particularly pharmaceutical care, has very discrete fixed dollar amounts attached to the provision of services. When deciding on which drugs to carry in a particular hospital or health system, analyses such as cost-benefit, cost-effectiveness, and cost-utility can help gauge the impact of various formulary decisions. All of these analyses attempt to determine the return on investment (ROI) or payback for the resources invested for a particular course of action. Similarly, the implementation of HIT is often put through a ROI methodology when evaluating vendors and conducting post-implementation analyses. However, the benefits sought from HIT are not easily quantifiable. Determining a ROI for implementing HIT has been one of the top significant barriers seen in past surveys of healthcare chief information officers (CIO).[9,10] Success in a healthcare initiative comes from more than direct financial returns of ROI calculations. Rather, benefits in areas such as customer satisfaction and internal business process improvements (i.e., patient safety improvements) should also be included in any evaluation of return on investments. The investments might not only include monetary expenditures but other inputs such as time of personnel or information.

One proposed method to determine the value of a change is the balanced scorecard (BSC) method. This method uses the multiple perspectives that drive a business process, past and future, and tries to align goals, talents, resources, and feedback in order to successfully manage a change process. BSC attempts to balance the financial and non-financial measures and not focus only on one area for a measure of success. An example of how the various elements work together in BSC is found in Figure 13-3. Organizations can choose their performance measures from the different areas that drive the business process. By balancing the financial with other important measures, no longer can the financial bottom-line overshadow successes in other critical areas.[8]

Evaluation: The Vendor

The marketplace for HIT is becoming a veritable "who's who" in technology today. Many companies that sell systems today may have not been in the marketplace 5 years ago and have entered on their own or merged with previous vendors. Given the volatility of the healthcare technology market, evaluation of the company selling a technology ranks almost as important as the technology itself. The relationship with a vendor goes beyond sales and installation and almost always

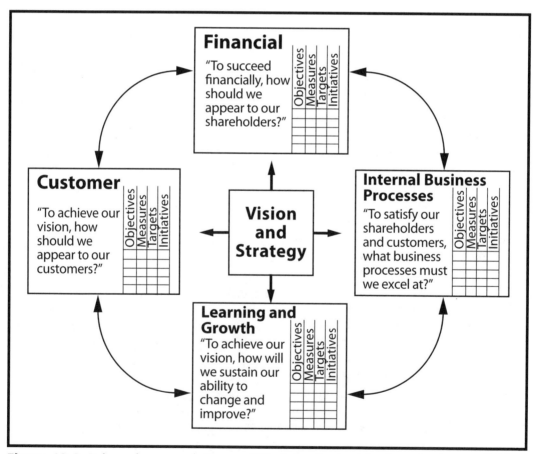

Figure 13-3. Balanced scorecard. *Source:* APO: Asian Productivity Organization. Available at: http://www.apo-tokyo.org/p-glossary_ images/image001.jpg.

includes a support relationship as well. This relationship can be a life-line or an anchor depending on the terms of the relationship.

The first contact most interested parties have with a vendor is the sales department. These individuals represent the frontline business aspect of the corporation. Although knowledgeable about their products, answers to specific questions from them need to be formal, written responses as the information gathering for evaluation begins. Questions to the vendor should reflect developed requirements and whether or not a system can meet specific technical and functional requirements should have written verification that will become useful in latter stages of evaluation. When entering a dialogue with a vendor, very often the sales team is included in discussions. Remember to distinguish what team each person represents in the company to know when the information needs further clarification. For example, answers to questions on capabilities of a system should include the engineers or other technical specialists as well the sales force. Relying only on the sales team might cause implementation of a system that does not meet requirements. The sales department can often provide a list of customers that use their system. This information could prove valuable as these contacts might provide new evaluation criteria suggestions, comments on past performance, additional requirements, or lessons learned in implementation.

Vendor maintenance and support constitute not only important criteria for selection of a vendor but will also serve as a key measure of vendor performance after system implementation. HIT, like any other system or machine will eventually have problems that need resolving. With technology this is accomplished commonly through a support and maintenance agreement. This agreement has defined periods and fees tied to them and dictate items such as when a vendor will come on site to assess problems, how phone or online support is provided,

spare parts, upgrades or updates to the system. Normally HIT needs as close to 100% availability as possible, but higher availability can carry higher cost for support. Lower availability carries a risk for interruption in service but higher rates of availability or performance might prove cost prohibitive. For example, for a system that is needed 365 days of the year, 24 hours a day, reducing the availability requirement from 99.95% to 99% adds 88 hours of unscheduled downtime per year. If the system is a critical system and needs support to ensure availability, then the expectations for amount support, both internal and external, for unscheduled downtime as well-scheduled downtime become important distinguishers for the different systems and vendors under consideration.

Evaluation: Technical Considerations

When implementing any new technology, there are, of course, technical aspects to consider. It is impossible to provide an all inclusive list of each one of them, especially since the growth in capabilities may soon make such a list somewhat incomplete. The considerations for implementing a new HIT, especially one that communicates with other systems, should at a minimum involve verification of security, authentication, authorization, interfaces, storage and messaging. One of the tenets of medicine, often attributed the Hippocratic Oath, is "do no harm." This tenet portrays the compassion of healthcare providers and the benevolent spirit of always protecting their patient's interests. Any technology used to treat patients must still ensure that the safety and care of the patients come first. One of the first ways a HIT can provide this assurance is through the highest standards of security, both physical and digital. The medical information stored and transmitted is extremely sensitive and protected by federal and state laws and standards. The most well known of the legal requirements is the federal Health Insurance Portability and Accountability Act (HIPAA) of 1996 which required the establishment of federal standards for the security (administrative, physical, and technical) of electronic health information.[11] Even though there are laws that mandates information security, it should not be assumed that all available systems are in compliance. With its notoriety, HIPAA compliance still remains in the top list of concerns for healthcare CIOs, over 10 years after inception.[9] The information sharing that is the lifeblood of good patient care could bring an organization to a standstill if information cannot be trusted when shared across or within systems or the security of the communications or transactions is suspect.

The utilization of information technology and electronic resources offer many more opportunities than existed with paper only records for violations of patients protected health information. For example, the installation of new pharmacy medication management system on a hospitals network could unintentionally open access points for unauthorized access to sensitive information if the new system is not properly examined and tested by a network security team. A common method of technical support by HIT vendors is through remote management. This requires that they have an ability to gain access to the system to diagnose problems when they occur. This support should occur through secure, encrypted connections and be monitored and managed by the organization, not the vendor. Every open network point on a healthcare network is a potential vulnerability even though it was established for a logical purpose. It is recommended that a potential buyer ask a vendor to provide verification that they can meet all relevant security requirements (federal, state, and institutional) prior to any installation. Additionally, hiring an independent contractor to evaluate the final list of candidates and their methodology may be helpful in some cases.

The care for patients relies on the transmission of messages. Historically, this transmission was through paper records and verbal exchanges. Increasingly today however, this transmission occurs through information systems technology such as EHRs and CPOE. Information systems are no different than people in that in order to have a good relationship, communication is the key. Any breakdown in communication adds time and possibly increases a chance for errors to occur.

HIT communications primarily utilize a message-based approach through translators known as interfaces which just like human interactions can sometimes lose messages in translation. A new HIT might need to interface with multiple separate systems, and the method and manner of interfaces could make or break the implementation. A system that utilizes industry standard messaging such as HL7 (www.HL7.org) messages would be a better choice than a system that utilizes proprietary interfaces.[12] Further, keeping the number of unique interfaces low reduces complexity in systems management since the number of interfaces grows quickly with increasing number of systems needing to be connected. A replicated data repository represents another method of integration that a vendor may utilize to keep interface complexity low. This physical data storehouse is translated to a common format from all the different sources and serves as the source data which other systems rely on for their functions. Finally, if one vendor under consideration already has one or more systems deployed that will require interfacing, then selecting a method of information exchange already in place could help reduce complexity and should be included in any analysis.

Evaluation: Bridging the Gaps

Many of the tools and devices used in modern healthcare settings have their roots in the business world where many of the information transactions occur in very well-defined areas. However, the workplace of a healthcare provider is not normally described as a closed work environment where all of the activities take place in a well-defined area. Thus over the past several years many of the Patient Care Information Systems (PCIS) appearing in healthcare environments now have adaptations for the mobile, multi-tasking members of today's healthcare teams. These systems have various form factors or sizes, communication techniques and capacities and software that coupled with deployed high speed broadband communications (i.e., Wi-Fi, WiMax, 3G cellular, etc.) liberate health care providers from working stationary at only one location inside the walls of a particular facility. This type of workflow provides added efficiencies by eliminating the need to walk to a central workstation at a hospital nursing station or use only a terminal located within a certain building to enter data. With mobile or handheld platforms a user can conduct their activities and transactions in nearly every patient care setting or externally with wireless data transmissions for data entry into the host system. This real data entry and retrieval can also improve patient safety if for example a drug interaction or the latest laboratory results are presented when a decision in a patient's treatment is made. However, these advances are not without risks and as often happen with technology development, the creation precedes policy and rules for the use of technologies that will change the workplace.

Healthcare information is considered sensitive, so healthcare transmissions sent need to be treated with the highest respect to avoid any negative effects. The wireless communications medium provides many great new benefits but also is the source of great risk that cannot be underestimated. Many devices now come equipped with one and in some cases multiple wireless communication techniques. The establishment of a wireless work environment also presents the potential for a rogue user or device to enter a wireless network. Some recommended actions by both a vendor and an organization to prevent unwanted damage from improper wireless communications are listed in Table 13-2.[13] Verifying if a vendor and your organization can meet all of the necessary steps for any system that might include mobile or wireless technologies can prevent a Pandora's box from being delivered and might eliminate candidates or cause a re-evaluation of your requirements to occur.

Evaluation: The Intangibles

An intangible is something whose importance is hard to sense or quantify. For an asset or activity, an intangible benefit often has quantifiable elements associated with them but the impact from them may equal more than the sum of the parts. For example, calculating the efforts undertaken by practitioners to prevent a negative event like a patient death or another morbid event may not adequately represent the true benefit or impact as measurable or tangible outputs in a healthcare delivery process. Nosocomial infections rates in the U.S. are one of the benchmarks for the Centers for Disease Control surveillance program, National Nosocomial Infections Surveillance System (NNISS). It is estimated that 5% of patients admitted to hospital each year get a nosocomial infection and from these infections over 26,000 deaths will occur. Nosocomial infections pose great risks to patients and in most cases can be prevented with simple adequate measures and precautions. So much so, that starting October 1, 2008, the Center for Medicaid and Medicare Services (CMS) will not reimburse for any diagnosis that stems from a preventable complication such as nosocomial infection.[14,15]

Efforts for treatments and precautions that prevent nosocomial infections represent tangible steps that have immeasurable intangible benefits on a patient's quality of life in preventing these infections. In the case

TABLE 13-2

Recommended Actions for Using Wireless HIT

Responsible Party	Activity
Vendor	Data encryption that meets or exceeds applicable standards
Vendor	Secure, encrypted data backup capability
Vendor	Role based security
Vendor	Two factor authentication of authorized users
Organization	Labeling and keeping inventory of all allowed devices on wireless network
Organization	Periodic security testing and monitoring of wireless network and devices
Organization	Educating all users of potential risks for wireless communications

Source: Adapted from reference 13.

of nosocomial infections, the environment and the healthcare practitioners can actually contribute to infections. The potential for healthcare technology, particularly mobile and/or handheld technology, to contribute to the infection rates of patients should not be overlooked. The surfaces of a HIT could harbor infectious agents that coupled with other factors such as multi-tasking providers going from multiple patient rooms and poor hand washing, could provide a vector mechanism for a nosocomial infection.[16] Evaluation of any new system expected to exist in or near a patient care setting should include a mechanism for cleaning or decontamination to reduce the potential for nosocomial infections. This evaluation should also include an executable plan on how and when to clean the devices that will not cause a negative impact on patient care and is not cost prohibitive.

The ability of a technology to work independently during network downtime and integrate information captured upon restoring normal communications deserves adequate attention when comparing different vendors and systems. The planning

for downtime from maintenance or other events, like natural disasters, should include discussion on which technology best supports these plans. The procedures required by personnel to complete their mission should support as little re-work as possible. For example, ideally all of the transactions in a pharmacy medication management system would integrate automatically and not require manually re-entry into a host system upon restoration of connections. Personnel that are dealing with an alternate way of doing business in a downtime scenario will appreciate the single entry of data and they will have less opportunity to commit entry errors as well.

Project Management

Installation

Once a determination to implement a system is made, the process known as project management really begins in earnest. Whether the new system replaces an existing one or is a completely new business process, it is important to forecast and identify the steps and resources needed to ensure success. Project management is simply the action end of change management and includes items such as schedules, goals, budgets, activities and the monitoring necessary to avoid delays in execution. A project management plan (PMP) should include the vendor as an integral part of the team creating the plan as they understand the requirements of their system and often have installed the system for many organizations. A good PMP provides a realistic set of deliverables for each contributor and must include buffers for unknown events and slippages in schedule. Many events depend on each other in a cascade fashion and cost overruns or service interruptions could occur without following a good PMP.

With any new HIT implementation, some amount of training should precede the use of the new system. Vendor conducted training usually comes with the acquisition but may not meet the needs of the organization. The individuals conducting the training may not have any experience as the intended user and thus can only address what the system can do but not truly understand the workflow impacts it represents. Vendor training often only reflects the ideal situation where a system performs as expected. However, it is also important to know what to do when the system does not perform as expected. One way of accomplishing this is to have a higher level of training in troubleshooting problems for pharmacy personnel as well as the IS department personnel. These personnel could attend a "mini boot camp" on the system and provide a first responder capability that could reduce the downtime spent waiting on a service call. In addition to the higher level of training, a small set of standard spare parts that are left in the department for fixing issues that arise could avoid shutting the system down for longer periods while awaiting parts that a trained super user can install.

Post-Installation

Now that the new toy is out of the box, the hard work does not end. The fallacy that the project management for a new HIT ends once installed leaves out a very important component of the change management process: measuring what changes actually occurred. The expectations and requirements for the installed system often precede the installation by months and sometimes years. What was once true about the organization and business processes might have changed. Even if no significant change has occurred, a good PMP requires some sort of evaluation of system performance in the actual environment.

The evaluation should compare the objectives or requirements for the system, the delivered capabilities, reliability of the system, impact on practices or processes, use of the system by target audience, and returns or gains made. Different evaluation methods will increase the knowledge of the system impact. Subjective methods such as user surveys provide opinions and behavioral information on the delivered product's.[4,17] Surveys are very often used to find human computer interaction (HCI) and other human factors issues with new technology.[18] The intense use of graphical user interfaces (GUI) and the potential to have a non-friendly, disruptive method of data entry, while although technically accurate for requirements, could create a barrier for use of a system. For example, a bad interface design might cause users to try and circumvent the new "nuisance" in their lives through workarounds or self created "fixes" and a survey becomes their outlet to describe the frustration. Besides subjective measures, objective measures decided upon prior to acquiring the technology, provide critical information. Objective measures determine if expected returns exist and could include the final direct and indirect costs in the implementation (money, personnel, time) in addition to meeting other expectations such as data security and other quality assurance metrics.[4,17]

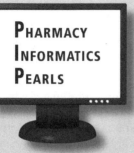

MANAGEMENT

PHARMACY INFORMATICS PEARLS

- Define the problem first then assess whether technology can provide a solution.
- List the attributes of a technology first before looking in the marketplace to see if it exists.
- List all of the actors in the play, especially the supporting cast, before assessing a technology.
- Make sure all of the actors have a voice in the decision and let them know they are heard.
- Develop a project plan sooner rather than later and stick to the plan, even a modified plan.
- Don't be afraid to change course or reverse course when trouble arises.
- Define measures of success before implementation and don't forget to measure and evaluate. Simply using a system does not mean it is a useful system.
- Even with a proven commercial system that others have deployed an issue can arise that no one saw coming. Remember to put downtime and support in the plan and expect the unexpected.
- Accepting change comes easier for some than others. Successful change involves knowing the organization, the business processes, and customer expectations, and maintaining productive relationships.
- A legacy system is a system that works.

Summary

Healthcare technologies today provide significant leverage for members of a healthcare team. The advances in communications and other computing capabilities do not come without costs in time, money, and personnel. With shortages in many sectors of professional communities, including healthcare and information technology, the decision to implement a technology cannot simply revolve around the technology itself or one group, such as the intended users. The process of proper project planning and the due diligence in vendor evaluation and selection offer an opportunity to help avoid costly mistakes in both execution as well as mistakes by the users of the technology. The different management issues that can arise from a technology, new or old, all lend themselves much easier to resolution if the set of plans for the system in question have well-defined "emergency exits" labeled in advance as a result of proper planning.

References

1. Monegain B. Report: Healthcare IT spending to grow to $39.5 billion by 2008. Healthcare IT News website. 2006. Available at: http://www.healthcareitnews.com/story.cms?id=4242 Accessed December 20, 2007.

2. Ford EW, Menachemi N, Phillips MT. Predicting the adoption of electronic health records by physicians: when will health care be paperless? *J Am Med Inform Assoc.* 2006;13:106–112.

3. Evidence Report/Technology Assessment. AHRQ Publication No. 06-E006. Costs and Benefits of Health Information Technology. April 2006.

4. Gremy F, Degoulet P. Assessment of health information technology: which questions for which systems? Proposal for a taxonomy, *Med Inform.* 1993; 18(3):185–193.

5. Ammenwerth E, Iller C, Mahler C. IT-adoption and the interaction of task, technology and individuals: a fit framework and a case study. *BMC Med Inform Decis Mak.* 2006;6:3.

6. Teich J. CPOE is tricky, but worthwhile. Ihealthbeat.org website. 2003. Available at http://www.ihealthbeat.org/articles/2003/1/29/CPOE-is-tricky-but-worthwhile.aspx?ps=1&authorid=. Accessed December 20, 2007.

7. Berg M. Implementing information systems in health care organizations: myths and challenges. *Int J Med Inform.* 2001;64:143–156.

8. Protti D. A proposal to use a balanced scorecard to evaluate Information for Health: an information strategy for the modern NHS (1998-2005), *Comp Biol and Med*. 2002;32:221-236.

9. The fourteenth annual HIMSS leadership survey sponsored by Superior Consultant. Health Information management Systems Society website. 2003. Available at http://www.himss.org/2003survey/. Accessed January 3, 2008.

10. The sixteenth annual HIMSS leadership survey sponsored by Superior Consultant. Health Information management Systems Society website. 2005. Available at http://www.himss.org/2005survey/. Accessed January 3, 2008.

11. Security Standard. Centers for Medicaid and Medicare Services website. 2007 http://www.cms.hhs.gov/SecurityStandard/. Accessed December 31,2007.

12. Grimson J, Grimson, W, Hasselbring W. The SI challenge in health care. *Comm ACM*. 2000;43(6):49–55.

13. Wireless Network Security. National Institutes of Standards and Technology website. Available at: http://csrc.nist.gov/publications/nistpubs/800-48/NIST_SP_800-48.pdf. Accessed January 10, 2008.

14. Rosenthal MB. Nonpayment for performance? Medicare's new reimbursement rule. *N Engl J Med*. 2007;357:1573–1575.

15. Nguyen QV. Hospital-acquired infections, eMedicine from WebMD website. August 21, 2007. Available at: http://www.emedicine.com/PED/topic1619.htm. Accessed January 10, 2008.

16. Doctors worried about hardware's infection risks. *Health Data Management*. December 2007:12.

17. Littlejohns P, Wyatt JC, Garvican L. Information in practice. *BMJ*. 2003;326:860–863.

18. Kuhn KA, Giuse DA. From hospital information systems to health information systems. *Meth Inform Med*. 2001;4:275–287.

Glossary

Adverse Drug Event—an injury resulting from a medication or lack of intended medication.

Affected Systems—identification of pharmacy information/ automation systems as well as hospital information systems that support pharmacy operations and the medication use process. These systems usually consist of the pharmacy information system (PIS), automated dispensing cabinets (ADM), pharmacy robot, TPN compounding machine, pharmacy's intranet and/or hospital's internet sites, admitting/registration system (ADT/registration) for patient access, financial systems, carousel inventory cabinets, bar code medication administration systems (BCMA), clinical decision support (CDS), computerized provider order entry (CPOE), electronic medication administration record (eMAR), clinical results/electronic healthcare record, laboratory information systems, etc.

Alert Fatigue—a state of irritability, exhaustion, or bewilderment triggered in clinicians who have been exposed to too many alerts, or alerts with a perceived history of irrelevance, which cause the user to ignore some or all of the alerts, thereby reducing the safety benefit of the decision support system.

Alert—an urgent notice generated by a computerized clinical decision support system (CDSS). These are usually in the form of a just-in-time, patient-specific message directed to one or more clinicians. It may be a warning regarding a clinician's documented action (or lack thereof) or a documented decision. Or it may be an urgent informational notification of a new clinical condition, circumstance, or change in patient status that requires immediate attention. Some alerts require a response before the clinician can continue.

American National Standards Institute (ANSI)—coordinates the development and use of voluntary consensus standards including Health Level Seven's (HL7) Arden Syntax standard.

Application—software written to work on a computer and designed to perform a specific task, in this context the PIS. It is what the user sees when he opens the PIS.

Arden Syntax Standard—an HL7 standard designed to allow clinicians to program medical logic into a clinical rule or guideline. The American Society for Testing and Materials first approved the Arden Syntax as a standard in 1992 (E-1460-92). Ownership was transferred to HL7 and ANSI in 1999 with the approval of version 2.0 of the standard. The Arden Syntax is the only approved standard for clinicians to encode medical logic into clinical rules known as medical logic modules (MLM).

ASC X12N—Accredited Standards Committee X12; creates standards for the cross industry electronic transmission of business information. ASC X12N standards are used for insurance eligibility and prior authorization communication.

Automated Dispensing Cabinets—secure storage cabinets typically located decentrally on patient care units capable of handling most unit-dose and some bulk (multiple-dose) medications due to storage limitations.

Automation—any technology, machine, or device linked to or controlled by a computer and used to do work. Automation is designed to streamline and improve the accuracy and efficiency of the medication use process.

Bar Code—a series of vertical lines and spaces of varying widths that encode data to be scanned and decoded through a computer.

Bar Code Medication Administration (BCMA)—an inpatient clinical decision support system to assist caregivers with the five rights of medication administration (right patient, right drug, right dose, right route, and right time). BCMA systems provide warnings if any of the five rights are compromised, and many BCMA systems require the nurse to enter an override reason if he/she chooses to proceed. In addition, BCMA systems promote right documentation (some hospitals call this the sixth right of medication administration).

Bar-coding at the Point of Care (BPOC)—a process in which the patient and various patient therapies are documented with a bar code scanner at the bedside.

Business Intelligence—an umbrella term that describes the strategic integration of technology and processes that allow organizations to leverage their data to make better decisions.

Carousel Automation—a medication storage cabinet with rotating shelves used to automate dispensing.

Centers for Medicare and Medicaid Services (CMS)—the federal healthcare programs for the elderly and indigent. For more information go to: http://www.cms.hhs.gov/

Centralized Robotic Dispensing System—centrally located devices designed to automate the entire process of medication dispensing including medication storage, distribution, restocking, and crediting of unit dose medications.

Change Management—a discipline in information systems service that seeks to ensure that standard methods and procedures are used when making changes to information technology infrastructure, attempting to balance the need for change with the potential negative impact changes can produce.

Clinical Advisory—a decision-making tool that is identified for a specific medication. Nursing guidelines are often created as an advisory. An example would be a suggestion by the pump to the user to use a 0.22-micron filter when administering a medication.

Clinical Decision Support (CDS)—providing clinicians or patients with clinical knowledge and patient-related information, intelligently filtered or presented at appropriate times, to enhance patient care. Clinical knowledge of interest could range from simple facts and relationships to best practices for managing patients with specific disease states, new medical knowledge from clinical research, and other types of information.

Clinical Decision Support System (CDSS)—a system (computer or otherwise) intended to provide CDS to clinicians, caregivers, and healthcare consumers. Automated CDSS are usually just-in-time, point-of-care messages in the form of an alert, reminder, recommendation, or informational notification regarding a patient. Automated CDS systems typically include a knowledge base (which contains stored facts and some method of algorithmic logic), an event monitor (to detect data entry or the storage of data from a laboratory or other system), and a communication system to the end user (unidirectional or bidirectional).

Clinical Informatics—the scientific study of the effective analysis, use, and dissemination of information in patient care, clinical research, and medical education.

Clinical Information System—a group of computers that run databases and software applications to effectively provide a comprehensive repository of patient-specific healthcare information. As a general term, this might be a laboratory, pharmacy, nursing documentation, or ordering system.

Clinical Pharmacy Technician—a highly skilled pharmacy technician or "pharmacist assistant" with advanced training and/or pharmacy technician certification completed.

Clinical Reminder—a context-sensitive electronic prompt to the provider to perform an intervention or procedure, based on the patient's specific clinical data as applied to a set of logical conditions.

Computerized Provider Order Entry (CPOE)—automated portion of a clinical information system that enables a patient's care provider to enter an order for a medication, clinical laboratory, radiology test, or procedure directly into the computer. The system then transmits the order to the appropriate department, or individuals, so that it can be carried out.

Corollary Orders—orders entered as adjuncts to a primary order, e.g., orders for laboratory tests to monitor effects of a medication order, orders for special diets in preparation for a medical procedure.

Cost of Downtime—associated costs including: (1) direct costs—staff salary, downtime equipment, lost revenue, downtime supplies, and (2) indirect costs—delays in medication delivery, increase in medication errors, staff stress levels, etc.

Dashboard—common report format used to quickly evaluate the performance of a business process. Dashboards commonly use visuals such as dials, gauges, or stoplights to represent results.

Data Integrity—the accuracy, completeness, consistency, and validity of data.

Data Mining—broad term that encompasses numerous methods used to identify patterns and relationships in data. Examples of data mining techniques include neural networks, rule induction, and genetic algorithms.

Data Warehouse—centralized repository of data from an organization's individual information systems that is organized into integrated subject domains for reporting or data mining. Data warehouses may be implemented with relational or dimensional data models.

Database—a large collection of data organized for rapid search and retrieval by a computer.

Database Query—general term to describe a "search" of a database that returns data for use in reporting or other analyses.

Dataset—the recommended parameters for each medication programmed into the smart pump software such as dose, dosing unit, rate, or concentration.

Dimensional Database Model—an approach to designing databases for the purpose of maximizing end-user friendliness and query performance as well as to preserve data history. These features stand in contrast to the strengths of the relational database model.

Dispenser—term that the Department of Health and Human Services Centers for Medicare & Medicaid Services uses to specify the pharmacy and pharmacist. It is assumed that this includes in addition to the dispensing of prescription medications that the appropriate verifications and patient education is provided by the dispenser.

Downtime—the period of time during which the healthcare facility's computer system is unavailable and electronic order entry is not possible.

Drug Library—list of medications programmed in the smart pump software. The library includes properties such as name, dose, and concentration for each medication listed.

e-Iatrogenesis—patient harm caused at least in part by the application of health information technology.

Electronic Health Record (EHR)—a longitudinal electronic medical record (EMR) of patient health information generated by one or more encounters in any care delivery setting. It contains episodes of care across multiple care delivery organizations (CDOs) within a community, region, or state.

Electronic Medical Record (EMR)—a computerized legal clinical record created in a CDO, such as a hospital or physician's office. It is an application environment composed of the clinical data repository (CDR), clinical decision support (CDS), controlled medical vocabulary (CMV), computerized provider order entry (CPOE), pharmacy, clinical documentation, and other ancillary applications.

Electronic Prescribing, or e-Prescribing—refers to the use of computing devices to enter, modify, review, and output or communicate drug prescriptions and medication regimens for patients. E-Prescribing is one component of CPOE systems.

eMAR—electronic medication administration record.

ePHI—electronically protected health information. Individually identifiable health information stored electronically by healthcare providers.

ePrescription—according to CMS, a prescription is not an ePrescription unless it is transmitted electronically in a standard format. Printed paper prescriptions and electronic faxes are not considered to be ePrescriptions by CMS rule.

Evaluation/Outcomes Measure—post downtime review to determine if existing policies and procedures, planning, and staffing worked, and what needs to be changed.

File Architecture—also referred to as the medication masterfile, a compilation of interconnected files and records that contain data elements that compose the medication and clinical information presented for use in an EHR system.

Fitness for Purpose—a property of data that is appropriate for a given use. In reporting or other data analysis, fitness for purpose is evaluated along dimensions of timeliness and relevancy for the task at hand.

Formulary—a health system's specific list of medications approved for use by its clinicians.

Hard Limit—a dose that serves as the absolute limit (high or low) for drug administration by the pump. Once this hard limit is reached, the dose cannot be overridden, serving as a warning to the pump user that the dose needs to be verified prior to drug administration.

Health Insurance Portability and Accountability Act (HIPAA)—law enacted in 1996 by the U.S. Congress in order to protect patient medical information. Title II of HIPAA, the Administrative Simplification (AS) provisions, requires the establishment of national standards for electronic health care transactions and national identifiers for providers, health insurance plans, and employers to address the security and privacy of health data.

Health Level Seven (HL7)—an important standards development organization for health information technology (HIT). For detailed information, see the HL7 website: http://www.hl7.org

Healthcare Information Technology (HIT)—any computer system designed to automate and/or enhance a healthcare process or workflow. HIT can be a small apparatus such as an IV infusion pump or a glucometer or a departmental information system such as a pharmacy or laboratory information system. It can be an institutional information system such as an admissions, discharge, and transfer (ADT) system, which may interface or interoperate with other departmental systems. HIT can also be a multi-institutional system, such as a regional health information organization (RHIO), or even a national health information network (NHIN).

Human Factors—physical, mental, or behavioral properties of people that may have critical influence on how people interact with technological systems, organizations, or their environment.

Imager—an electronic device similar to a scanner that analyzes an image, including linear and two dimensional bar codes, and digitally converts it into data.

Implementation—the execution of a plan that, when referring to a technology system, generally encompasses requirements analysis, determination of project scope, integration plan, user training, policy development, and delivery.

Improper Dose Error—administration to the patient of a dose that is greater than or less than the amount ordered by the prescriber or administration of duplicate doses to the patient, i.e., one or more dosage units in addition to those that were ordered.

Informaticist—someone who applies information technology to a specific discipline (e.g., pharmacy informaticist).

Information Systems (IS)—(1) Computerized systems for workflow management such as a pharmacy computer system, or an information retrieval system such as a library. The defining characteristic is a database and specialized features and functions for a dedicated purpose. (2) A department of HIT or computer professionals. When designating a department, IS usually stands for Information Services.

Informational Notice—may be a patient-specific automated rule, such as an MLM, to inform of a change in patient status. This type of informational notice may be urgent (e.g., to report a change in renal function) or non-urgent (e.g., to report a hospital admission of a potential study patient). An informational notice may also be product-specific such as a pop-up box during order entry to announce a look-alike, sound-alike (LASA) drug.

Infusion Pump—a device that administers drugs or nutrition to a patient through intravenous, subcutaneous, intramuscular, intrathecal, epidural, or intra-arterial routes. Infusion pumps can administer fluids in very controlled amounts.

Integrated Systems—when information systems that perform different functions share the same database, application space, and often hardware. They are usually provided as a single solution.

Integration—in information technology, the physical or functional linking of two separate systems in order to achieve a desired new functionality or capability, often through the use of interfaces. (Note: The definition is still a matter of debate in the informatics community.)

Interfaced Systems—when separate information systems (with separate databases) are built to communicate with one another. This requires the development of an interface to normalize information for interpretation by both systems.

Interface—internal communication between two separate entities (i.e., hardware or software) that allows information and resources to be shared without affecting how external entities (i.e., a user) interacts with each system.

IOM—the Institute of Medicine.

Knowledge Base—a collection of stored facts, rules, algorithms, heuristics, and models for problem solving. Knowledge base data may be organized in a database or even a simple table in

which explicit relationships exist. Familiar examples of commercial knowledge bases that incorporate databases are drug-drug interaction and drug allergy alerting systems.

Levels of Downtime—duration of downtime that will require different activation of the downtime plan to maintain pharmacy operations, for example: (1) short duration—up to 2 hours, (2) medium duration—2 to 7 hours, and (3) long duration—greater than 8 hours.

Linear Symbology—a one-dimensional bar code consisting of vertical lines and spaces.

Logical Observation Identifiers Names and Codes (LOINC)—a standard to facilitate the exchange of clinical laboratory results. The Regenstrief Institute, Inc., maintains the LOINC database of about 41,000 terms, and its supporting documentation.

Look-Alike, Sound-Alike (LASA)—a medication safety designation to prevent confusion between drugs with similar spelling or pronunciation.

Maintenance—work that must be done to a software program to ensure that the system is updated and accurate.

Medical Logic Module (MLM)—a rule for an Arden Syntax based clinical rules engine. HL7 defines a MLM as an encoded clinical rule that contains enough logic to make a single clinical decision. MLMs in use today have been developed for many purposes, such as clinical alerts, recommendations, reminders, informational notices, interpretations, diagnosis, quality assurance functions, continuous quality improvement, bio-surveillance, administrative support, and for clinical research.

Medication Error—any preventable event that may cause or lead to inappropriate medication use or patient harm while the medication is in the control of the health care professional, patient or consumer.

Medication Management System—an automated system that is often connected to other healthcare systems, that supports patient safety, and that improves the quality of care by reducing practice errors and misuse. A medication management system does so by providing access to medications only by authorized personnel and (usually) only if a validated order exists within the system.

Medication Masterfile—compilation of records that individually contain data elements that compose the medication information presented for use in an EHR system.

Medication Reconciliation—the process of identifying the most accurate list of all medications a patient is taking, including name, dosage, frequency, and route, and using this list to provide correct medications for patients anywhere within the health care system. Reconciliation involves comparing the patient's current list of medications against admission, transfer, and/or discharge orders.

Medication-Use System—a complex system involving multiple individuals, processes and technology to manage the ordering, verifying, procurement, preparing, distribution, monitoring, and education of medication therapy.

Monitoring Error—failure to review a prescribed regimen for appropriateness and detection of problems, or failure to use appropriate clinical or laboratory data for adequate assessment of patient response to prescribed therapy.

NCPDP—National Council for Prescription Drug Programs; an organization that creates and promotes standards for the transfer of data to and from the pharmacy services sector of the healthcare industry. NCPDP is an ANSI-accredited standards development organization that has over 1450 members representing all areas of pharmacy services. NCPDP has developed standards for provider identification and telecommunication standards for pharmacy claims. It has also developed SCRIPT, which consists of multiple standards supporting prescription communication and processing.

National Council for Prescription Drug Programs (NCPDP) Script—is a standard for ambulatory prescription messaging between pharmacies and third party payers. The NCPDP standard has been in use for decades. In 2004, HL7 had started its own efforts to develop a standard for institutional prescription messaging, and decided to create a harmonized mapping between NCPDP's script and HL7's RX messages. Their intention is to ensure interoperability of prescription information across the entire healthcare information environment.

Notification—a patient- and context-sensitive prompt to the ordering provider, attending physi-

cian, primary provider, or care team to alert them of new information (i.e., abnormal lab result) or tasks in need of completion (i.e., unsigned order or note).

Omission Error—failure to administer an ordered dose to a patient before the next scheduled dose, if any.

On Line Analytical Processing (OLAP)—a class of applications to support complex queries and analysis across multiple dimensions. OLAP systems often implement a dimensional data model and are closely related to data warehouses.

On Line Transaction Processing (OLTP)—a class of applications designed to support transaction based operational processes such as order entry or packaging. OLTP systems often rely on databases that implement a relational data model.

Open Database Connectivity (ODBC)—standard interface for accessing modern database systems.

Order Menu—a listing of orders from which clinicians may select individual orders, organized to support a specific purpose, ordering environment, or type of order.

Order Set—compilation of medication and procedure orders that can be accessed and ordered from a single source in the EHR. These are analogous to paper pre-printed order forms.

Patient Care Information System (PCIS)—technology system used by a health care professional for the provision of care to a patient, either directly through decision support or in a support role such as informational storage or management of information function. PCIS supports the provision of care for patients.

PDP—Medicare Prescription Drug Plan (PDP) is the prescription drug plan that was created with the Medicare Prescription Drug, Improvement and Modernization Act of 2003.

Personal Health Records (PHR)—an Internet-based set of tools that allows people to access and coordinate their lifelong health information and make appropriate parts of it available to those who need it.

Pharmaceutical Care—the responsible provision of drug therapy for the purpose of achieving outcomes that improve a patient's quality of life.

Pharmacy Information System (PIS)—a system that provides pharmacy staff the necessary application environment to practice the profession of pharmacy; often includes the ordering, procurement, preparation, dispensing, and monitoring portions of the medication use process.

Prescriber—the health practitioner who has the legal authority for ordering ambulatory medications.

Prescribing Error—incorrect drug selection (based on indications, contraindications, known allergies, existing drug therapy, and other factors), dose, dosage form, quantity, route, concentration, rate of administration, or instructions for use of a drug product ordered or authorized by physician (or other legitimate prescriber); illegible prescriptions or medication orders that lead to errors that reach the patient.

Profile—unique set of options and best practice guidelines for a specific patient population.

Protected Health Information (PHI)—this is information about a person that must remain secure, as defined by Health Insurance Portability and Accountability Act (HIPAA).

Quick Order—a pre-configured order in which the components (e.g., medication, dose, route, schedule, amount, number of refills, etc.) are specified, allowing for faster order entry and limiting opportunities for entry errors. These are sometimes referred to as order sentences and may be maintained and standardized across an institution or created by individuals as personal quick orders, user preferences or preference lists. transcribed into the receiving systems. Few current ePrescribing installations currently realize this goal.

Radio Frequency Identification (RFID)—a computerized chip or tag with an antenna capable of storing data in conjunction with a receiving module for purposes of product identification or tracking.

Recommendation—an automated rule, such as an MLM, that suggests a course of action. For example, a patient-specific dosage or a suggestion for a laboratory test. Ideally, all recommendations are evidence-based and institutionally approved.

Recovery Period—time period post downtime for entry of data generated during downtime to update pharmacy information/automations systems that were affected during downtime.

Regional Health Information Organization (RHIO)—proposed definition by the Department of Health and Human Services, BearingPoint, and the National Alliance for Health Information and Technology. A governance entity comprising separate and independent healthcare-related organizations that have come together to improve the quality, safety, and efficiency of healthcare for communities in which it operates and for which it takes responsibility to develop transparent, inclusive processes that enable the interoperable exchange of health information in a manner that protects the confidentiality

Relational Database Model—an approach to designing databases based on mathematical set theory. Proper application of the model helps ensure data integrity is maintained during transactions that update, add, or remove data.

Reminder—an automated rule, such as an MLM, that suggests the clinician has overlooked or forgotten to perform an action such as documenting a decision, event, or finding.

Reporting—the concise presentation of relevant operational or clinical data for decision making or performance review purposes.

RXNORM—a clinical drug nomenclature standard produced by the National Library of Medicine.

Scanner—an electronic device that analyzes an object, such as a linear bar code, and digitally converts it into data.

Scheduled Downtime—system outage that is scheduled for pharmacy information/automation systems allowing for prospective downtime planning; most common reasons include planned hardware or software upgrades.

Server—the heart of a network of computers, providing a centralized and organized location for the PIS, database, and application.

Smart Pump—a computerized infusion device that can be programmed to include a specific set of data.

Soft Limit—similar to hard limits but can be overridden and a dose can be programmed for delivery.

Structured Query Language (SQL)—standard language used to query and manage databases. Pronounced "sequel."

Supply Chain Management—the management of the pharmaceutical order-to-pay process including management of inventory and distribution of supplies throughout the medication use process.

Switch—a company that provides a communication network to support claims adjudication, eligibility checking and electronic prescribing for pharmacies.

Symbology—the pattern represented in a bar code that encode data and allow it to be converted into information with the use of a scanner or imager. A symbology is similar to a computer language.

Systematized Nomenclature of Medicine Clinical Terms (SNOMED CT)—a comprehensive clinical terminology, originally created by the College of American Pathologists. For more information, see the National Library of Medicine Unified Medical Language System website: http://www.nlm.nih.gov/research/umls/Snomed/snomed_main.Html

Technology—anything that is used to replace routine or repetitive tasks previously performed by people, or which extends the capability of people.

Two-dimensional (2D) Symbology—a bar code that may use dots or lines arranged on the vertical and horizontal axes that can contain up to several thousand characters.

Unauthorized Drug Error—administration to the patient of medication not authorized by a legitimate prescriber.

Unscheduled Downtime—system outage that is not scheduled for pharmacy information/automation systems, resulting in no prospective downtime planning. Most common reasons include unplanned hardware or software failures, power outages, and extreme weather conditions.

Workstation—the computer in the pharmacy that a staff member uses to interact with the PIS.

Wrong Dosage-Form Error—administration to the patient of a drug product in a different dosage form than ordered by the prescriber.

Wrong Drug-Preparation Error—drug product incorrectly formulated or manipulated before administration.

Wrong Time Error—administration of medication outside a predefined time interval from its scheduled administration time (this interval should be established by each individual health care facility).

Index